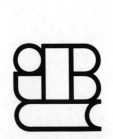

HEALTH ISSUES
in the
BLACK
COMMUNITY

RONALD L. BRAITHWAITE
SANDRA E. TAYLOR
editors

foreword by
LOUIS W. SULLIVAN, M.D.
Secretary of the U.S. Department
of Health and Human Services

HEALTH ISSUES
in the
BLACK
COMMUNITY

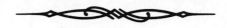

Jossey-Bass Publishers · San Francisco

For sales outside the United States, contact Maxwell Macmillan
International Publishing Group, 866 Third Avenue, New York,
New York 10022.

Manufactured in the United States of America

Library of Congress Cataloging-in-Publication Data

Health issues in the Black community / [edited by] Ronald L.
 Braithwaite, Sandra E. Taylor. — 1st ed.
     p.   cm. — (The Jossey-Bass health series)
   Includes bibliographical references and index.
   ISBN 1-55542-477-5 (alk. paper)
   1. Afro-Americans—Health and hygiene.   I. Braithwaite, Ronald
L., date.   II. Taylor, Sandra E., date.   III. Series.
   [DNLM: 1. Blacks—United States.   2. Health Promotion—United
States.   3. Health Status.   4. Social Problems—United States.   WA
300 H433855]
RA448.5.N4H395   1992
362.1'089'96073—dc20
DNLM/DLC
for Library of Congress   92-20174
                                                                CIP

FIRST EDITION
HB Printing   10 9 8 7 6 5 4 3 2 1   *Code 9276*

The Jossey-Bass Health Series

CONTENTS

Foreword   xiii
*Louis W. Sullivan, M.D., Secretary of the U.S. Department of
Health and Human Services*

Preface   xvii

The Editors   xxi

Contributors   xxiii

Part I: Health Status in Social Context

1. African-American Health: An Introduction   3
   Ronald L. Braithwaite, Sandra E. Taylor

2. A Demographic Profile of African Americans   6
   Christiane B. Hale

3. The Mental Health Status of Black Americans: An Overview   20
   Sandra E. Taylor

4. The Health Status of Black Women   35
   Byllye Y. Avery

Part II: Critical Health Topics

5. AIDS/HIV Epidemics in the Black Community   55
   Bill Jenkins

6. Prevention, Intervention, and Treatment of
    Chemical Dependency in the Black Community   64
    Donnie W. Watson

7. Alcoholism and the African-American Community   79
    Creigs C. Beverly

8. Heart Disease, Stroke, and Hypertension in Blacks   90
    Carolyn J. Hildreth, Elijah Saunders

9. Cancer and Black Americans   106
    Claudia R. Baquet, Tyson Gibbs

10. Diabetes and the Black Community   121
    Frederick G. Murphy, M. Joycelyn Elders

11. Homicide and Violence: Contemporary Health Problems
    for America's Black Community   132
    Deborah Prothrow-Stith, Howard Spivak

Part III: Infants, Youth, and Late Adulthood

12. Homeless Women with Children   147
    Aisha Gilliam

13. "Too Soon, Too Small, Too Sick": Black Infant Mortality 165
    Virginia Davis Floyd

14. Lead Poisoning: A Modern Plague Among
    African-American Children   178
    Wornie L. Reed

15. Sickle Cell Anemia and African Americans   192
    Charles F. Whitten

16. Adolescent Pregnancy in the African-American Community 206
    Joyce A. Ladner, Ruby Morton Gourdine

17. Elderly Issues in the African-American Community   222
    Mary S. Harper

Part IV: Health Education and Resource Development

18. Health Education and Black Health Status   241
    Rueben C. Warren

Contents

19. Indigenous Community Health Workers in the 1960s
    and Beyond   255
    Doris Y. Wilkinson

20. Health Promotion and Disease Prevention Strategies
    for African Americans: A Conceptual Model   267
    Collins O. Airhihenbuwa

21. Effective Intervention Strategies for Producing Black
    Health Care Providers   281
    Moses K. Woode, Kathleen Bodisch Lynch

Part V: The Future of Health for African Americans

22. Reproductive Rights and the Challenge for
    African Americans   301
    Faye Wattleton

23. Health Policies and the Black Community   315
    Bailus Walker, Jr.

24. Coalition Partnerships for Health Promotion
    and Empowerment   321
    Ronald L. Braithwaite

25. The Health of the Black Community in the Twenty-first
    Century: A Futuristic Perspective   338
    Stephen B. Thomas

    Afterword   351
    David Satcher

    Name Index   355

    Subject Index   365

FOREWORD

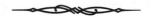

The founding fathers of this country cited life, liberty, and the pursuit of happiness as inalienable rights for each citizen. Yet the quality of life—a healthy life—is, in the 1990s, still not assured for far too many black Americans.

Over most of the 1980s, the gap between life expectancy of black and white Americans increased. White Americans are living longer, while the average life span of blacks declined from a high of 69.7 years in 1984 to 69.2 years in 1988. While preliminary data suggest that the gap has begun to narrow, the disparity still remains.

This disparity is mirrored in disproportionately higher mortality from many causes. Cancer, heart disease and stroke, cirrhosis, diabetes, infant mortality, unintentional injuries, and homicide were identified as the largest contributors to an estimated 60,000 excess black deaths in this country by the Secretary's Task Force on Black and Minority Health in 1985. Since then, AIDS has also emerged as a serious health threat to black Americans. The number of excess deaths has continued to increase, reaching 80,000 in 1988, according to Christiane B. Hale in the second chapter of this book. Other statistics confirm this sobering depiction of black health in America. Black men are nearly twice as likely to die from cancer as the general population. Blacks are 33 percent more likely to have high blood pressure than whites and are more likely to suffer strokes at an earlier age and with more severe results. Black babies are twice as likely as white babies to die before their first birthday. Young black males are the leading killers of young black males. Black males fifteen to twenty-four years old experience a homicide rate 700 percent higher than that of white males in the same age group. The rate of AIDS among blacks is more than triple that of whites.

We know that poverty and limited access to health services are partly accountable for these grim statistics. Medical care alone will not eliminate the devastating impact of chronic disease on the disadvantaged, nor will it reduce, as much as we would like, the rate of infant mortality or the burden of homicide and violence or many of the other health problems that are borne by the poor in our society alone.

If every citizen is to enjoy an equal opportunity for health, both individual and collective action will be needed. Taking control of one's own fate and assuming personal responsibility is one aspect of this effort. What I have called a "culture of character" is a way of thinking and being that actively promotes responsible behavior and the adoption of life-styles that are conducive to good health. The "culture of character" by no means applies only to black Americans, nor does it rely solely on a heightened sense of personal responsibility. It seeks to empower all Americans to reduce their own health risks, and it also seeks community empowerment to mobilize all our social, economic, and political institutions to support healthier citizens and communities. I believe this combination of individual responsibility and community empowerment is vital to improving the health status of black Americans.

We are fortunate in having a framework to help guide our efforts. Healthy People 2000 is a nationwide collaborative effort involving health professionals and other citizens, private organizations, and public agencies at all levels. It is led by the U.S. Public Health Service. Based on the report *Healthy People 2000: National Health Promotion and Disease Prevention Objectives*, the initiative seeks to reduce preventable death and disability, enhance the quality of life, and greatly reduce disparities in health status among Americans. The 300 objectives present in Healthy People 2000 challenge us to work in our personal and professional capacity toward whichever specific targets are most appropriate for our situation. Healthy People 2000 also directs our attention toward another area where special efforts are needed for blacks, namely, clinical preventive services. These services—immunizations, screening for early detection of disease or risk factor, and patient counseling—are vital to good health. Many barriers limit the access of minorities and disadvantaged populations to preventive services, including poor geographic distribution and lack of health insurance. Public officials and health professionals must work to reduce these barriers, but individuals must also recognize that they have a responsibility to seek and obtain appropriate preventive services for themselves and their families.

By no means am I advocating that we should wait until the year 2000 for measurable gains in the health status of minorities. This is why I have also developed program directions that articulate near-term objectives for improving minority health status. These objectives range from increasing access to health services to reducing the risk of disease and injuries among minorities.

The issue of black health in America is both urgent and complex. Those of us who are black health professionals may be particularly touched because we know family members, friends, and patients who fall into the statistics previously cited. This personal connection sustains our determination to combat these problems. One of the great merits of this book is its comprehensive and sensitive exploration of the avenues by which we can achieve significant health improvements for blacks. Working together, we can make the lives of all Americans longer, happier, more productive, and more fulfilling.

Washington, D.C.   Louis W. Sullivan, M.D.
August 1992   *Secretary of the U.S. Department*
                                                      of Health and Human Services

To all in the Healthy People struggle
for the year 2000

PREFACE

Health Issues in the Black Community evolved from the editors' concern about the many diseases and other health-related problems affecting the African-American population. It is intended to meet the need for a readily accessible resource on these topics. The book addresses current health problems confronting African Americans and discusses relevant strategies and policy implications. While it is not intended to be a comprehensive treatment of all pertinent health problems affecting blacks, the twenty-five chapters included provide information on some of the more salient health concerns. Though the contributors present information from perspectives unique to their disciplines and experiences, a common theme is the necessity for change if the black community is to achieve significantly improved health in the twenty-first century.

The purpose of the book is threefold: (1) to provide a forum for stimulating discussion on culturally relevant strategies and models for the prevention of disease in black communities, (2) to provide a futuristic perspective on black health issues for students, academicians, public policy makers, and health administrators in public health sciences and related disciplines, and (3) to document selected health problems and advance strategies for alleviating them. The multidisciplinary emphasis allows for applicability across a wide range of areas. The disciplines of health education, public health, allied health, community health, nursing, psychology, medical sociology, medical anthropology, human services, social policy, and social welfare are all represented in the book. Many of the contributors are foremost experts in their fields.

Overview of the Contents

Part One, "Health Status in Social Context," sets the stage by providing an overview of some general health issues of African Americans. Chapter One

xvii

furnishes an introduction to the breadth of health issues covered. Chapter Two presents a demographic profile of black health status. In Chapter Three, issues pertaining to black mental health are covered. Chapter Four surveys women's health status.

Part Two, "Critical Health Topics," focuses on issues viewed as particularly significant for African Americans. Included in this section are chapters on the AIDS/HIV epidemic (Chapter Five), chemical dependency (Chapter Six), alcoholism (Chapter Seven), heart disease, stroke, and hypertension (Chapter Eight), cancer (Chapter Nine), diabetes (Chapter Ten), and violence (Chapter Eleven). These are all problems that disproportionately contribute to "excess" deaths in the black community.

Part Three, "Infants, Youth, and Late Adulthood," addresses health problems that affect age-specific populations. The chapters in this section provide insight into the impact of socioeconomic and other factors on these age-specific groups. Chapter Twelve focuses on homeless women with children. The subject of Chapter Thirteen is infant mortality. Chapter Fourteen examines the problem of lead poisoning. Sickle cell anemia is the topic of Chapter Fifteen. In Chapter Sixteen, the social and medical consequences of adolescent pregnancy are explored. Chapter Seventeen discusses issues related to the elderly. Each of these areas can be viewed as representing a grave health problem in the black community.

Part Four, "Health Education and Resource Development," explores selected strategies for general health promotion. Chapter Eighteen establishes an overall context in which to place subsequent chapters. Chapter Nineteen focuses on the usefulness of community health care workers. In Chapter Twenty, a conceptual model for health promotion and disease prevention is presented. Chapter Twenty-One addresses strategies for increasing the number of minority health care professionals. Collectively, these chapters advance knowledge on health and human resource development.

Part Five, "The Future of Health for African Americans," offers suggestions for facilitating planned change. Dealing with both the psychological and the physiological "self," this section addresses how African Americans can make progress in the health arena through implementation of self-determined strategic initiatives. It argues in favor of social policies that are culturally relevant and sensitive to the specific population served. Chapter Twenty-Two discusses initiatives in the area of reproductive rights. Chapter Twenty-Three focuses on the formulation of health policy. Community organization and empowerment are explored in Chapter Twenty-Four. Chapter Twenty-Five recapitulates the importance of social, political, and economic variables for advancing the health agenda in the black community in the late twentieth and early twenty-first centuries.

A note is in order regarding the use of *black* versus *African American*. Both terms appear throughout the work based on the individual preferences of the authors. The terms are used interchangeably in some chapters. While some changes were made for enhanced readability, every effort was made to honor the authors' preferences.

The chapters included in this volume were not intended to be fully integrated. Rather, they are "stand-alone" contributions, consistent with the nature of the book as a reference or reader. It should also be noted that the individual chapters represent the views of their particular authors and in no way should be construed as representing a consensus of opinion or the position of the respective affiliated organization or agency.

Acknowledgments

The compilation of this volume is the result of many dedicated persons believing in a single mission of uplifting the health status of African Americans. We would like to first thank our contributing authors who worked assiduously in the submission and revision of drafts. Recommendations from colleagues facilitated the completion of the project. We especially acknowledge the input of Drs. John Austin, Daniel S. Blumenthal, Nelson McGhee, Wilbur H. Watson, and anonymous reviewers throughout various stages of the project. We also appreciate the encouragement of our students, friends, and families, who provided moral support from the beginning.

We are particularly indebted to Angela D. Wimes, who served as coordinating assistant for this effort, and Mary Holiday for clerical support during the preparation of the manuscript. We also express sincere appreciation to Rebecca McGovern and Xenia Lisanevich at Jossey-Bass who expedited the book's progress at every stage.

This book was supported in part through the generosity of the Henry J. Kaiser Family Foundation, which has long been a champion of the improved health of disenfranchised populations. Finally, we acknowledge our home institutions, the Morehouse School of Medicine/Emory University School of Public Health and Clark Atlanta University, for providing an environment conducive to carrying out this project.

Atlanta, Georgia Ronald L. Braithwaite
August 1992 Sandra E. Taylor

THE EDITORS

Ronald L. Braithwaite is visiting professor at the Emory University School of Public Health, Office of Public Health Practice, as well as adjunct professor in the Department of Community Health and Preventive Medicine at the Morehouse School of Medicine (MSM). Formerly, he served as director of MSM's Health Promotion Resource Center. He received his B.A. degree (1967) in sociology and his M.S. degree (1969) in rehabilitation counseling from Southern Illinois University. He received his Ph.D. degree (1974) in educational psychology from Michigan State University, where he was a National Institute of Mental Health fellow. He was later a postdoctoral fellow at Yale University and at the University of Michigan's Institute for Social Research and School of Public Health.

Presently, Braithwaite serves as a consultant to the W. K. Kellogg Foundation and various federal government health agencies, including the National Institutes of Health (NIH), the National Institute of Mental Health (NIMH), and the National Institute of Drug Abuse (NIDA). His most recent research emphasis is on community organization and development for health promotion. He also serves as an editor for the *American Journal of Health Promotion*. His published works appear in the *Journal of the American Medical Association, Health Education, Journal of Health Care for the Poor and Underserved*, and *Public Health Reports*.

Braithwaite was formerly director of the Norfolk Area Health Education Center and associate professor in the Department of Psychiatry at Eastern Virginia Medical School. Braithwaite has held faculty appointments at Hampton University, Howard University, and Virginia Commonwealth University. He has received awards from the National Association of Medical Minority Educators and the National Society of Allied Health.

Sandra E. Taylor is associate professor and chairperson of the W.E.B. Du Bois Department of Sociology at Clark Atlanta University, where she formerly served as assistant director of the Center on Health and Aging. She received her B.A. degree (1977) in sociology from Norfolk State University, her M.A. degree (1978) in sociology from Atlanta University, and her Ph.D. degree (1983) in sociology from Washington University. She was a National Institute of Mental Health postdoctoral fellow at the University of Michigan's School of Public Health, and the Program for Research on Black Americans at the Institute for Social Research. She has studied abroad in what was formerly East Germany and West Germany. Some of Taylor's recent publications are in the fields of social psychology and medical sociology, including articles in *Psychology: A Journal of Social Behavior*, *Journal of the Black Nurses' Association*, and *Journal of Social and Behavioral Sciences*.

Her current research interests are in the areas of qualitative evaluation of health and illness programs and health promotion for minority populations. She currently serves as a consultant to local, state, and federal government health agencies, including the National Institutes of Health and the U.S. Alcohol and Drug Administration and Mental Health Administration (ADAMHA). She also serves on several advisory boards, including the Stanford University Health Promotion Resource Center Film Project on Substance Abuse Prevention.

Both editors have lectured widely on a variety of health topics, nationally and abroad. They have held visiting lectureships at universities in Ghana and Cameroon, serving as Fulbright-Hays scholars, as well as in the Caribbean and other Third World countries. They recently conducted workshops in conjunction with the American Public Health Association (APHA), the American Evaluation Association (AEA), and the federal Office for Substance Abuse Prevention (OSAP).

CONTRIBUTORS

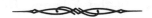

Collins O. Airhihenbuwa is an associate professor of health education and affiliate faculty member of the Black Studies Program at Pennsylvania State University. He received his B.S. degree (1980) in health care administration and planning from Tennessee State University. He received his M.P.H. degree (1981) in health care planning and administration and his Ph.D. degree (1983) in public health education, both from the University of Tennessee in Knoxville. He is a consultant to several national and international agencies, including USAID and the World Health Organization.

Byllye Y. Avery is a women's health care activist. She received her B.A. degree (1959) in psychology from Talledega College and her M.Ed. degree (1969) in special education from the University of Florida. She is founding president of the National Black Women's Health Project, headquartered in Atlanta, Georgia. Avery also cofounded the Gainesville Women's Health Center and Birthplace, an alternative birthing center. She is a MacArthur Foundation Fellow and is the recipient of two honorary degrees.

Claudia R. Baquet is associate director and chief of special populations of the Cancer Control Science Program for the National Cancer Institute's Division of Cancer Prevention and Control. She received her B.S. degree (1973) in zoology from Pomona College/Claremont College; her M.D. degree (1977) from Meharry Medical College; and her M.P.H. degree (1983) from Johns Hopkins University School of Hygiene and Public Health. She has been the recipient of awards from such organizations as the American Cancer Society, the National Medical Association, and the International Black Women's Health Congress for her work on blacks and cancer.

Creigs C. Beverly is professor of social work at Wayne State University, where he is also project administrator of two major grants from the W. K. Kellogg

Foundation in partnership with the Detroit Public School System. Beverly received his B.A. degree (1963) in sociology and psychology from Morehouse College, his M.S.W. degree (1965) from Atlanta University, and his Ph.D. degree (1972) in urban education from the University of Wisconsin. He has been a Fulbright Fellow and Carnegie Fellow. He has received national recognition for his work in dropout prevention, community development and empowerment, and substance abuse.

M. Joycelyn Elders is director of the Arkansas Department of Health. She earned her B.A. (1952) in biology from Philander Smith College. She received her M.D. degree (1960) and M.S. degree (1967) in biochemistry from the University of Arkansas Medical School. Elders has served as a research fellow at the University of Arkansas Medical School as well as an assistant professor of pediatrics. She has authored or coauthored almost 150 papers that have appeared in scholarly journals.

Virginia Davis Floyd is director of the Family Health Services Section (maternal and child health), Georgia Division of Public Health. Programs under her direction include the Women, Infants and Children Program (WIC), Child and Infant Health, Immunization, Women's Health, Family Planning, Children's Medical Services, Genetics, and state offices of Nutrition and Dental Health. She studied biology at Spelman College and Sophia University in Tokyo, Japan, and earned early admittance to medical school. She received her M.D. degree (1976) from Howard University and her M.P.H. degree (1987) from Emory University.

Tyson Gibbs is assistant professor in the Department of Anthropology at Georgia State University in Atlanta. He received his B.A. degree (1973) in anthropology from Dartmouth College. He received his M.A. degree (1977) in cultural anthropology and his Ph.D. degree (1979) in medical anthropology from the University of Florida. He also has a certificate in gerontology from the University of Florida. Formerly Gibbs was program director of the National Cancer Institute, Special Populations Studies Branch, in Bethesda, Maryland.

Aisha Gilliam is associate professor of health education in the Department of Physical Education and Recreation at Howard University. She received her B.A. (1972) and M.A. (1973) degrees in educational psychology from Clark University and her Ed.D. degree (1982) in health education from Columbia University. Gilliam has additional certification in parent effectiveness training, reality therapy, AIDS education, elementary education, and school psychology.

Ruby Morton Gourdine is supervisor of Social Work Services and coordinator of the Childfind Program in the District of Columbia Public Schools. She received her B.A. degree (1969) in sociology from Howard University, her M.S.W. degree (1975) from Atlanta University, and her D.S.W. degree (1984) from Howard University. She is a board member of the Metropolitan Chapter of the National Association of Social Workers and a member of the Mayor's Teenage Pregnancy Prevention Panel.

Christiane B. Hale is chief of the Office of Community Assessment, Tacoma-Pierce (Washington) Health Department, and clinical professor in the Department of Health Services, School of Public Health and Community Medicine, University of Washington. She received her B.A. degree (1971) in history from Auburn University, her M.P.H. degree (1974) in epidemiology from the University of Alabama Medical Center, and her Ph.D. degree (1978) in social psychology and demography from the University of Cincinnati. Hale was formerly professor of epidemiology and director of the Maternal-Child Health Training Program at the School of Public Health, University of Alabama at Birmingham.

Mary S. Harper is research, policy, and development director for the 1993 White House Conference on Aging. She is also coordinator of Long Term Care Programs for the Mental Disorders of the Aging Research Branch, National Institute of Mental Health. She received her B.S. degree (1950) in nursing education/secondary school education, and her M.S. degree (1952) in psychiatric mental health nursing/educational psychology from the University of Minnesota. She received her Ph.D. degree (1963) in sociology/clinical psychology from St. Louis University. Harper has published extensively in the area of mental health and the elderly and is the author of *Mental Illness in Nursing Homes: An Agenda for Research* (1986), the first book published on this topic in the United States.

Carolyn J. Hildreth is assistant professor of medicine at Johns Hopkins University and a faculty member in the Department of Medicine, Division of Ambulatory and Internal Medicine, at Sinai Hospital in Baltimore, Maryland. She received her B.A. degree (1978) in biology from Vassar College and her M.D. degree (1982) from the University of Illinois. She is board certified in internal medicine and completed her residency at Cook County Hospital in Chicago.

Bill Jenkins is an epidemiologist in the Division of Sexually Transmitted Diseases for the Centers for Disease Control. Previously, he served as manager of the National Minority Organization's HIV Program at the Centers for Disease Control as well as chief of the Research/Evaluation Section, Division of Sexually Transmitted Diseases. He received his B.A. degree (1967) in mathematics from Morehouse College and his M.S. degree (1974) in biostatistics from Georgetown University. He received his M.P.H. degree (1977) and his Ph.D. degree (1983) in epidemiology from the University of North Carolina–Chapel Hill School of Public Health.

Joyce A. Ladner is professor of social work and vice president for academic affairs at Howard University. She is the coeditor of *Adolescence and Poverty* (1991) and author of *Tomorrow's Tomorrow: The Black Woman* (1971) and *Mixed Families: Adopting Across Racial Boundaries* (1977). She received her B.A. degree (1964) in sociology from Tougaloo College. She received her M.A. degree (1966) and Ph.D. degree (1968), both in sociology from Washington University in St. Louis.

Kathleen Bodisch Lynch is assistant professor of medical education at the University of Virginia School of Medicine, where she is also assistant director for research and evaluation in the Office of Student Academic Support. She received her B.A. degree (1973) in psychology from LaSalle College, her M.A. degree (1975) in clinical psychology from West Virginia University, and her Ph.D. degree (1986) in educational research and evaluation from the University of Virginia. Lynch has conducted program evaluations and research on minority medical education programs since 1986.

Frederick G. Murphy is a program analyst and commissioned officer in the U.S. Public Health Service, Centers for Disease Control. In addition, he consults with staff at the Morehouse School of Medicine in the identification and development of community intervention and prevention strategies appropriate for use among low-income and minority populations nationwide. He received his B.A. degree (1974) in psychology from Oakwood College and dual M.S. degrees (1977) in public hygiene and international affairs from the University of Pittsburgh Graduate Schools of Public Health and Public International Affairs.

Deborah Prothrow-Stith, an expert on violence, is assistant dean for government/community programs and lecturer for the Department of Health Policy and Management at the Harvard University School of Public Health. She has served as commissioner of public health for the Commonwealth of Massachusetts and as a staff physician for the Boston City Hospital. She received her B.A. degree (1975) in mathematics from Spelman College and her M.D. degree (1979) from the Harvard University Medical School. She recently coauthored a book on teenage violence titled *Deadly Consequences* (1991).

Wornie L. Reed is professor of sociology and director of the Urban Child Research Center at Cleveland State University. Prior to assuming those positions, he was director of the William Monroe Trotter Institute and chair of the Department of Black Studies at the University of Massachusetts at Boston. He received his B.S. degree (1959) in education (science and mathematics) from

Alabama State University. He received his M.A. degree (1974) and Ph.D. degree (1976), both in sociology from Boston University.

Elijah Saunders is associate professor of medicine, head of the Division of Hypertension, and clinical director of the Hypertension Center at the University of Maryland School of Medicine in Baltimore. He also serves as vice president for Graduate Medical Education and Affiliations at the University of Maryland Hospital. Saunders received his B.S. degree (1956) in chemistry from Morgan State University and his M.D. degree (1960) from the University of Maryland School of Medicine. He has written extensively on the subjects of heart disease, stroke, and hypertension, particularly as they affect special populations.

Howard Spivak is chief of the Division of General Pediatrics at the New England Medical Center/Floating Hospital for Infants and Children and associate professor of pediatrics at Tufts University School of Medicine. He received his B.A. degree (1969) in biology and M.D. degree (1973) from the University of Rochester. He also served as deputy commissioner of the Massachusetts Department of Public Health from 1988 to 1990.

Stephen B. Thomas is associate professor of community health in the Department of Health Education and director of the Minority Health Research Laboratory at the University of Maryland in College Park. He received his B.S. degree (1980) in school health education from Ohio State University, his M.S. degree (1981) in health education from Illinois State University, and his Ph.D. degree (1985) in community health education from Southern Illinois University. His areas of expertise include community health advocacy, for which he has been nationally recognized.

Bailus Walker, Jr., is dean of the College of Public Health at the University of Oklahoma's Health Sciences Center, where he is also codirector of the Center for Epidemiologic Research. He received his B.S. degree (1954) in biology and chemistry from Kentucky University, his M.P.H. degree (1959) in occupational and environmental health from the University of Michigan, and his Ph.D. degree (1975) in public health from the University of Minnesota. He has authored numerous manuscripts on occupational and environmental health.

Rueben C. Warren is the assistant director for minority health at the Centers for Disease Control (CDC) and Agency for Toxic Substances and Disease Registry (ATSDR) in Atlanta, Georgia. He serves as chief adviser to the director of CDC and ATSDR on minority health. He is also a clinical professor at the Morehouse School of Medicine. Warren is board certified in dental public health. He received his B.A. degree (1968) in biology from San Francisco State University and his D.D.S. degree (1972) from Meharry Medical College.

He also received his M.P.H. (1973) and Dr.P.H. (1975) degrees from the Harvard University School of Public Health.

Donnie W. Watson is an associate professor of psychiatry, a licensed clinical psychologist, and director of the Cork Institute on Black Alcohol and Other Drug Abuse at the Morehouse School of Medicine. He received his B.A. degree (1978) in psychology from St. Olaf College. He received his M.A. (1980) and Ph.D. (1982) degrees in clinical psychology with a concentration in alcohol studies from Vanderbilt University. His expertise is in the area of evaluation and treatment of substance abuse and chemical dependency among adolescents and adults.

Faye Wattleton was president from 1978 to 1991 of Planned Parenthood Federation of America, the nation's oldest and largest voluntary reproductive health care organization. She is a prominent spokesperson for the reproductive health and rights movement. She received her B.S. degree (1964) in nursing from Ohio State University and her M.S. degree (1967) in maternal and infant care from the Columbia University School of Nursing, where she also earned a C.N.M. in midwifery.

Charles F. Whitten is distinguished professor of pediatrics and associate dean for curricular affairs at Wayne State University, where for eighteen years he has been director of the Comprehensive Sickle Cell Center, sponsored by the National Institutes of Health. He received his A.B. degree (1942) from the University of Pennsylvania in zoology and his M.D. degree (1945) from Meharry Medical College. He is founder and president of the Sickle Cell Detection and Information Program, which conducts a model statewide comprehensive sickle cell program. In addition, he is founder and president of the National Association for Sickle Cell Disease, Inc.

Doris Y. Wilkinson is professor of sociology at the University of Kentucky, where she is also research director for a national medical history project on early African-American physicians. Wilkinson received her B.A. degree (1958) in social work and English from the University of Kentucky. She received her M.A. degree (1960) in sociology and anthropology and her Ph.D. degree (1968) in medical sociology, both from Case Western Reserve University. She received her M.P.H. degree (1985) in health policy/public health from Johns Hopkins University. She has written numerous articles and books and conducted extensive research on the African-American experience, including issues related to race, gender, class, and clinical decision making as well as ethnic customs, life-styles, and life chances.

Moses K. Woode is associate dean for academic support at the University of Virginia School of Medicine. He is also associate professor of medical education and associate professor of obstetrics and gynecology. He has been active in minority medical education programs for the past fifteen years and directs all of the School of Medicine's academic enrichment programs for minority and disadvantaged students. He earned his B.S. degree (1972) and his M.S. degree (1976) in chemistry from the University of Ghana. He received his Ph.D. and D.I.C. degrees (1978), also in chemistry, from the Imperial College of Science, Technology, and Medicine at the University of London.

HEALTH ISSUES
in the
BLACK
COMMUNITY

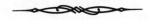

PART I

Health Status
in Social Context

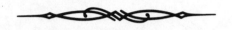

1

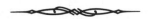

African-American Health:
An Introduction

Ronald L. Braithwaite
Sandra E. Taylor

This book was motivated by scholars sensitized to Afrocentric perspectives on the politics of health in America. It grew out of a need to articulate thinking and interpretation of scientific data related to the issues of health and disease in the black community. The contents represent a convergence of contemporary thought on an array of health conditions affecting black Americans. By taking a broad, contextual approach, the book's contributors depart from the usual disease-model perspective. These authors, through a multidisciplinary strategy, propose tangible changes in health delivery systems to combat the debilitating health conditions characterizing the black populace.

A Call to Action

In many ways, this book is a call to action by those concerned with the widening gap in health status between blacks and nonblacks. There is little utility in calling attention to the disparities in health status between blacks and other racial/ethnic groups without offering practical solutions. Recommendations have included organized community effort to prevent disease and promote health as a valuable and effective strategy (Institute of Medicine, 1988). But it is useful to point out that approximately 80,000 more minority persons than whites die each year. Recent estimates suggest that this statistic has increased by 20,000 since it was reported in the 1985 *Report of the Secretary's Task Force on the Status of Black and Minority Health*. This book seeks in part to serve as a resource for the community of health care providers, researchers, educators, students, and policy makers by analytically addressing the widening gap in health status between blacks and whites. It also seeks to offer functional approaches to raising the political consciousness about strategies for redress. It does not purport to be an exhaustive inventory of all health problems in black America. For example, many important issues—

such as nutrition, sexually transmitted diseases, asthma, language disorders, obesity, and health behaviors—are only tangentially addressed in this work. These health concerns, however, are acknowledged as pertinent areas where disparities exist between black and nonblack populations. Moreover, chonic conditions, including cirrhosis, stroke, and cardiovascular and kidney disease, are examined to varying degrees in context with other disease entities.

We employ a broad definition of health in this work to include social, economic, psychological, and environmental variables related to health outcomes. Health is a state characterized by the following attributes: anatomical integrity; the ability to perform personally valued family, work, and community roles; the ability to deal with physical, biological, and social stress; a feeling of well-being; and freedom from the risk of disease and untimely death (Stokes, Noren, & Shindell, 1982). This definition is preferable to others, among other reasons because it more readily allows for measurement and is less idealistic than other alternatives (Last, 1987, 1986).

Health is of crucial importance to people in all walks of life. Factors such as income, education, occupation, environment, and access to services impact health status. The disparity between black and white health has been linked to these factors, both individually and collectively. Perhaps the most common link is that the disadvantage in health for blacks is largely due to their overrepresentation in lower income groups (Jaynes & Williams, 1989). The combination of factors accounting for this disparity cannot exclude racial bias. As demonstrated in many of the chapters, being black in America has significant costs.

Major health problems can be identified within the black community; such problems result in a shorter life expectancy for blacks in comparison to their white counterparts. The death rate for black Americans is approximately one and one-half times that of whites and black life expectancy is declining (Leffall, 1990). This statistic, however, is a conservative estimate. According to Nickens (1991), black mortality rates are about 50 percent higher than those for whites. Farley and Allen (1989, p. 35) state, "there is an unambiguous trend toward lower mortality rates, but there are persistent and substantial differences between the races." Chronic conditions, years of productive life lost, and "excess" deaths within the black community all point to the distinct health disparity between blacks and whites. These and other conditions are discussed in this volume from the general perspective that structured reform is necessary if black America is to experience a positive shift in health status in the twenty-first century. Various chapters suggest strategies for dealing with specific health concerns and provide prescriptions for change. They may also serve as a means for generating hypotheses in the testing of viable health paradigms.

An exhaustive examination of health problems confronting the black community is next to impossible. This is due, in part, to the multitude of health problems that may be apparent at any given time. We make this point, however, as a backdrop to the identification of still another health problem we are compelled to address. The issue of pollution in relation to ecological conservation has taken on increasing importance in recent years. The environmental crisis in urban America—notably the location of superfund waste sites—affects blacks disproportionately. Closely related to this problem is that of infrastructure (including water supply, wastewater treatment, and waste disposal systems), which contributes to the list of health risks to blacks (Bullard, 1992).

Conclusion

For the reasons just mentioned and in light of other health issues discussed throughout the book, one might readily conclude that the health status of the African-American community is imperiled. A real challenge lies before us. Regardless of the particular health issue or its antecedents, immediate and deliberate actions will be required for positive systemic change. We make such a call for the thirty million African Americans living within these United States.

References

Bullard, R. D. (1992). Urban infrastructure: Social, environmental, and health risks to African Americans. In B. J. Tidwell (Ed.), *The state of black America 1992* (pp. 183–196). New York: National Urban League.

Farley, R., & Allen, W. R. (1989). *The color line and the quality of life in America.* Oxford: Oxford University Press.

Institute of Medicine. Committee for the Study of Public Health, Division of Health Care Services. (1988). *The future of public health.* Washington, DC: National Academy Press.

Jaynes, G. D., & Williams, J.R.M. (Eds.). (1989). *A common destiny: Blacks and American society.* Washington, DC: National Academy Press.

Last, J. M. (Ed.). (1986). *Maxcy-Rosenau public health and preventive medicine* (12th ed.). Norwalk, CT: Appleton-Century-Crofts.

Last, J. M. (1987). *Public health and human ecology.* Sydney, Australia: Appleton and Lange.

Leffall, L. D. (1990). Health status of black Americans. In J. Dewart (Ed.). *The state of black America 1990* (pp. 121–142). New York: National Urban League.

Nickens, H. W. (1991). The health status of minority populations in the United States. *Western Journal of Medicine, 155,* 27–32.

Stokes, J., Noren, J. J., & Shindell, S. (1982). Definition of terms and concepts applicable to clinical preventive medicine. *Journal of Community Health, 8,* 33–41.

U.S. Department of Health and Human Services. (1985). *Report of the Secretary's Task Force on Black and Minority Health* (Vol. 1, Executive Summary). Washington, DC: U.S. Government Printing Office.

2

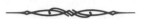

A Demographic Profile of African Americans

Christiane B. Hale

In 1990, African Americans made up 12.3 percent of the U.S. population and were disproportionately represented among the young, the poor, the home- less, and those with indicators of poor health status. Median age was 27.5 years, compared with 33.5 years for whites; median household income was $18,098, 55 percent of the white median family income. Rates of home- lessness among African Americans were two to three times their proportion in the population. African-American births were at least twice as likely as white births to be high risk, but almost 11 percent of African-American mothers received late or no prenatal care, compared with 4.9 percent of white mothers. African-American age- and gender-specific mortality rates exceeded those of white Americans so much that one-third of African- American deaths in 1988 — more than 80,000 — were excess in terms of the age- and gender-specific mortality of comparable white groups. Seventy percent of the excess mortality occurred before the age of sixty-five, and 40 percent occurred before the age of forty-five. African-American death rates in infancy and from homicide, stroke, cirrhosis, diabetes, and acquired im- mune deficiency syndrome (AIDS) were two or more times greater than those of whites. Socioeconomic disparities account for only some of this excess mortality. Almost one-third of African Americans lack private health insur- ance, and nearly as many live in states that provide minimal support for Medicaid. Considerable evidence suggests that, independent of socio- economic status or insurance status, African Americans are less likely to be included in appropriately designed prevention or detection programs or to receive early treatment for chronic conditions.

In its 1985 report, the Secretary's Task Force on Black and Minority Health analyzed 1979–81 data and reported that African Americans were generally 1.5 times as likely to be sick and die as whites (U.S. Department of Health and Human Services, 1985). These excess risks may have worsened during the 1980s (Centers for Disease Control, 1990; Griffith & Bell, 1989; Kapantais & Powell-Griner, 1989; National Research Council, 1989).

This chapter was written to provide a statistical background against which to examine this troubling phenomenon. It consists of three sections comparing demographic information about African Americans and whites. In the first, the two groups are compared in terms of age and gender composition, marital status, socioeconomic status, and place of residence. In the second, the fertility and mortality experience of the two groups are contrasted. In a third section, evidence is examined suggesting that African Americans—because of their socioeconomic position and their patterns of residence in certain states—may be overrepresented among those who lack health insurance and therefore may experience difficulty gaining access to health care.

Sociodemographic Characteristics

By 1990, African Americans were the nation's second-largest population group. The U.S. Bureau of the Census estimated that of 248.1 million people, 30.3 million (12.3 percent) were African Americans (U.S. Bureau of the Census, 1989c). Non-Hispanic whites comprised about 74 percent of the population, and Hispanics made up about another 10 percent. In the remainder of this chapter, the term *whites* or *white Americans* is used to mean non-Hispanic whites.

Age Composition

The age composition of a population influences its birth and death rates. Population groups are often described as "young" or "old," referring to their average age. In 1990, the median age of the U.S. white population was estimated to be 33.2 years, while the median age among African Americans was 27.5 years (U.S. Bureau of the Census, 1989c). Young populations generally have higher birth and fertility rates; as will be seen later, this is true for African Americans. But young populations should also have lower death rates, and, as will also be seen, African Americans do not.

Gender Composition

Demographers measure the gender composition of populations in terms of their gender structure, or the ratio of males per 100 females. The gender ratio of most populations' births is between 95 and 105. At virtually every age, males are more likely to die than females. Because the risk of dying also increases with age, the gender ratio begins to fall in older age groups.

White and African Americans have very different gender ratios, especially in the young adult age groups. In 1990, the gender ratio in the youngest white age group was 105; the ratio was persistently above 100 until age forty to forty-four and fell steadily thereafter. Among African Americans at the youngest ages, the gender ratio was 103. But, in contrast to the pattern among whites, by age twenty to twenty-four, it had fallen to 95, and by thirty to thirty-four, it was below 90. Put another way, the gender ratio among African Americans in this last age group is about equal to that of sixty- to sixty-four-year-old whites.

Household Composition

Populations with gender ratios outside normal limits often show patterns of family formation and household composition that also do not conform to the dominant model (Guttentag & Secord, 1982). This is the case for African Americans. In 1987, 51.3 percent of African-American families were comprised of married couples, and 35.4 percent were headed by women (U.S. Bureau of the Census, 1989a). Comparable figures for white families were 83.2 percent and 12.9 percent, respectively.

Socioeconomic Status

The concept of *socioeconomic status* is used to designate position in a hierarchical organization of society; outside the United States, the concept is called *social class*. Both are derived from the notion of a stratification of people from lower to higher in terms of access to power, prestige, and property. These abstractions are generally operationalized by using measures of education, occupation, and income, and that practice is followed here.

On each of these measures, African Americans rank lower than whites (Table 2.1). Although African Americans have made substantial educational gains during the past twenty years, they still lag behind whites in terms of median years of education and the proportions completing high school and college. The high school completion rates of African Americans in 1988 were comparable to those of whites in the early 1970s. The rate of college graduation among females was about equal to that of white females in 1975, but college graduation levels among African-American males were about where they were among whites in 1960 (U.S. Bureau of the Census, 1988).

Patterns of income and occupation echo the differences in education. The 1987 median household income of whites was 1.6 times that of African Americans; among those living below poverty, income differences were minor but did exist. Among those employed, half as many African Americans as whites held managerial or professional positions, but nearly three times as many worked in service jobs. There were no differences in the proportions employed in technical occupations.

Closely related to socioeconomic status is the concept of poverty or having a family income below the federally designated poverty level. (This measure varies with family size and is calculated in terms of the dollars needed to purchase food; see O'Hare, 1985.) In 1987, 9.1 percent of white families and 31.8 percent of African-American families were living below this poverty threshold (U.S. Bureau of the Census, 1989a). Female-headed families

Table 2.1. Measures of Socioeconomic Status, by Race, 1987.

	African-American	White
Median years of education	12.3	12.7
Percent completing high school		
Males	63.0	76.5
Females	63.7	75.9
Percent completing college		
Males	11.0	24.5
Females	10.4	16.9
Median household income		
All households	$18,098	$32,529
Those below poverty	$5,419	$5,908
Occupation		
Managerial/professional	14.9	29.0
Technical	22.7	22.5
Service	24.1	8.2

Source: Data extracted from U.S. Bureau of the Census, 1988, Table 12, p. 74; 1989b, Table 16, pp. 60–87.

were particularly likely to be living in poverty, and 29.5 percent of white families were female headed compared to 54.8 percent of African-American ones (U.S. Bureau of the Census, 1989a).

Place of Residence

Nearly 80 percent of Americans live in one of the country's 283 metropolitan areas (Frey, 1990), which are defined as cities with at least 50,000 population plus those living in adjacent communities economically linked to these cities. Metropolitan residence is slightly more common among African Americans. In 1987, 82.7 percent of African Americans lived in metropolitan areas, compared with 75.6 percent of whites.

The Census Bureau categorizes metropolitan places as either central city or ring; the latter is synonymous with suburban areas. During the 1970s and 1980s, middle-class people tended to move from the central cities to suburbs, resulting in a concentration of poor people in many central cities. At the same time, jobs in the central cities decreased as they followed population movement. The result was a diminution in the tax base available to fund public services increasingly needed by the changing central city populations (Kasarda, 1988). African Americans were more likely than whites to be affected by these trends: in 1987, 57.7 percent of African Americans but 25.5 percent of whites resided in central cities (U.S. Bureau of the Census, 1989b).

State and Regional Distribution. African Americans are found in virtually every state, but over half live in the thirteen states usually categorized as southern (Maryland, Virginia, North Carolina, South Carolina, Georgia,

Florida, Alabama, Mississippi, Tennessee, Kentucky, Louisiana, Arkansas, and Texas) (U.S. Bureau of the Census, 1990). About one of five African Americans lives in South Carolina, Georgia, Alabama, Mississippi, or Louisiana. These five states are among the poorest in the country in terms of income, and they have historically ranked lowest in terms of per capita appropriations for education, health, and other human services.

The Homeless. African Americans are disproportionately represented among the homeless: In New York about 25 percent of the population is black, but black Americans comprise 73 percent of the city's homeless people (Institute of Medicine, 1988). Similarly, they make up 7.5 percent of Ohio's population and 11 percent of that state's homeless.

Demographic Processes

There are three major demographic processes: birth, death, and migration. This chapter focuses on the first two. Although migration patterns of African Americans have been complex and are well studied, a discussion of them would add little to our understanding of health differentials between white and African Americans.

Before comparing patterns of fertility and mortality, one limitation to these comparisons must be noted. Demographic trends are often described by rates, which measure events in terms of some population aggregation, such as deaths per 1,000 people. Rates are as accurate as is the count of events (which comprises the rate's numerator) and of the population (the rate's denominator). Rates calculated for African Americans are less accurate than those describing whites because population counts—derived from the decennial U.S. census—are less complete for African Americans than for whites.

In the 1970 census (the first one for which census accuracy could be thoroughly assessed), the white underenumeration rate was less than two percent, while the African-American rate was 7.5 percent, or nearly four times higher. African-American males age twenty to thirty-nine were most often missed; their underenumeration rates exceeded 17 percent. Despite efforts to improve the accuracy of the 1980 census, patterns of underenumeration among African Americans were roughly identical to those seen in 1970 (Fay, Passel & Robinson, 1988).

Most published statistics—including many in this chapter—use unadjusted population counts or their derivatives in the denominators (H. Rosenberg, personal communication, August 1990). When denominators are too low, rates will be higher than reality. Thus, up to about 15 percent of differences between African-American and white fertility and mortality rates could be explained by differential accuracy of the denominators. However, this problem does *not* explain the persistence of fertility and mortality differentials across time (because the underenumeration appears constant), nor does it account for interracial variations in rates substantially greater than 15 percent often reported in the following sections.

Birth and Fertility Rates

The most frequently used measure of births is the *birth rate*, or the number of births per 1,000 people. If two groups have dissimilar birth rates but also have dissimilar age structures, it becomes difficult to determine whether the birth rates are truly different or merely appear so because one population has more young people (who are more likely to be having children) than the other does. This issue can be resolved by using *fertility rates*, measures which have as their denominator the number of births per 1,000 women age fifteen to forty-four (the general range of childbearing years). There are several ways of computing fertility rates, but the one most sensitive to population age structures is the total fertility rate, which estimates the number of children an average group of 1,000 women would have if the age-specific fertility rates at one point in time were to prevail throughout their childbearing years. Because each of these measures conveys somewhat different—but equally important—information about fertility trends, both are used in the comparisons here.

In 1988, the birth rate among African Americans was 22.2 as compared to 14.7 births for every 1,000 people, and the total fertility rate per 1,000 women was 2,402 for African Americans as compared to 1,814 for whites (see Table 2.2). In developed nations such as the United States, a total fertility rate of 2,100 children per 1,000 women is considered the level needed for population replacement. The white total fertility rate fell below replacement level in the early 1970s and, although some modest increase occurred after 1984, it has not yet returned to that level. In contrast, the total fertility rate among African Americans fell less precipitously and has been persistently above replacement level. The 1988 African-American fertility rate (2,402) is not only 1.3 times above the 1988 white fertility rate (1,814), but it is slightly above the 1970 white rate of 2,385.

Demographic Characteristics of Births. Certain demographic characteristics of mothers or their infants have been identified as "risk factors." Mothers and infants with such characteristics are more likely than average to

Table 2.2. Birth and Total Fertility Rates, by Race, 1988.

	African-American	White
Births per 1,000 people	22.2	14.7
Total fertility rate per 1,000 women	2,402	1,814

Source: Data extracted from National Center for Health Statistics, 1990b, Tables 1 and 4, pp. 15, 18, 19.

experience health and/or social problems consequent to birth. Important maternal risk factors include the following: age younger than twenty, and especially younger than eighteen; being unmarried; and not having completed high school. Other significant risk factors are late prenatal care (care that began after the sixth month of pregnancy) or none at all and low infant birthweight. Birthweights less than 2,500 grams (about 5.5 pounds) and especially less than 1,500 grams (about 3 pounds) are risk factors for either death or, among survivors, significant handicap (Institute of Medicine, 1986).

Table 2.3 shows the proportion of white and African-American births with one or more of these demographic characteristics in 1988. For each one, significantly more African-American births were high risk. African-American mothers were twice as likely as whites to be eighteen or nineteen years old, to have had less than twelve years' education, or to have had late or no prenatal care. They were 3.6 times more likely to be unmarried. Their infants had more than two times the risk of weighing less than 2,500 grams at birth and experienced nearly three times the risk of weighing less than 1,500 grams.

Mortality Rates

Mortality rates vary by age; the very young and the very old are biologically more likely to die than are those between the two extremes. Mortality rates also vary by gender, with males at each age more likely to die than females. Because of these biological risks, mortality rates are computed both by age ("age-specific mortality rates") and by gender. When populations differ in their age structure, as do white and African Americans, age-adjusted death rates are computed, in effect, to erase the impact of age composition.

On all measures, mortality rates in the United States vary dramatically by race, as Table 2.4 illustrates. Age-adjusted rates (line 1 of Table 2.4) show that white females have the lowest mortality rates, followed, in order, by African-American females, white males, and African-American males.

Table 2.3. Percent of Births That Were High Risk, by Race, 1988.

	African-American	White
Maternal age		
< 18 years old	7.2	3.6
18–19 years old	12.3	6.9
Unmarried mother	63.5	17.7
Maternal education < 12 years	30.7	17.3
Late or no prenatal care	10.5	4.9
Infant birthweight		
< 2,500 grams	13.0	5.6
< 1,500 grams	2.8	0.9

Source: Data extracted from National Center for Health Statistics, 1990b, Tables 2, 18, 22, 29, and 30, pp. 16, 32, 37, 40, 41.

Table 2.4. Selected Mortality Rates, by Race, 1987.

	African-American		White	
	Male	Female	Male	Female
Age-adjusted death rate (per 100,000 people)	1,037.8	593.1	664.3	384.4
Life expectancy at birth[a]	64.9	73.4	72.3	78.9
Infant mortality rate (per 1,000 live births)	19.0	16.1	9.5	7.4
Neonatal mortality rate	12.5	10.4	5.9	4.8
Postneonatal mortality rate	6.6	5.8	3.6	2.7
Years of potential life lost (per 1,000 people <65 years old)	133.8	71.3	66.1	34.6

[a] 1988 provisional data.

Source: Data extracted from National Center for Health Statistics, 1990a, Tables 1, 13, and 4, pp. 14, 32, 16; 1990c, Tables 14 and 25, pp. 106, 125–126.

African-American males have a particularly disadvantageous mortality experience. Their age-standardized risk of death is 1.6 times that of white males and 1.8 that of African-American females. In comparison, African-American females have 1.5 times the age-standardized mortality risk of white females.

Yet another way of measuring mortality is to compute life expectancy, or the number of years an individual born in a given year could expect to live if the age-specific mortality rates observed that year were unchanged through his or her lifetime. Line 2 of Table 2.4 shows provisional 1988 life expectancies in the United States. Within each racial group, females lived longer than males. Within each gender, life expectancy for whites exceeded that of African Americans; the difference was 5.5 years for females and 7.4 years for males. Life expectancies for both white groups and African-American females are within the range of those seen in other developed nations, but those of African-American males are at levels more often seen in less developed nations (Population Reference Bureau, 1990).

The next three rows of Table 2.4 list infant mortality rates, or the number of deaths that occur per 1,000 live births. These rates are among the most frequently used mortality measures because they are also sensitive indices of societal well-being (Hale, 1990; Yankauer, 1990). In addition to showing the infant death rate, Table 2.4 displays rates of neonatal mortality, deaths occurring during the first four weeks of life, and postneonatal mortality—deaths from 28 to 365 days of life. Neonatal mortality occurs primarily as a result of low infant birthweight, while postneonatal mortality has long been considered a more direct indication of socioeconomic inequities (Antonovsky & Bernstein, 1977). In 1988, as in earlier years, African-American infant and neonatal mortality rates for both males and females were 2.1 times the white rates, and the postneonatal death rate was 2.0 times greater.

The last line of Table 2.4—the years of potential life lost before age sixty-five per 1,000 people—is one approach to measuring preventable death. Consistent with other mortality measures, this figure is lowest for white females, higher for white males and African-American females, and highest for African-American males. Within each racial group, males lose about 1.9 times the number of years of potential life that females do. Within gender, African Americans lose about twice as many years of potential life as whites.

Estimation of Excess Mortality. A more refined approach to calculating preventable deaths is to calculate "excess mortality," or the difference between the actual number of African Americans who died in a given year and the number who would have died had their age- and gender-specific mortality rate been the same as that of whites (U.S. Department of Health and Human Services, 1985, pp. 63–75). That method was used to estimate excess deaths in 1988 for this chapter by applying the age- and gender-specific mortality rates for whites in 1988 reported by the National Center for Health Statistics to population estimates generated by the U.S. Bureau of the Census (National Center for Health Statistics, 1990a, 1990b, 1990c, 1990d).

Results of these analyses indicate that 80,786 of the 263,922 African-American deaths in 1988 (30.6 percent) were excess—33 percent of deaths in males and 27.7 percent of female deaths (Table 2.5). Forty percent of all excess deaths occurred before age forty-five: approximately 45 percent of male deaths and one-third of female deaths. For both groups, another 35 percent of excess deaths occurred before age sixty-five. Thus, more than 80 percent of excess deaths in African-American males and 70 percent of excess deaths in females occurred before age sixty-five.

The Secretary's Task Force found that 80 percent of excess deaths in 1979–81 arose from six causes: homicide/accidents, infant mortality, cancer, cardiovascular and cerebrovascular diseases, substance abuse (measured by

Table 2.5. Excess Mortality[a] Among African Americans, by Age and Gender, 1988.

Age Group	Total		Males		Females	
	Number	Percent	Number	Percent	Number	Percent
All ages	80,786	100.0	47,623	100.0	33,163	100.0
<1	7,097	8.8	3,814	8.0	3,283	9.9
1–14	1,437	1.8	806	1.7	631	1.9
15–24	2,779	3.4	2,234	4.7	545	1.6
25–44	21,027	26.0	14,354	30.1	6,673	20.1
45–64	28,354	36.3	17,558	36.9	11,796	35.6
≥65	19,092	23.6	8,857	18.6	10,235	30.9

[a] See text.

Source: White age- and gender-specific mortality rates from National Center for Health Statistics, 1990a, Table 2, p. 15 were applied to Series 14 (middle series) population estimates in U.S. Bureau of the Census, 1989c, Table 4, pp. 38–43.

deaths from cirrhosis), and diabetes. More recently, acquired immune deficiency syndrome has been added to the list of major causes of excess death: although African Americans comprised about 12 percent of the population, they accounted for 22 percent of AIDS-related deaths (Kapantais & Powell-Griner, 1989).

Excess deaths from these seven causes in 1988 were estimated using relative risks and compared with those reported for 1980 (U.S. Department of Health and Human Services, 1985, Table 2.5, p. 67). The results suggest that the higher risk of dying (compared with whites) observed among African Americans in 1980 had not improved by 1988 and may actually have increased for many causes (Table 2.6).

African-American males experienced an increase in their overall risk of death. There were no changes in their relative risk of death from cancer and stroke, and their relative risk of death from cirrhosis actually dropped. More than offsetting that decrease were increases in their relative risk of death as infants and from homicide, accidents, heart disease, and diabetes.

Table 2.6. Age-Adjusted Death Rates by Selected Causes, Gender, and Race, 1980 and 1988.

	Males			Females		
	African-American	White	Relative Risk	African-American	White	Relative Risk
1980						
All causes	1,112.8	745.3	1.5	631.1	411.1	1.5
Infant mortality	2,586.7	1,230.3	2.1	2,123.7	962.5	2.2
Homicide	71.9	10.9	6.6	13.7	3.2	4.3
Accidents	82.0	62.3	1.3	25.1	21.4	1.2
Cancer	229.9	160.5	1.4	129.7	107.7	1.2
Heart disease	327.3	277.5	1.2	201.1	134.6	1.5
Stroke	77.5	41.9	1.9	61.7	35.2	1.8
Cirrhosis	30.6	15.7	2.0	14.4	7.0	2.1
Diabetes	17.7	9.5	1.9	22.1	8.7	2.5
1988						
All causes	1,037.8	664.3	1.6	593.1	384.4	1.5
Infant mortality	2,167.7	930.5	2.3	1,821.5	782.2	2.3
Homicide	58.2	7.7	7.6	12.7	2.8	4.5
Accidents	69.0	49.9	1.4	22.2	18.8	1.2
Cancer	227.0	157.6	1.4	131.2	110.1	1.2
Heart disease	286.2	220.5	1.3	181.1	114.2	1.6
Stroke	57.8	30.0	1.9	46.6	25.5	1.8
Cirrhosis	20.7	12.1	1.7	9.3	5.0	1.9
Diabetes	19.8	9.6	2.1	22.1	8.4	2.6
AIDS	31.6	9.9	3.2	6.2	0.7	8.9

Source: 1980 figures are from U.S. Department of Health and Human Services, 1985, Table 5, p. 67; 1988 figures were calculated from National Center for Health Statistics, 1990a, Tables 1, 2, 12, and 25, pp. 14, 15, 30–31, 43.

African-American females experienced no change in their overall relative risk of deaths and in their relative risk of death from accidents, cancer, and stroke. There was a substantial decrease in their relative risk of death from cirrhosis. Like African-American males, however, their relative risk of death as infants or from homicide, heart disease, and diabetes rose substantially during the 1980s. Earlier data for AIDS deaths are not available, but in 1988 the relative risk of dying from AIDS was 3.2 among African-American males and 8.9 among females.

Demography and Health of African Americans

African Americans are particularly vulnerable to inequities inherent in U.S. policies, which historically have expressed the view that health care is a private rather than public good. With this definition, the U.S. government has removed itself from any significant role in guaranteeing access to that care. Health insurance is the basic mechanism determining access, and, over time, health insurance has been linked with employment (Williams & Torrens, 1988). Unemployment and underemployment are more common among African Americans; thus, lack of insurance is especially marked among them. While 17.4 percent of Americans younger than age sixty-five are estimated to lack health insurance in any form, that figure includes 32.9 percent of African Americans but only 14.2 percent of whites (Butler, 1988; Short, Monheit, & Beauregard, 1988).

Medicaid is the federally funded program that provides health insurance for certain categories of poor and uninsured people. About 6 percent of whites and about 30 percent of African Americans are covered by this program (Gold, Kenney, & Singh, 1987). Each state must participate in Medicaid or create some other option that insures eligible groups, but each state may also establish eligibility ceilings within broad guidelines. As a result, interstate variations in coverage have been marked. For example, in 1986, a poor mother with three children in Alabama was ineligible for AFDC and thus Medicaid, if the annual household income was more than $1,764 per year, but that same family in California was eligible for Medicaid provided household income was *below* $10,600 annually (Gold & Kenney, 1985; Gold, Kenney, & Singh, 1987). While some action has been taken to reduce these extremes, interstate variations persist. African Americans are most likely to feel the negative impact of these variations because they are concentrated in states that define Medicaid eligibility in the most restrictive terms.

Conclusion

African Americans are sociodemographically distinct from the white population. They are younger, on average, and are more often female and unmarried. The African-American community is disproportionately concentrated in central cities or Southern states. African Americans are also poorer than whites. They are less likely to graduate from high school or college or to hold professional or managerial positions. Median family income for African Americans is half that of whites, and nearly one-third of African Americans live below the poverty threshold.

African Americans are twice as likely as whites to have high-risk births. Elevated risk also characterizes the mortality patterns of African Americans, especially males, whose life expectancy of less than sixty-five years is more typical of that seen in developing nations. One measure of the excess mortality experienced by African Americans is the finding that in 1988, one-third of all deaths — more than 80,000 — were excess; in other words, the numbers of people dying exceeded expectations based on the age- and gender-specific mortality of comparable white groups. Three-quarters of the excess mortality occurred before the age of sixty-five, and 40 percent occurred before the age of forty-five. Much of the excess mortality can be explained by higher death rates in infancy and from homicide, stroke, cirrhosis, diabetes, and AIDS.

African Americans appear less likely than whites to have benefited from public health initiatives designed to reduce the risks of a poor pregnancy outcome, or to lessen the incidence of death from preventable conditions, or to detect and treat chronic diseases. For example, in 1988 nearly 11 percent of African-American women received late or no prenatal care, compared to 4.9 percent of white women. Part of the explanation lies in their lack of health insurance, which controls access to health care. One-third of African Americans have no private health insurance, and nearly that many live in states that historically have limited access to Medicare (and to other social services). The persistent association between race and the lack of care utilization — even within the same socioeconomic stratum — suggests that discrimination is a plausible explanation for the poorer health status indicators observed in African Americans.

References

Antonovsky, A., & Bernstein, J. (1977). Social class and infant mortality. *Social Science and Medicine, 11*(3), 453–470.

Butler, P. A. (1988). *Too poor to be sick: Access to medical care for the uninsured.* Washington, DC: American Public Health Association.

Centers for Disease Control. (1990, July). CDC Surveillance Summaries: Reports on selected racial/ethnic groups, special focus: maternal and child health. *Morbidity and Mortality Weekly Report, 39*(3).

Fay, R., Passel, J., & Robinson, J. G. (1988). *The coverage of population in the 1980 census* (U.S. Bureau of the Census Publication No. PHC80-E4). Washington, DC: U.S. Government Printing Office.

Frey, W. H. (1990, July). Metropolitan America: Beyond the transition. *Population Bulletin, 45*(2).

Gold, R. S., & Kenney, A. M. (1985). Paying for maternity care. *Family Planning Perspectives, 17*(3), 103–111.

Gold, R. B., Kenney, A. M., & Singh, S. (1987). *Blessed events and the bottom line: Financing maternity care in the United States.* New York: Alan Guttmacher Institute.

Griffith, E.E.H., & Bell, C. C. (1989). Recent trends in suicide and homicide among blacks. *Journal of the American Medical Association, 262*(16), 2265–2269.

Guttentag, M., & Secord, P. F. (1982). *Too many women? The sex ratio question.* Newbury Park, CA: Sage.

Hale, C. B. (1990). Infant mortality: An American tragedy. *Population trends and public policy* (No. 17). Washington, DC: Population Reference Bureau.

Institute of Medicine. (1986). *Preventing low birthweight.* Washington, DC: National Academy Press.

Institute of Medicine, Committee on Health Care for Homeless People. (1988). *Homelessness, health, and human needs.* Washington, DC: National Academy Press.

Kapantais, G., & Powell-Griner, E. (1989). Characteristics of persons dying from AIDS: Preliminary data from the 1986 National Mortality Followback Survey. *Advance data from vital and health statistics* (No. 173). Hyattsville, MD: National Center for Health Statistics.

Kasarda, J. D. (1988). Jobs, migration, and emerging urban mismatches. In M. G. McGeary & L. E. Lynn, Jr. (Eds.), *Urban change and poverty.* Washington, DC: National Academy Press.

National Center for Health Statistics. (1990a). Advance report of final mortality statistics, 1988. *Monthly Vital Statistics Report* (Vol. 39, No. 7, Suppl.). Hyattsville, MD: Public Health Service.

National Center for Health Statistics. (1990b). Advance report of final natality statistics, 1988. *Monthly Vital Statistics Report* (Vol. 39, No. 4, Suppl.). Hyattsville, MD: Public Health Service.

National Center for Health Statistics. (1990c). *Health, United States, 1989.* Hyattsville, MD: Public Health Service. ˙

National Center for Health Statistics. (1990d). *Vital statistics of the United States, 1987* (Vol. 2, Pt. B, Mortality). Hyattsville, MD: Public Health Service.

National Research Council. (1989). *A common destiny: Blacks and American society.* Washington, DC: National Academy Press.

O'Hare, W. P. (1985, June). Poverty in America: Trends and new patterns. *Population Bulletin, 40*(3).

Population Reference Bureau, U.S. Department of Labor. (1990). *World population data sheet, 1990.* Washington, DC: U.S. Government Printing Office.

Short, P. F., Monheit, A., & Beauregard, K. (1988, October). *Uninsured Americans: A 1987 profile.* Paper presented at the annual meeting of the American Public Health Association, New Orleans, LA.

U.S. Bureau of the Census. (1988). Educational attainment in the United States: March 1987 and 1988. *Current Population Reports* (Series P-20, No. 428). Washington, DC: U.S. Government Printing Office.

U.S. Bureau of the Census. (1989a). Household and family characteristics,

March 1988. *Current Population Reports* (Series P-20, No. 437). Washington, DC: U.S. Government Printing Office.

U.S. Bureau of the Census. (1989b). Poverty in the United States, 1987. *Current Population Reports* (Series P-60, No. 183). Washington, DC: U.S. Government Printing Office.

U.S. Bureau of the Census. (1989c). Projections of the population of the United States, by age, sex, and race: 1988–2080. *Current Population Reports* (Series P-25, No. 1018). Washington, DC: U.S. Government Printing Office.

U.S. Bureau of the Census. (1990). Projections of the populations of states, by age, sex, and race: 1989 to 2010. *Current Population Reports* (Series P-25, No. 1053). Washington, DC: U.S. Government Printing Office.

U.S. Department of Health and Human Services. (1985). *Report of the Secretary's Task Force on Black and Minority Health* (Vol. 1, Executive Summary). Washington, DC: U.S. Government Printing Office.

Williams, S. J., & Torrens, P. R. (Eds.). (1988). *Introduction to health services* (3rd ed.) New York: Wiley.

Yankauer, A. (1990). What infant mortality tells us. *American Journal of Public Health, 80*(6), 653–654.

3

The Mental Health Status
of Black Americans:
An Overview

Sandra E. Taylor

There is no paucity of research on general aspects of mental health in the black community. A 1991 computerized search on the topic accessed over 1,600 works within the scientific body of literature since 1980 alone. But despite this high volume of research, much remains to be learned about the psychological state of African Americans in comparison to other racial and ethnic groups. While countless studies have focused on various aspects of the mental health of African Americans, many gaps in our knowledge still exist. This chapter provides an overview of black mental health in the identification of research and policy considerations.

Mental health connotes different things to different people. There is considerable variation among definitions within and between the major disciplines and professions. Because of the difficulty in defining this concept and since varying definitions prevail in the literature, it is important to make clear the use of the term in this chapter. Borrowing a relatively comprehensive definition from Gary and Jones (1978, pp. 6–7), the following forms the working definition of *mental health* in this chapter: the ability of an individual to control or modify his or her environment so that he or she is able to (1) exercise sound and realistic judgment and strategies for dealing with problems, (2) satisfy basic biological and basic human needs, (3) establish meaningful physical and emotional relationships with others, (4) take responsibility for personal feelings and actions, (5) have a functional integrated self-image with an awareness of how freedom, autonomy, and morality relate to one's image, and (6) support efforts to promote the growth and development of one's own cultural or social group. While this definition has its own limitations, as Gary and Jones (1978) concede, it is appropriate for the discussion in this chapter.

Social Trends in Black Mental Health

Almost a decade ago, Poussaint (1983) discussed the deteriorating mental health of African Americans in the context of socioeconomic and racial

factors. Unfortunately, blacks in the United States continue to suffer disproportionately from low socioeconomic status and institutional racism, leaving
them overrepresented in some categories of mental disorder. For example,
Brown, Eaton, and Sussman (1990) found that blacks tend to have higher
rates of phobic disorder than whites even when specific demographic, socioeconomic, and sociocultural factors are controlled. According to the *Diagnostic and Statistical Manual of Mental Disorders* (DSM-III), the essential feature
of phobic disorder is persistent and irrational fear of a specific object,
activity, or situation that results in a compelling desire to avoid the dreaded
object, activity, or situation. The fear is recognized by the individual as
excessive or unreasonable in proportion to the actual dangerousness of the
object, activity, or situation (American Psychiatric Association, 1980, p. 225).
Using data from a large community-based survey (2,340 black and 3,936
white respondents), the authors found that being female, young, and having
low educational attainment were also among significant risk factors for
recent phobia (defined as meeting DSM-III criteria within the month before
the interview). Moreover, contemporary social problems such as homelessness and drug addiction, which affect blacks disproportionately, are
clearly linked to mental disorders. Particularly in the instance of homelessness, persons with mental disorders constitute a significant subgroup;
recent NIMH-supported studies indicate prevalence ranges from 28 to 37
percent (Tessler, 1990). Although the prevalence of mental disorders has been
found to be less dramatic among persons with various drug addictions, a
high degree of psychiatric disorder is found in this population as a result of
alcohol and other substance abuse.

Poussaint's (1983, p. 234) contention that "there appear to be no safety
nets that protect the health or psyche of the Afro-American from institutional racism, poverty, high unemployment, and a stagnant economy" is still
valid despite national initiatives for improved mental health. While the
problem of meager financial resources is likely to pose a mental threat to
anyone affected, the problem of racism uniquely affects the nonwhite population. This problem, coupled with the fact that higher proportions of blacks
are adversely impacted by poverty, unemployment, and recessionary periods,
places the African-American community at tremendous risk for diminished
mental health. The avoidance of or delay in seeking professional help for
mental disorders poses a further problem. It is not surprising that many
nonwhite populations are reluctant to turn to the mental health system. Such
reluctance is partially due to an attitude of fear and suspicion. Similarly,
stigma plays a role in resistance to services. The tendency to rely more on the
medical than the mental health system often leads blacks to the hospital
emergency room as the gateway to mental health care (Rosenthal & Carty,
1988).

Mental Health Utilization and Treatment

Blacks constituted 18.4 percent of all hospital admissions in 1980, including
state and county mental hospitals, private psychiatric hospitals, nonfederal

general hospitals, and Veterans Administration (VA) medical centers (Manderscheid & Barrett, 1987). Comparative figures were 79.9 percent for the
white population and 1.6 percent "other," including Asians, Native Americans, Alaskan Natives, and Pacific Islanders. Given that blacks constituted
only 12 percent of the U.S. population during this same period, their
overrepresentation is clear. It is important to note, however, that utilization
rates are not an accurate measure of incidence of disorders.

Although utilization and treatment are inextricably linked to race/
ethnicity, other factors impact the breadth of mental health services received
by black clients. Cleary (1989) points out that mental health utilization
patterns are influenced by psychological and cultural factors as well as the
availability, organization, and financing of care. Moreover, the effect of removing financial barriers to care is better understood within the context of the
psychological and cultural factors that play an important role in determining who seeks care and how it is actually sought (Cleary, 1989). The cultural
factor in utilization and treatment is significant. Rosenthal and Carty (1988)
indicate that patterns of utilization that show lower use of services by ethnic
group members tend to diminish when physical and cultural barriers to
adequate community-based services are removed.

The idea that black mental health disorders must be examined in a
cultural context is certainly not new. Thomas and Comer (1973) clearly
articulated the importance of cultural spheres to mental health almost
twenty years ago. Despite this demand for greater recognition of the client's
particular culture, however, there is still a tendency to assess the mental
health of blacks without regard to their cultural background.

Research shows that blacks and other minorities receive less than
adequate treatment in most community mental health programs (President's
Commission on Mental Health, 1978). Experiences with mental health professionals that translate into doubt, fear, or suspicion in black patients lead to
their rejection of services. Problems related to minorities who are underserved, misdiagnosed, segregated, and overinstitutionalized are a serious
concern and are often influenced by factors outside the purview of the
mental health system (Rosenthal & Carty, 1988).

The mental health of blacks has historically been underemphasized in
American society, in part because of the stereotype that they are not easily
susceptible to depression or related disorders. Instead of being viewed as
experiencing the same kinds of conditions provoked by stressful life events
that the larger white population experiences, blacks have been adversely
labeled in ways that reflect a belief in inherent pathology. Nonwhites have
been found to be diagnosed with more serious mental illnesses than whites
and are more often discharged as schizophrenics, while whites are classified
as having depressive disorders (Bell, Bland, Houston, & Jones, 1983). Data on
admission for inpatient psychiatric services during 1980 show that 31 percent of blacks received diagnoses of affective disorders, compared to 44
percent of whites. However, 36 percent of blacks were diagnosed with schizophrenia, compared to 19 percent of whites (Manderscheid & Barrett, 1987).

Baker's (1988) concise historical account of African Americans places in context factors which impact diagnosis and treatment. When therapy includes an examination of the client's heritage and cultural background, misdiagnosis and improper labeling are reduced.

Labeling can be a self-fulfilling prophecy. Persons diagnosed as mentally ill may become victims of that very label. One specific argument is that diagnoses of mental illness should be considered suspect since there is profit to be had in the labeling process. According to Szasz (1960, p. 118), mental illness is a convenient myth that serves "to obscure the everyday fact that life for most people is a continuous struggle [for human value]." Stereotypes and erroneous impressions negatively influence diagnoses of black clients. Various discussions point to the failure to diagnose depression among this population as a result of such preconceived notions (Bell, Bland, Houston, & Jones, 1983; Poussaint, 1983).

Although improvements have occurred within the mental health profession, impediments to the successful treatment of nonwhites, particularly blacks, still exist. There continues to be a need for addressing black mental health concerns in a more systematic as well as a more culturally sensitive manner. While the tendency to diagnose patients as "schizophrenic" may be reduced, the communication of culturally insensitive professionals with black patients is still too often characterized by narrowly defined ideas as to the components of mental health. Misconceptions about blacks interfere with therapeutic successes.

A growing body of research focuses on formulating concepts and strategies necessary to comprehend the dimensions of black mental health care (Lyles & Carter, 1982). Today's mental health professional must be knowledgeable about strategies for treating diversified populations (Ruiz, 1990). For Lyles and Carter, the context of the black familial structure and its adaptive strengths offers a framework by which therapists can gain valuable insights into the functioning of blacks. Similarly, Baker (1987) views black family strengths and the role of the extended family throughout the life cycle as providing a key supportive thread. She identifies five mental health issues resulting from maladaptive strategies: (1) black-on-black homicide, (2) teenage pregnancy, (3) attempted suicide, (4) substance abuse, and (5) postincarceration adjustment. Informed strategies related to the black client's familial and other important institutional contexts (for example, religion) are more likely to lead to positive outcomes. In short, treating the client from a holistic perspective is critical for nonwhite clients.

The general idea that blacks have higher rates of mental illnesses than whites do is captured via findings on use of treatment facilities. Because data are much more readily available on public than private facilities, and since blacks are more likely than whites to utilize such facilities, the statistics tend to depict lowered mental health status among blacks in comparison to their white counterparts. Greater proportions of blacks than whites receive treatment for mental disorders in public facilities and are subject to less intensive care than those receiving treatment from private centers. This includes shorter therapy sessions, greater incidences of visits with inexperienced therapists, and drug therapy with minimal psychiatric treatment (Cannon & Locke, 1977).

The earlier mentioned statistics and other recent data that show a higher proportion of black hospital admissions are well established (U.S. Bureau of the Census, 1991; Manderscheid & Barrett, 1987; Manderscheid & Sonnenschein, 1990). These data do not differ drastically from earlier findings, which show rates of mental illness and hospital admissions for blacks of all ages as being higher than comparable rates for whites (President's Commission on Mental Health, 1978). National data indicate that black men are hospitalized at a rate 2.8 times greater than white men; black women are hospitalized at a rate 2.5 times greater than white women (Manderscheid & Barrett, 1987). It is important to understand that these data, in part, reflect socioeconomic factors that feed into the dual health care delivery system characterizing American society.

Impact of Racism

It is generally recognized that the effects of racism can be a hazard to mental health. Stressors related to alienation and other adverse conditions as a result of racial discrimination pose psychological threats to even the most confident of blacks (Benjamin, 1991). Additionally, nonwhites are further burdened by unmet mental health needs (Jones & Korchin, 1982; Rosenthal & Carty, 1988). These factors combine in reducing the overall life chances of minority group members. This is acutely apparent among blacks despite modest gains toward greater political and socioeconomic parity. Discrimination continues to plague America's racial and ethnic minorities in immeasurable ways. Perhaps the worst is the psychological harm caused by racist attitudes and discriminatory behaviors. Thus, regardless of the adaptive behavioral responses blacks employ to combat such prejudices, they are subjected to much greater psychological hazards than their white counterparts.

In light of the adverse effects of racism on blacks, one might contend that the impact of discrimination alone provides a clue to the status of black mental health vis-à-vis that of whites. It would follow that since whites are not subjected to racial discrimination, they experience better mental health as a result of their symbolic shield — skin color. Given the various stresses caused by discrimination, blacks are at an undeniably greater risk for reduced mental health. But despite the multiple effects of discrimination, blacks are apparently finding ways to resist debilitating stressors and are not succumbing to the various disorders that threaten their very existence. From this perspective, rather than unequivocally accepting conclusions that blacks have lowered levels of mental health than whites, one might instead ask why the gap between indicators of mental health for blacks and whites is not even greater.

Gary (1991) recommends caution in interpreting current findings on black mental health (in light of the lack of conceptual frames, appropriate methodologies, and other resources to guide systematic research). From another standpoint, Akbar (1991) discusses the disservice of allowing mental health professionals from alien cultures to define those with disorders. He identifies four classes of disorders: (1) the alien-self disorder, (2) the antiself disorder, (3) the self-destructive disorder, and (4) the organic disorder. His perspective emphasizes "universal mental health—that which fosters and cultivates survival of itself" (Akbar, 1991, p. 342). A major implication of this approach is that until the African-American community can effectively define what is normal for it, black mental health will continue to be stifled.

This discussion underscores the vagueness of the term *mental health*, as well as the difficulty of measuring it. To categorically conclude that mental health is lower for blacks than for whites ignores the existence of strength and conviction among African Americans—qualities that historically have helped to sustain them, both physically and mentally. Additionally, socioeconomic status must be examined in deriving conclusions. Studies on the effects of race and socioeconomic status on mental health are inconsistent. Analysis of the Epidemiologic Catchment Area (ECA) study data ($n = 16,436$) found that blacks in general did not have a higher prevalence of major depression than whites (Somervell et al., 1989). Findings from this study found no significant interaction of race with socioeconomic status. A recent study including 804 subjects (Cockerham, 1990) found that while blacks did not have significantly more distress than whites, low-income subjects did show greater tendencies toward psychological distress.

Socioeconomic Status

Just as there are competing hypotheses for why blacks have lower levels of mental health in comparison to whites, similar hypotheses can be observed relative to socioeconomic status. It has often been observed that persons from lower socioeconomic backgrounds suffer higher rates of mental disorder than persons who are more economically advantaged. Some of the earliest studies corroborating this hypothesis include Faris and Dunham (1939), Dunham (1959), and Dohrenwend and Dohrenwend (1965). While findings tend to be consistent in reporting a disproportionately high degree of mental disorders among low-income populations, there is far less consistency in the explanations offered. Many have argued in favor of an inverse relationship between socioeconomic status and mental disorders, theorizing that this pattern is caused by social stress or social selection.

The social stress explanation views psychological problems as a common consequence of high levels of environmental stress (Antunes, Gordon, Gaitz, & Scott, 1974). Emphasis is placed on the concentration of stress in the low-income person's environment and the lack of social and economic resources to effectively cope with the various stressors. This explanation has as its rival a social selection hypothesis, which emphasizes social mobility and assumes that the causes of mental disorders are independent of socio-economic status.

In a study of the relationship between the joint influence of race and socioeconomic status on mental health, Ulbrich, Warheit, and Zimmerman (1989) found that socioeconomic status interacts with race to increase psychological symptoms of distress. Additionally, they report that blacks from lower socioeconomic backgrounds were more vulnerable to the impact of economic problems than their white counterparts. Extrapolation from this study suggests that the coupling of racism with the effects of low socio-economic status makes low-income blacks especially vulnerable to mental disorders.

Just as there are problems associated with the operationalization of mental health in general, there too is a problem with defining social class. Attempts have been made to address this problem; however, methodological concerns still remain and could account for the inconsistency in findings. Whether socioeconomic status is defined in terms of household income, occupational status, or education, past studies have tended to conclude that mental health problems correlate with a decline in socioeconomic status. Kessler (1979) found that persons from low-income backgrounds are more disadvantaged than their more affluent counterparts by the greater degree of stressful experiences encountered, as well as by life events that affect their emotional functioning more severely. The impact of negative life experiences coupled with the susceptibility to economic problems poses a threat to much of the African-American community.

Regardless of the particular explanation that may account for the relationship between socioeconomic status and mental health, low-income persons (and therefore a substantial number of blacks) have been found to be more vulnerable to psychological distress. This finding has led to broad and overgeneralized negative ideas about the black population. Smith (1978) points out the fact that research has concentrated on the prevalence of mental disorders among low-income blacks, as if the black population were monolithic. Many researchers sensitive to the dynamics of varying behaviors and different cultures have emphasized the need to define concepts in terms of neutrality and all-inclusiveness, as opposed to conformity with white, middle-class norms (Lyles & Carter, 1982; Nobles, 1973; Spurlock, 1982; Williams, 1981; Willie, Kramer & Brown, 1973; Smith, 1978). While strides have been made to address deficiencies in the operationalization of concepts related to black mental health and socioeconomic status, much remains to be done in this area.

Issues of Gender

It is commonly believed that the rates of mental illness are higher for women than men. This assumption is, in part, due to long-standing stereotypes that continue to link women with expressive and men with instrumental traits.

Men are often portrayed as having strong attributes of character, while women tend to be seen as emotionally weak and easily upset. These characterizations lead to "commonsense" notions that men possess greater mental stability. Research, however, suggests a different picture.

National data for minority populations reveal a greater use of mental health facilities by men (Rosenstein, Milazzo-Sayre, & Manderscheid, 1990). However, since women have been found to be more likely to express a need for help and because this has been used as an indicator of mental disorder, women are sometimes construed as having lowered degrees of mental health stability in comparison to their male counterparts. What is not captured in these kinds of interpretations are affected persons who do not seek help.

It has been demonstrated that women are more likely than men to seek professional help when faced with a serious personal problem (Neighbors & Howard, 1987), while men tend to shun help and respond to their problems in a more internalized way. For example, although studies show that women are more likely to attempt suicide, more men actually succeed in committing suicide (Cleary, 1989). This discrepancy has been explained in terms of females' intentions to call attention to the need for help, while males tend to be more instrumental and typically have a different outcome in mind. The pattern of suicide by method (for example, firearms and poisoning) varies little by race but substantially by gender (Rosenberg et al., 1987). National data show that the suicide rate for blacks aged 15 to 24 increased by 40 percent among females from 1986 to 1991, and 49 percent among males from 1984 to 1989 (National Center for Health Statistics, 1992). The lower rate for females could be associated with seeking help before the onset of major mental health problems. Generally, men are more likely to be hospitalized and women to be outpatients (Clausen, 1979). The literature is relatively consistent in showing more reported depression among women than men.

Black Women: Multiple Roles, Multiple Stresses

Since black women experience a double disadvantage in living in a society that values both "whiteness" and "maleness," they are vulnerable to mental disorders often precipitated by prejudices and discriminatory practices. Moreover, given that a large proportion of black women are also economically disadvantaged, they are especially prone to various stressors related to everyday life. Copeland (1982) illuminates the situation of black low-income women, pointing out that stereotypes and prejudices have adversely affected their self-concepts and feelings of adequacy. The combined effects of being poor, black, and female tend to create an array of health hazards, physical as well as mental. In addition, the chances of receiving adequate mental health care are small, since prevalent gender, race, and class biases are likely to be reflected at the institutional level as well as in the therapeutic encounter (Olmeda & Parron, 1981).

The research on black women and mental health is sketchy. However, it is known that reaching out for help, although sometimes with negative consequences, is a common response. Self-defeating behavior is often a mechanism of attention. The higher rate of attempted suicide among women in comparison to men has been documented. Baker (1984) studied the charts of fifty-six African Americans between the ages of sixteen and twenty-nine who attempted suicide and were admitted to a university hospital. Thirty-nine of these subjects were female and seventeen male. Results indicate that females were younger than males and were less likely to have severe diagnoses. Of the thirty-nine females who attempted suicide, 54 percent had made a prior attempt. It has been documented that the suicide attempts of black women are precipitated by strong feelings of hopelessness, powerlessness, and overall depression. The high levels of stress can be a result of the multiple roles assumed (Copeland, 1982; Smith, 1981). In an earlier study of 1,345 suicide attempts, Pederson, Awad, and Kindler (1973) found that among nonwhites (primarily black), women outnumbered men six to one. This compared to a ratio of three to one for whites (Pederson, et al., 1973). In either case, the higher number of attempted suicides by women can be interpreted as a desperate cry for relief from their problems.

Similarly, black women have increasingly turned to alcohol and other drugs as a reprieve. Black women have been found to have higher rates of heavy drinking than white women, although they also comprise higher rates of abstainers. The heavy drinking of black women often found in the data tends to be a way of temporarily forgetting troubles, as manifested in weekend escapades. According to the President's Commission on Mental Health (1978), alcoholism was the third leading diagnosis for admissions to state and county hospitals; rates for black and white women were 50.1 and 12.4 per 100,000, respectively.

The problem of alcoholism requires special assessment, treatment, and prevention approaches that take into account unique sociocultural factors inherent in the life experiences of minority women (Olmeda & Parron, 1981). These indicators suggest that the coping mechanisms of black women are different from those of their white counterparts. Particularly in the case of low-income black women, the effects of racism, sexism, and/or classism take a heavy toll. Additionally, older low-income black women may find themselves in "quadruple jeopardy" (Jackson, 1973, p. 207). Strategies used by black women in coping with stressors include various forms of support from fellow black women. Shared feedback has been found to be especially therapeutic in coping with racism and sexism (Myers, 1980).

It is interesting that while black women are faced with higher rates of more serious mental disorders than whites, they have lower rates than black men. The report of the President's Commission on Mental Health (1978) shows that black women were diagnosed more often than white women with higher rates of schizophrenia (118.2 compared to 42.8 per 100,000) and lower rates of depressive disorders (10.2 versus 23.1 per 100,000). The difference in mental health status is substantial when black women are viewed in comparison to their white counterparts; when black women are compared to black men using other indicators, however, this latter group fares even worse.

The Special Case of Black Males

Data in Table 3.1 show that males represented a larger percentage of minority admissions than females did in 1986. It should be noted that specific rates for blacks cannot be discerned from these data. Past studies, however, show that black males were almost consistently higher in rates of mental disorder when compared to their female counterparts (President's Commission on Mental Health, 1978; Manderscheid & Barrett, 1987). Additionally, admission figures should not be confused with those for persons undergoing treatment or otherwise under a physician's care. Specific rates are also shown for persons under care; the pattern showing higher rates for males holds except for the partial-care category. These higher rates for black men are consistent with other status indicators of black men in America (for example, employment, school dropout, and crime rates). Data from a 1990 national sample indicate a higher number of cocaine-related emergency room episodes for black males (27,745) in comparison to white males (15,515), and black and white females (14,833 and 8,331 respectively) (National Center for Health Statistics, 1992). The data point to this group's dire condition and underscore the importance of attempts by black organizations to reverse this trend. One example is a Morehouse College effort that seeks to provide a social science research base for policies and other actions directed toward resolving the problem.

The complexities surrounding black men in America cannot be diminished in any diagnosis of their mental health. Their vulnerability to mental disorders is connected to a wide range of conflicts. Jones and Gray (1983) identify racism as a major culprit. Hilliard (1985) reminds counselors of black males that their environment is also characterized by other cultural

Table 3.1. Minorities as a Percent of Admission and Under-Care Populations[a] by Sex and Program Type, 1986.

	Inpatient Services		Outpatient Services		Partial-Care Services	
	Admissions	Under Care	Admissions	Under Care	Admissions	Under Care
Total (both sexes)	24.5	28.7	15.2	15.5	19.5	24.1
Male	27.1	33.4	15.6	17.9	20.4	22.8
Female	21.0	21.9	14.6	13.2	18.3	25.7

[a] Includes state and county mental hospitals, private psychiatric and nonfederal general hospitals, VA medical centers, multiservice mental health organizations, and freestanding outpatient clinics.

Source: Adapted from Rosenstein, Millazzo-Sayre, Manderscheid, 1990.

and sociopolitical forces that must be understood. Included among these forces are hosts of varying networks that tend to operate differently by gender.

For example, friend and family networks tend to function differently for black males than for black females. Research on the black elderly suggests that friendship assumes a more important role in the total well-being of black women than black men (Taylor, 1985–1986). Similarly, aspects of social support have been found to reduce mental distress in black women but not in black men (Brown & Gary, 1987). Past research recommends studies to determine which aspects of social support might help improve the mental health of black males. In the specific instance of gender differences in drug use and affective distress, biopsychosocial explanations have been proposed (Brunswick, 1988).

Conclusion

This chapter examined aspects of social trends, treatment and utilization, racism, socioeconomic factors, and gender issues in an overview of the mental health status of blacks. Since mental health has been defined in varying ways, a cross-sectional view of the literature would seem to provide the clearest picture of the situation. This makes it possible to uncover varying indicators of the mental health status of blacks.

The difficulty of treating mental disorders is compounded by factors of race/ethnicity and socioeconomic status. For blacks and/or low-income populations, obvious drawbacks include race and class prejudices resulting in discriminatory treatment. Similarly, the gender factor makes the situation more acute in some ways for black women. Their multifaceted roles leave them vulnerable to various stressors. Black men, however, are more likely to be diagnosed with higher rates of mental disorders. Such findings, when combined with other indicators, confirm that the black male in America is indeed plagued with multiple risks. Williams (1986), for instance, discusses problematic experiences of young black males with the educational and criminal justice systems, sustained unemployment, and the high prevalence of alcoholism, all of which may lead to mental disorders. While available data tend to project a negative outlook for young black males, Myers (1989) argues that a shift in the thrust of mental health thinking, research, and intervention is a start in positively impacting the situation. This conceptual approach — an urban stress model — is not restricted to young black males, but is designed to encompass young black females and children as well (Myers, 1982).

As with other illnesses that disproportionately affect African Americans, concentrated efforts must be made to resolve the problem. The improved mental health of the African-American community will require, minimally, a three-dimensional thrust. The identification of (1) treatment needs, (2) research needs, and (3) societal needs (with a focus on reducing stressors contributing to mental disorders) is crucial. Certain recommendations in the promotion of black mental health have previously been made in the literature but are reiterated in this work, since not enough has been done to implement them. For example, with respect to the need for services, the number of minority mental health professionals must be increased and they must be placed strategically after training to reach the numbers of blacks in need of effective treatment.

Major research needs include increased studies on the causes of mental disorder among blacks, with special analyses focused on socioeconomic and gender differences. These studies will require analyses of nationally representative data on the model of recent research (Jackson, 1991) that sheds light on black mental health and other dimensions of African-American life. Additionally, two related areas where data are especially needed include the mental health needs of blacks and their access to services. Finally, structural changes in American society—including affordable health care and the removal of barriers to full employment—are necessary toward promoting black mental health. Our national commitment to enhancing the mental health of African Americans can be bolstered through concentrated attention in these areas.

References

Akbar, N. (1991). Mental disorder among African Americans. In R. L. Jones (Ed.), *Black psychology* (pp. 339–352). Berkeley, CA: Cobb & Henry.

American Psychiatric Association. (1980). *Diagnostic and statistical manual of mental disorders* (3rd ed.). Washington, DC: Author.

Antunes, G., Gordon, C., Gaitz, C. M., & Scott, J. (1974). Ethnicity, socioeconomic status, and the etiology of psychological distress. *Sociology and Social Research, 58,* 361–368.

Baker, F. M. (1984). Black suicide attempters in 1980: A preventive focus. *General Hospital Psychiatry, 6*(2), 131–137.

Baker, F. M. (1987). The Afro-American life cycle: Success, failure, and mental health. *Journal of the National Medical Association, 79*(6), 625–633.

Baker, F. M. (1988). Afro-Americans. In L. Comas-Diaz & E.E.H. Griffith (Eds.), *Clinical guidelines in cross-cultural mental health* (pp. 151–181). New York: John Wiley & Sons.

Bell, C., Bland, I., Houston, E., & Jones, B. (1983). Enhancement of knowledge and skills for the psychiatric treatment of black populations. In J. Chunn, P. Dunston, & F. Ross-Sheriff (Eds.), *Mental health and people of color* (pp. 205–238). Washington, DC: Howard University Press.

Benjamin, L. (1991). *The black elite.* Chicago: Nelson-Hall.

Brown, D. R., Eaton, W. W., & Sussman, L. (1990). Racial differences in prevalence of phobic disorders. *Journal of Nervous and Mental Disease, 178*(7), 434–441.

Brown, D. R., & Gary, L. E. (1987). Stressful life events, social support networks, and the physical and mental health of urban black adults. *Journal of Human Stress, 13*, 165–174.

Brunswick, A. F. (1988). Drug use and affective distress: A longitudinal study of urban black youth. In A. R. Stiffman & R. A. Feldman (Eds.), *Advances in adolescent mental health* (pp. 101–125). Greenwich, CT: JAI Press.

Cannon, M. S., & Locke, B. Z. (1977). Being black is detrimental to one's mental health: Myth or reality? *Phylon, 38*(4), 408–428.

Clausen, J. A. (1979). Mental disorder. In H. E. Freeman, S. Levine, & L. G. Reeder (Eds.), *Handbook of medical sociology* (pp. 97–112). Englewood Cliffs, NJ: Prentice-Hall.

Cleary, P. D. (1989). The need and demand for mental health services. In C. A. Taube, D. Mechanic, & A. Hohman, *The future of mental health services research* (DHSS Publication No. ADM 89-1600, pp. 161–184). Washington, DC: National Institute of Mental Health.

Cockerham, W. C. (1990). A test of the relationship between race, socio-economic status, and psychological distress. *Social Science and Medicine, 31*(12), 1321–1326.

Copeland, E. J. (1982). Oppressed conditions and the mental health needs of low-income black women: Barriers to service, strategies for change. *Women & Therapy, 1*(1), 13–26.

Dohrenwend, B. P., & Dohrenwend, B. S. (1965). The problem of validity in field studies of psychological disorder. *Journal of Abnormal Psychology, 70*, 52–69.

Dunham, H. W. (1959). *Sociological theory and mental disorders*. Detroit, MI: Wayne State University Press.

Faris, R.E.L., & Dunham, H. W. (1939). *Mental disorders in urban areas*. Chicago: University of Chicago Press.

Gary, L. E. (1991). Mental health of African Americans: Research trends and directions. In R. L. Jones (Ed.), *Black psychology* (pp. 727–745). Berkeley, CA: Cobb & Henry.

Gary, L. E., & Jones, D. J. (1978). Mental health: A conceptual overview. In L. E. Gary (Ed.), *Mental health: A challenge to the black community* (pp. 1–25). Philadelphia: Dorrance.

Hilliard, A. G. (1985). A framework for focused counseling of the African American man. *Journal of Non-White Concerns in Personnel & Guidance, 12*(2), 72–78.

Jackson, J. J. (1973). Black women in a racist society. In C. V. Willie, B. M. Kramer, & B. S. Brown (Eds.), *Racism and mental health* (pp. 185–268). Pittsburgh, PA: University of Pittsburgh Press.

Jackson, J. S. (Ed.). (1991). *Life in black America: Findings from a national survey*. Newbury Park, CA: Sage.

Jones, B. E., & Gray, B. A. (1983). Black males and psychotherapy: Theoretical issues. *American Journal of Psychotherapy, 37*(1), 77–85.

Jones, E. E., & Korchin, S. J. (1982). Minority mental health: Perspectives. In

E. E. Jones & S. J. Korchin (Eds.), *Minority mental health* (pp. 3–36). New York: Praeger.

Kessler, R. C. (1979). Stress, social status, and psychological distress. *Journal of Health and Social Behavior, 20,* 259–273.

Lyles, M. R., & Carter, J. H. (1982). Myths and strengths of the black family: A historical and sociological contribution to family therapy. *Journal of the National Medical Association, 74*(11), 1119–1123.

Manderscheid, R. W., & Barrett, S. A. (Eds.). (1987). *Mental health, United States 1990* (DHHS Publication No. ADM 87–1518). Washington, DC: National Institute of Mental Health.

Manderscheid, R. W., & Sonnenschein, M. A. (Eds.). (1990). *Mental health, United States 1990* (DHHS Publication No. ADM 90-1708). Washington, DC: National Institute of Mental Health.

Myers, H. F. (1982). Stress, ethnicity, and social class: A model for research with black populations. In E. E. Jones & S. J. Korchin (Eds.), *Minority mental health* (pp. 118–148). New York: Praeger.

Myers, H. F. (1989). Urban stress and mental health in black youth: An epidemiologic and conceptual update. In R. L. Jones (Ed.), *Black adolescents* (pp. 123–152). Berkeley, CA: Cobb & Henry.

Myers, L. W. (1980). *Black women: Do they cope better?* Englewood Cliffs, NJ: Prentice-Hall.

National Center for Health Statistics. (1992). *Health, United States, 1991.* Hyattsville, MD: Public Health Service.

Neighbors, H., & Howard, C. (1987). Sex differences in professional help seeking among adult black Americans. *American Journal of Community Psychology, 15,* 403–417.

Nobles, W. W. (1973). Psychological research and the black self-concept: A critical review. *Journal of Social Issues, 29*(1), 11–31.

Olmeda, E. L., & Parron, D. L. (1981). Mental health of minority women: Some special issues. *Professional Psychology, 12*(1), 103–111.

Pederson, A. M., Awad, G. A., & Kindler, A. R. (1973). Epidemiological differences between white and nonwhite suicide attempters. *American Journal of Psychiatry, 130*(10), 1071–1076.

Poussaint, A. F. (1983). The mental health status of blacks—1983. In J. D. Williams (Ed.), *The state of black America 1983* (pp. 187–239). New York: National Urban League.

President's Commission on Mental Health. (1978). *Report of the Task Panel on Minority Mental Health.* Washington, DC: U.S. Government Printing Office.

Rosenberg, M. L., Smith, J. C., Davidson, L. E., & Conn, J. M. (1987). The emergence of youth suicide: An epidemiologic analysis and public health perspective. *Annual Review of Public Health, 8,* 417–440.

Rosenstein, M. J., Milazzo-Sayre, L. J., & Manderscheid, R. W. (1990). Characteristics of persons using specialty inpatient, outpatient, and partial care programs in 1986. In R. W. Manderscheid & M. A. Sonnenschein (Eds.),

Mental health, United States 1990 (DHHS Publication No. ADM 90-1708, pp. 139–172). Washington, DC: National Institute of Mental Health.

Rosenthal, E., & Carty, L. A. (1988, June). *Impediments to service and advocacy for black and Hispanic people with mental illness.* Paper prepared for the National Institute of Mental Health as partial fulfillment of a contract to the Mental Health Law Project. Washington, DC.

Ruiz, D. S. (Ed.). (1990). *Handbook of mental health and mental disorder among black Americans.* New York: Greenwood Press.

Smith, E. J. (1981). Mental health and service delivery for black women. *Journal of Black Studies, 12*(2), 126–141.

Smith, S. H. (1978). Research on the mental health of black people. In L. E. Gary (Ed.), *Mental health: A challenge to the black community* (pp. 314–359). Philadelphia: Dorrance.

Somervell, P. D., Leaf, P. J., Weissman, M. M., Blazer, D. G., & Bruce, M. L. (1989). The prevalence of major depression in black and white adults in five United States communities. *American Journal of Epidemiology, 130*(4), 725–735.

Spurlock, J. (1982). Black Americans. In A. Gaw (Ed.), *Cross-cultural psychiatry* (pp. 163–178). Boston: John Wright.

Szasz, T. S. (1960). Myth of mental illness. *American Psychologist, 15,* 113–118.

Taylor, S. E. (1985–1986). Older persons' perceptions of health and well-being: An examination of life satisfaction for male and female elderly. *Journal of Minority Aging, 10*(2), *11*(1), 54–73.

Tessler, R. (1990). What have we learned to date? Assessing the first generation of NIMH-supported research studies on the homeless mentally ill. In P. Morrissey & D. L. Dennis (Eds.), *Homelessness and mental illness: Toward the next generation of research studies* (pp. 9–18). Proceedings of a conference sponsored by the National Institute of Mental Health. Bethesda, MD: U.S. Department of Health and Human Services.

Thomas, C. S., & Comer, J. P. (1973). Racism and mental health services. In C. Willie, B. Kramer, & B. Brown (Eds.), *Racism and mental health* (pp. 165–181). Pittsburgh, PA: University of Pittsburgh Press.

Ulbrich, P. M., Warheit, G. J., & Zimmerman, R. J. (1989). Race, socioeconomic status, and psychological distress: An examination of differential vulnerability. *Journal of Health and Social Behavior, 30,* 131–146.

U.S. Bureau of the Census. (1991). *Statistical abstract of the United States: 1991* (111th ed.). Washington, DC: U.S. Government Printing Office.

Williams, D. H. (1986). The epidemiology of mental illness in Afro-Americans. *Hospital and Community Psychiatry, 37*(1), 42–49.

Williams, R. L. (1981). *The collective black mind: An Afrocentric theory of black personality.* St. Louis, MO: Williams & Associates.

Willie, C. V., Kramer, B. M., & Brown, B. S. (1973). *Racism and mental health.* Pittsburgh, PA: University of Pittsburgh Press.

4

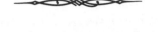

The Health Status
of Black Women

Byllye Y. Avery

"We are sick and tired of being sick and tired" was the battle cry of African-American women in the 1980s. We understood fully the words of our Mississippi freedom fighter Fannie Lou Hamer. These words have been whispered silently in the minds of many women, and voice was again given to that silent protest in 1983 at the historic First National Conference on Black Women's Health Issues. The conference—convened at Spelman College in Atlanta in June 1983—attracted more than 2,000 women, nearly all women of color.

This conference was certainly not the first on African-American health concerns, but it was the first to say to African-American health care consumers that we must come together, share our health issues and problems, and develop our own perspectives and approaches. This initial meeting signaled to millions of African-American women that our health status is in crisis, but even more critically that the solutions to our problems lie within our own power. We ourselves will find workable individual solutions and will work collectively to impact our health situation as African-American women.

The Impact of U.S. Society on Black Women's Health Status

The National Health and Nutrition Examination Surveys (NHANES) indicates that over half of the African-American women surveyed between the ages of eighteen and twenty-five reported that they live in a state of psychological distress (National Center for Health Statistics, 1979). These women rated their distress greater than white women of the same age who were diagnosed with mental disorder. Thus, an examination of the context of our lives

Note: In this chapter, the author frequently uses the first person plural to convey the sense of ownership and responsibility African-American women have begun to feel toward these health problems and also to reject the objectifying language that so often has been used toward black women by the scientific and medical community.

becomes essential in determining the etiology of illness and appropriate health promotion strategies.

Deeply ingrained racism and classism have relegated many women to low-paying jobs or no jobs. It is particularly important to examine the lives of women who are surviving on lower incomes, since it is their lives and health that suffer most in this country. The same inhibiting factors have led to significantly reduced educational opportunities for women. And sexism has played a major role in robbing women of self-esteem. Even as old stereotypes are diminished, women are continually viewed and used as sex objects. Racism further exacerbates and reinforces negative feelings about women and their ability to achieve (Copeland, 1982). For many women, much of this occurs even in the midst of working and caring for their families. Home-lessness, poor education, drug abuse, and increased crime have dispropor-tionately plagued the lives of people forced to live on low incomes, many of whom are women. The reality of the fragility of their lives makes it difficult to focus on the monumental task of preventive health.

The National Center for Health Statistics reports that African Ameri-cans are far more likely to be assessed in fair or poor health than any other racial groups, and this relationship holds regardless of age (Ries, 1990). In fact, the rate of disease among African Americans is almost double the rates for other races.

In examining health statistics for African-American women, the focus must continue to include analyses of sexism, racism, and classism as well as other contributing factors such as structural unemployment and illiteracy. The degrading and dehumanizing manner in which African Americans entered the United States continues to affect their health statistics, as inade-quate educational opportunities, unemployment, underemployment, sub-standard housing, and racist attitudes keep advancement at a virtual stand-still for this population.

Violence and Abusive Behavior

The effects of violence in the lives of African-American women have emerged recently as a pressing issue. Quite often, incidents of domestic and sexual violence are underreported and accepted as "women's lot." For many years, American culture has virtually ignored the high incidence of beatings, incest, and rape that women suffer. Similarly, women's silence has been passed on for generations. The behavior of men has been blamed on the seductiveness or disobedience of women and girls. In the early 1970s, white women started to speak out about domestic violence. These actions led to the establishment of battered women's shelters that housed African-American, Latina, and white women. At the First National Conference on Black Women's Health Issues in 1983, many African-American women talked about their experi-ences. One woman stated that she thought that only white women were victims of abuse because "that's who I heard talk about it."

African-American culture is riddled with frustration, hopelessness, powerlessness, and alienation. African Americans are faced with a "hydra-headed" oppression that often leads to anger turned inward; such individuals often strike out at those physically closer and most vulnerable. For example, in 1986 homicide was the leading cause of death for all blacks age fifteen through thirty-five, but 19 of every 1,000 African-American women were murdered. Every hour women are victims of domestic violence (Straus, Gelles, & Steinmetz, 1981). The cycle of abuse damages not only the victim but the perpetrator as well. This behavior tends to be repeated by affected children in turn.

Men are often hesitant to intervene with family members or friends and learn to consider this atrocity as "family business." This is one example of how sexism is perpetuated, and it hurts all parties, by destroying women's lives and disrupting the family and community structure. The models of male violence and misogyny prevalent in the dominant white society and saturating the images available in the media must also be acknowledged as a strong influence on all youth, male and female, in the United States today. Additionally, public education programs consistently fail to expose the frequent links between violence and alcohol or substance abuse. We must also educate community members and health workers alike to the fact that many women are beaten by their partners for the first time when they become pregnant.

We need to encourage the use of community-based treatment centers for both violent abusers and their victims. It is essential that the African-American community as a whole, including the religious community, take responsibility and leadership in the development and implementation of its own relevant, easily accessible programs. The African-American community at times may seem headed on a path of self-destruction. Under our own committed leadership, we have it within our power to turn this dynamic around into something positive. Specifically, as African-American women, we must start rearing boys who respect themselves and women. It is also necessary that girls be reared to respect themselves more and expect the very best from their male counterparts. We must stop "loving" our sons and "raising" our daughters and give both the love they need for responsible self-respect. It is also necessary that African-American men start assuming the role of modeling respectful behavior toward themselves and women. We must believe that with guidance and modeling in how to handle frustration, anger, and conflict nonviolently, young black men can learn to take pride in their restraint rather than in violent reaction.

Drugs and Antisocial Behavior

Many people surviving in American society are in constant pain. The struggle to make ends meet, the effort to find some meaning in our lives, and the sense of alienation and loneliness all have led to habitual use of drugs in the

African-American community. This is partly because they are readily available and because the dominant culture promotes "quick-fix" solutions to the pain and struggle of living. Many people are victims of various legal drugs, including alcohol, tobacco, food, and sex; others have fallen victim to illegal drugs. The "drug culture" has invaded the African-American community and is already taking a toll on the next generation. The American medical system — which provides drug cures in treating almost everything — has aided society in looking for solutions to all of life's problems in a bottle, pill, or shot. The medical community has been singularly ineffective in developing useful therapies for alcohol or drug addiction. The few successful community-based treatment programs for women, especially African-American women, have been seriously undervalued and underfunded; often they are not designed with women's needs in mind (Women's Health Care Forum, 1991).

While women traditionally have not been the primary users of mood-altering substances in our communities, African-American women are being drawn increasingly into these habits as part of the broader American drug culture. There is a tremendous need for reliable research findings on the incidence of illegal drug use. Its illegal nature makes it very difficult to gather "hard" data on its use. Drug abuse and the concomitant problems associated with the consumption of alcohol and other substances have paralyzed our legal system, stunned our costly health care system, and overcrowded our already ineffective penal system. While it is necessary to focus on stopping the flow of drugs, equal emphasis must be placed on eliminating the conditions that lead to massive drug use.

Reproductive Health Issues

As teenage pregnancy and high infant mortality become national dilemmas, reproductive health for all African-American women assumes critical importance. For many women who are young, single, and poor, reproductive health must be defined within the context of basic survival and quality-of-life issues. By reconceptualizing the issue of reproductive rights to include the impact of race, gender, and class on the lives of African-American women, a new perspective on the situation of African-American women is gained. This new perspective provides the appropriate framework for closing the gaps in our knowledge of the impact of multiple oppressions on life and health decision-making processes. There is a continuing need for African-American women to identify all of the issues relevant to our sexual activity and to redefine female sexuality and reproduction within our own historical and contemporary experiences.

Pertinent to this discussion are other important questions, including the following: How does a person, long denied, begin to believe she has a right to certain information? How do African-American women in particular begin the process of empowerment that must be thoroughly integrated into everyday life experiences and situations? How does the ability to assume control benefit African Americans and African-American women in particular? How do feelings of powerlessness translate into action or inaction on African-American women's reproductive health issues? How do parents transmit information about sexuality and relationships to children? In the discussions of "sexual activity," how much do we truly understand about what causes so much "sexual passivity" among all women, especially poor women and women of color? As part of a white-dominated, racist, and sexist society, many African Americans may themselves fail to understand how that society often creates positive incentives for young women of color to engage in sexual risk-taking behavior at every level and to "choose" too-early parenthood as their best life option (Dash, 1986).

Cultural and societal dynamics in the African-American community have had a direct impact on the decisions African-American women make about sexuality and reproduction. Most African-American women have not acknowledged or shared with one another information on the interconnection of their emotional, sexual, and reproductive experiences. Historically, repressive attitudes toward sexuality and reproduction, rooted in group value systems and practices and manipulated by racism and sexism, have created an atmosphere of reticence, fear, evasion, and silence (although much of this is also American culture-specific and class-specific, not unique to the African-American community). Early and frequent pregnancies recurring cyclically within families often meet a general, fatalistic acceptance within the African-American community. Yet frequently these infants and young children represent unique sources of hope and renewal within the community and across the generations within families.

African-American Infant Mortality and Women's Health

The health of one's mother begins with her mother's mother. The intergenerational cycle of poverty and near poverty makes it difficult for African-American families to enter into preventive health care habits. The impact of these intergenerational health patterns is most significant when we examine infant mortality statistics. Most African-American families are unaware of the pervasiveness of the problem in this area, much less understand the causes.

Only 61 percent of African-American women receive prenatal care in the first trimester of pregnancy (U.S. Department of Health and Human Services, 1990). In 1986, 18 of every 1,000 African American babies born died in the first year of life, and 12.5 percent of all births were of low birthweight. These rates are nearly double the white rates—a pattern that has existed for almost forty years. It must be pointed out that there were improvements in the African-American infant mortality rate throughout the 1970s; however, there was a leveling followed by an increase in the 1980s. This rise has been attributed in part to federal programs cuts, which have affected African-

American women disproportionately. Technological advances aimed at survival for low-birthweight and premature babies once born have not improved the situation; these babies still die at an alarming rate.

These infant mortality data suggest that African Americans constitute an almost entirely separate class of people in this country, and that this de facto segregation is a violation of basic human and civil rights. Innovative public health programs that place high priority on women's health needs must be created. Such strategies will need to challenge the notion that health care is a privilege. Most health care providers realize that the best pregnancy outcomes occur when basic needs are met long before birth and even pregnancy, and that women who seek prenatal care early tend to have better outcomes.

Historically, the U.S. government has not provided free maternal and child health services to all its citizens, despite repeated attempts by progressive forces to get Congress to pass and sustain such legislation (Mulligan, 1976). This shortcoming, in stark contrast to most European and other modern industrial countries, is one root cause of the poor standing of the United States in the world's infant mortality rankings (Straus, Gelles, & Steinmetz, 1981). But it should be clear that it is not simply the presence of so many poor people of color in the American population that elevates the infant mortality rate, as some contend. Even when people of color are removed from the comparative pool, most other industrialized countries still do better, mainly because their social support improvements are swifter and go much farther than those in the U.S. (World Health Organization Regional Office for Europe, 1985).

This situation is also one of the root causes of the persistent gap between African-American and white infant mortality rates, since African Americans are overrepresented among the poor. African-American families, women especially, are also overrepresented among the uninsured and those judged ineligible for publicly funded programs (Cronin & Hartman, 1989).

Aside from the fact that care is unavailable to many women, poor women who do seek care are often inconvenienced by public services designed for provider convenience. Large prenatal clinics require women to wait considerable lengths of time to see the health care provider for a very brief encounter. Visits are often missed because women misunderstand the relevance of a clinic visit that lasts less than fifteen minutes and requires two or three hours' waiting time. Often women are turned away at the end of the session without seeing anyone. Many African-American women are employed in jobs that allow little or no time for prenatal visits and may provide little or no employer coverage for prenatal or maternity care. For low-income working women who are not able to use sick time, the lost wages make prenatal waiting time an expensive endeavor.

The unacceptably high infant mortality rate among African Americans is a social problem that is being handled as a medical problem. If basic social supports were put in place to reduce the infant mortality rate, a reduction in the rates of many life-threatening diseases among African Americans might also occur later in adulthood. The purpose of preventive public health programs is to reach the most vulnerable groups with early interventions. The American public health system has failed to address the contribution of other sectors (education, employment, housing, sanitation, and so on) to health outcomes in its preventive health programs. It has also allowed the investments that are made in prevention programs to be voluntary rather than mandated or systematic and subject to local and national political whims. As a result, only a fraction of the most vulnerable African-American women ever benefit from first-rate public health programs; only a fraction of those eligible are even enrolled in such programs.

In the case of African Americans and their families, this situation has remained basically unchanged in many parts of the country for more than four decades, despite pockets of improvement (National Center for Health Statistics, 1990). In the last five years, conditions have worsened, so that levels of poverty and the associated higher infant mortality rates among African Americans are now worse in some areas than they were before the "Great Society" programs of the 1960s.

When U.S. policy is compared to that of Europe, it becomes clear that Europeans recognize that providing generous benefits and incentives to all women and children is the most cost-effective way to reduce health and medical care costs in the long run (Wagner, 1989). American policy makers, on the other hand, tend to blame women for failing to care for themselves and for not obtaining prenatal care. Not only do some policy makers impede benefits and social supports for poor women and families, they are particularly punitive toward poor African-American women, who are characterized as abusive for such problems as drug addiction during pregnancy and have their civil rights violated during pregnancy and birth more frequently than other women (Curriden, 1990; Kolder, Gallagher, & Parsons, 1987).

The issue of infant mortality in the African-American community also needs to be more clearly linked to women's health, nutrition, and other aspects of reproductive health care, such as high rates of both intended and unintended pregnancy among young unmarried women, the unavailability of government-funded abortion services, high rates of government-funded sterilization (sometimes involuntary), and many birth control programs isolated from comprehensive, community-based health services. The bleakness depicted by U.S. infant mortality rates can be interpreted as women (historically marginalized and ignored in major societal sectors) being neglected by society and their lack of resources to bear and rear the next generation. For too long, maternal and child health programs have focused on the developing fetus and on the newborn and developing child and their needs, as if women were invisible or had no needs except to nurture children. All of us must begin to see infant mortality as primarily a woman's health issue, and to recognize that it will not be possible to reduce African-

American infant mortality without making a firm and unqualified commitment to meeting the critical needs of women. When that is done, babies will
begin to not just survive, but to thrive in American society.

Teenage Pregnancy

Three million pregnancies occur each year in the United States due to either
contraceptive failure or the lack of use of contraceptives. African-American
teenagers tend to wait an average of one year between initiating sexual
intercourse and first using a prescription method of contraception. Some
analysts suggest that five out of every six pregnancies are unintended (Trussel,
1988). Other reports suggest that many teen pregnancies are consciously
intended (Dash, 1986). Because many young women are faced with uncertain
and dismal futures, peer pressure, and low self-esteem, having a baby becomes an empowering experience. Most young people are unable to concep-
tualize the difficulties they will encounter caring for themselves and a child.
Eighty percent of pregnant teenagers become high school dropouts. Seventy-
one percent of female-headed families living below the poverty level are
headed by African-American women (Wilson, 1987). These staggering numbers are disturbing because it is very difficult to gain support, education, and
employment once pregnancy has occurred too early. The financial hardship,
paired with the powerlessness that develops, contributes to the cycle of
poverty that grips many families. Interestingly, because of the intense focus
on pregnant teens in the African-American community, it is labeled a problem of the black community in the public imagination, obscuring the fact
that teen pregnancy rates are even higher for U.S. whites, and that U.S. teens
overall have the highest industrial world rates (Alan Guttmacher Institute,
1981).

    Millions of African-American women and children escape these cir-
cumstances in spite of all odds seemingly against them. With adequate
support from the start, these families might have achieved even greater
heights. The health and social service systems of this nation have studied our
failures endlessly and have even built lifetime careers on them. We have not
learned very much at all about how those who have changed and improved
their situations actually accomplished it, especially African-American
women who are single parents or single heads of households. This must
become a priority in the women's health research agendas that are established in the future.

Sexually Transmitted Diseases

Most African-American families do not have a legacy of open discussions
about sexuality or sexual behaviors. Most people avoid direct conversations,
despite the fact that society is full of nuances and sexuality is used extensively
to promote and sell products. The lack of information and insensitivities

compound the problem. The presence of sexually transmitted disease can carry a stigma and the connotation of promiscuous behavior. Quite often if one does seek treatment for a sexually transmitted disease, it means being ignored and treated impersonally and rudely by health care workers. African Americans also carry the burden of being seen as excessively sexual beings, which is a product of both racist and sexist oppression. Family traditions and communications barriers make education and attitudinal changes in all these areas difficult and challenging. Sexually transmitted diseases have been taught, if taught at all, by subject rather than in the context of sexual behavior and transmission or protective practices that will apply to other situations. Health promotion and prevention efforts have largely centered on educating women, but it is crucial that efforts to educate men develop to include grass-roots community involvement that will encourage men to talk with one another about their sexual behavior and the impact of their practices on the rest of the population.

Life grows dim early for many African-American youth. It is difficult to be young and not be into drugs, alcohol, and sex. For many, school has been a boring and sometimes painful experience. The cost of college makes it prohibitive, and it is difficult to earn a living or a minimum wage with only a high school diploma. Rampant unemployment, homelessness, and violent conditions in some communities function in such a way that the idea of practicing safer sex appears irrelevant. Many women worry about questioning men about their sexual behaviors or whether or not they practice safer sex. The fear of rejection and of being alone provokes anxiety that delays the conversation or prevents it from taking place.

AIDS

Acquired immune deficiency syndrome (AIDS) has disproportionately affected the African-American community. The National Center for Health Statistics reports that in 1986, African Americans accounted for 2,063 AIDS deaths (22 percent of the total) while constituting only 12 percent of the total population. Eleven percent of reported deaths were caused by heterosexual contact with drug abusers who shared or used contaminated needles. Women, especially African Americans and Latinas, are now the fastest growing group at risk for HIV infection (Centers for Disease Control, 1990). Most observers believe that this is a direct result of contact with men whose histories or present life-styles include drug abuse and needle sharing. Estimates show 52 percent of female AIDS cases are listed as "black, non-Hispanic"; 20.5 percent are Hispanic and 26.5 percent are "white, non-Hispanic."

There are many situations that African-American women must be especially careful of and demand protection from, because of the high percentage of black men who are, or have been in, America's prisons. Men who are imprisoned are at high risk for AIDS due to homosexual contact while incarcerated. For example, in Georgia prisons, 6 to 7 percent of the inmates are estimated to be HIV infected (Georgia Department of Human Resources, 1987). These men do not think of themselves as "gay" and continue to have sexual relations with women after their release. Given this situation, safe practices on the part of men who have been in prison could greatly reduce the risk factors for HIV infection and other sexually transmitted diseases in women. The prison population rarely receives health education and wellness promotion information. African-American infant mortality rates are exacerbated as many infected women give birth to babies who are HIV positive. As these high rates of HIV-infected newborns in the African-American community are publicized, the tendency has been to focus only on the babies, rather than realizing that an epidemic among women is being revealed simultaneously. There is even less publicity about the hospital testing, often without the mother's knowledge or consent, that produces this information and that is a clear violation of the mother's rights. When a pregnant woman does know she is HIV positive, she is often under extreme pressure to undergo an abortion.

Many women are unaware and afraid to talk about so-called "safer sex" practices. African-American women are no exception. This type of "take-charge" practice requires considerable education and support, which are rarely available. Also, there are enormous barriers involved in condom use for many African-American women, ranging from power imbalances in the sexual relationship to the symbolic negative meanings that are attached to the use of this device in many communities (Worth, 1989).

Malnutrition and Undernutrition

Inexpensive, fat-filled, low-nutrition food is prevalent in the African-American community, promoted through the media as a source of psychological comfort, pleasure, and reward. For many African Americans, it may also symbolize a way of "belonging" to mainstream American life. It is often very expensive to eat a healthy diet in a poor community, and for many trying to achieve minimum health by obtaining healthy food, it is also an inconvenience.

Stores carry what people buy. This means that some stores may reinforce poor eating habits because individuals buy what stores carry. Food shopping and eating habits are most difficult to change. The battle to overcome many dietary problems are won and lost in the kitchen.

Many African Americans are caught in a cultural crossfire, wanting to take on the eating styles of modern urban America and at the same time yearning for familiar, hard-to-obtain foods from the cultural past. For some African Americans, a lot of foods connote "love," especially for those who remember with fondness the holiday tradition of chitterlings (pork fat), greens, dry rice, beans, sweet potato pie, and all of the warm, wonderful memories associated with such a meal. For many, it is hard to give these up, particularly since food is often the only avenue for enjoyment, good times, and fulfillment. But malnutrition is only part of the story. Statistics are virtually nonexistent on the most severe childhood undernutrition and deprivation in African-American communities in the past, which may only show up today as greater vulnerability to disease or early death in adults. While childhood nutrition for African Americans has improved somewhat recently, that improvement is not nearly as great as for the white community. This fact is reflected both in the infant mortality gap between the races and also in the high rates of low birthweight babies among African Americans. Clearly, the nutritional needs of young, childbearing African-American women are not being met, either before or during pregnancy.

Exercise

The poor health status of African-American women is influenced by poor health habits and unbalanced attitudes toward work, exercise, and relaxation. The effects of economic struggle, little time, and few choices for recreational activities have contributed to the idea that exercise, often viewed as "playing," is a luxury that few can afford. Children play, adults work, and when work is done, rest is the rewarding activity. For African-American women, as for women almost everywhere in the world, time for rest is often less than half that available to men.

Sedentary occupations and life-styles lead to high numbers of health problems, and societal and work-related stress affects all organs of the body. Women who work at home taking care of families and/or residing in public housing facilities have very little incentive to participate in health promoting exercises. Young girls in high school participate in exercise activities, generally as a requirement. Although they are exposed to several recreational activities, there is very little carryover to their lives outside of school or as adults. This is due in part to the practices of one's family and peers. Certain kinds of physical activities are more readily available to some ethnic groups, or to males only, and this promotes excellence in some areas for a few individuals. In order for African-American women to interrupt the intergenerational patterns of behavior with regard to exercise, both attitudinal and life-style changes must occur.

Diabetes

According to the Office of Minority Health, diabetes affects African-American women disproportionately. The high incidence demonstrates a relationship between nutrition, obesity, and social class. This disease is evident in the African-American community by the prevalence of women amputees and those who are insulin dependent. Since the economic conditions of many women influence this statistic, it often remains unchanged and is passed on to the next generation because of the difficulty of modifying life-style and other behaviors. Often the condition first appears in pregnancy and then recurs later in life. New studies on women athletes indicate that adequate exercise, especially early in life, may be an important factor in preventing diabetes. Systematic studies remain to be done to determine the significance of this as a preventive factor for African-American women.

Hypertension and Cardiovascular Diseases

High blood pressure is a major health problem in the African-American community. Hypertension affects about 7.5 million people, and half of African Americans over the age of fifty have this disease. Hypertension is the leading cause of kidney failure and hypertension-related and end-stage renal disease and is a major contributor to heart disease and stroke, according to the *Report of the Secretary's Task Force on Black and Minority Health* (U.S. Department of Health and Human Services, 1985). While heart disease and related circulatory conditions remain the leading cause of death for all Americans, African Americans are overrepresented in these statistics. Compared with African-American men, African-American women experience excess deaths from coronary heart disease (U.S. Department of Health and Human Services, 1985). Any analysis of hypertension and circulatory or cardiovascular diseases must take into aocount the stress people of color face. The invalidation of one's culture and one's race carries a heavy toll. These basic indicators of identity are nonchangeable and should be seen by society as enhancing rather than invalidating factors. The prevalence of all these diseases must be viewed as related to stressors in African-American culture.

Heart disease and stroke remain the leading causes of disability and death among all American women over fifty-five years old. Experts disagree on the most significant contributing factors; some favor a physiological/biological model, while others believe the causes are partly psychological. Only in recent decades have experts in these disease areas begun to focus more systematically on the damage attributable to social habits such as smoking and alcohol, on the effects of diet and exercise, and on the contributions of social and psychological stress associated with poverty, violence, racism, and lack of opportunity. Other neglected elements in the analysis of these diseases among African-American women must include the effects of undiagnosed and/or untreated childhood diseases such as measles and rheumatic fever, and childhood undernutrition or malnutrition, which contribute directly to kidney diseases and heart conditions.

The experts' slowness in recognizing the etiology of these diseases in the general population as well as within the African-American community is further complicated by the absence of appropriate and adequately controlled research on women's health in the United States (Society for Women's Health Research, 1991).

Cancer

According to the American Cancer Society, cancer incidence is higher for African Americans than for whites, and the death rate from cancer is also higher. Cancer sites that show increases among African Americans include breast, lung, colon-rectum, prostate, and esophagus.

Cervical Cancer

The incidence of invasive cancer of the cervix dropped in both African-American and white women in the past fourteen years, although the incidence in African-American women is still double that in white women. Conventional medical wisdom about cervical cancer has tended to focus on women and their behavior, suggesting that their promiscuity is the cause. Racism among health care providers has compounded this sexist prejudice (*Taking Our Bodies Back*, 1974). More recent studies point out that it may be males who are transmitting viruses and other organisms to women, and that their promiscuity may be the source of infection in monogamous women (Robinson, 1984). The medical community has shown little or no initiative in promoting prevention of cervical cancer—through condom use, for example—or in encouraging screening. The absence of PAP smear screening programs in convenient, affordable, and acceptable settings remains a problem for many women in the African-American community.

Breast Cancer

It is estimated that one of every nine American women will develop breast cancer in her lifetime. Women whose mothers or sisters have had breast cancer are up to four times as likely as other women to develop or have the disease themselves. (However, this risk factor only applies to those mothers or sisters whose breast cancer appeared before menopause. Also, black women are less likely than white women to report one or more primary relatives with breast cancer.)

The National Center for Health Statistics reports that 29 of every 100,000 deaths among African-American women were due to breast cancer in 1986. Although fewer African-American women get breast cancer than white women, the survival rates are lower: 64 percent versus 76 percent. In attempting to explain this apparent increased vulnerability, researchers are just beginning to disentangle the influence of poverty from that of race. Cancer is a relationship between a host and an invader. Inadequate attention has been focused on those social, environmental, and nutritional factors, beginning in childhood, that may lead to a weakened immune system in many African-American women throughout life.

It is currently accepted that a reduction in dietary fat will probably contribute to lower rates of heart disease and cancer and that exercise in some young women reduces the incidence of breast cancer in later life (Frisch, Wyshak, Albright, Albright, & Schiff, 1989). African-American women will certainly not be harmed by acting on these suggestions now. It is also important to reduce or eliminate smoking and alcohol use—factors that have been found to be contributors to increased breast cancer rates.

There is a pressing need for preventive education and services for African-American women at risk of breast cancer. Mammography makes it possible for breast cancer to be detected at an early stage and can save lives in women over fifty, although the benefit for younger women has not yet been demonstrated, even though many professional physician groups recommend mammography screening at younger ages. However, this preventive intervention is not readily available, and a large number of African-American women are not knowledgeable about the procedure. Many cancer experts feel that preventive care should include a yearly clinical examination, appropriate mammography, and monthly breast self-examinations. African-American women may eventually be shown to benefit more from earlier and more frequent mammography screening and examinations, but the studies have not yet been done that conclusively show this benefit. As the agenda for new women's health research is being developed, this area is an appropriate one for inclusion.

Lung Cancer

Mortality rates for lung cancer among African-American women are twice as high as for nonminority women (National Cancer Institute, 1989). This discrepancy can be attributed to many factors. Tobacco companies conduct advertising campaigns that target the African-American community. Billboards are plentiful and link good times, fun activities, peer acceptance, adult status, and many other attributes with smoking. Nicotine addiction, like alcohol and drug addiction, fills a void. The "fear of death" approach to smoking cessation is ineffective because the rates of death from a myriad of other, more immediately lethal causes are so staggeringly high. Dipping snuff once was prevalent among older black women, even though documentation of this practice is not readily available. This activity has apparently become much less common in the last thirty years; today, it is socially unacceptable. Sadly, dipping snuff has been replaced by drugs and other additions that are more systemic and destructive.

Organizing for Change

Using the self-help approach to program development among a broad-based constituency of African-American women, the National Black Women's Health Project (NBWHP) (1990) provides safe and supportive environments for black women to express the full range of their attitudes and feelings about sexuality and life's experiences. Freedom for African-American women to speak out in an atmosphere that validates their experiences and accepts them as individuals capable of assuming control of and transforming their lives is necessary and long overdue. The NBWHP offers such an environment, a place where African-American women are not "deviant," not "other," but the norm, despite artificial age, class, and life-style barriers. Since the 1980s,

African-American women have started looking critically at factors affecting the quality of their lives and affecting their health status. The concept of self-help groups organized around no specific disease entity makes the NBWHP's approach novel. When we dialogue with women of the African diaspora worldwide, we are able to understand the implications of complex economic and sociopolitical factors influencing our health outcomes.

Conclusion

There is clear evidence that many of the most severe health problems facing African-American women are primarily caused by poverty, racism, and lack of opportunity. We must continue our struggle against these barriers. At the same time, we can target some issues more specifically:

1. We need research that will identify more precisely how and why African-American women are overrepresented in disease categories such as heart disease, hypertension, cancer, diabetes, and AIDS. The women's health research agenda now being developed at the National Institutes of Health must make certain that sufficient attention is paid to race and social-class factors.
2. We must hold the existing health and medical care system accountable so that it is not an instrument of further racism, stress, and punitiveness in African-American women's lives.
3. We must begin to redefine basic problems such as the high U.S. infant mortality rate as women's health issues as well as social, legal, and economic issues, and not as technical medical problems.
4. When treatment programs are being developed, we must insist that people who will be making use of these services help to design them and that services appropriate to women's needs are made available.
5. We must develop the leadership and commitment from within our own communities to address violence — especially violence and the silence that surrounds our sexual and reproductive life — so that we have positive models to offer future generations.
6. We must create new opportunities for preventive, life-saving information to be given in an atmosphere of trust.
7. We must investigate and celebrate the remarkable successes that so many women and families have created, despite enormous obstacles, and learn from them.

To redefine our status, African-American women will require opportunities and safe settings, and social supports (including child care) in steps toward enhanced health. Before African-American women will be able to take these steps in large numbers, we will require vocal and committed leadership from our own community. But we are not waiting for that commitment before beginning to organize for needed health opportunities.

References

Alan Guttmacher Institute. (1981). *Teenage pregnancy: The problem that hasn't gone away*. New York: Author.

Centers for Disease Control. (1990). *DC HIV/AIDS Surveillance Report*. Atlanta, GA: Author.

Copeland, E. (1982). Oppressed conditions and the mental health needs of low-income black women: Barriers to service, strategies for change. *Women & Therapy, 1*(1), 13, 25–26.

Cronin, C., & Hartman, R. (1989, December). *The corporate perspective on maternal and child care*. Washington, DC: Washington Business Group on Health.

Curriden, M. (1990, March). Holding mom accountable. *American Bar Association Journal, 76,* 50–53.

Dash, L. (1986, January 26–31). At risk: Chronicles of teenage pregnancy. (A six-day series). *Washington Post*, Jan. 26 (52), pp. A1, A12, A13; Jan. 27 (53), pp. A1, A8, A9; Jan. 28 (54), pp. A1, A8, A9; Jan. 29 (55), pp. A1, A18; Jan. 30 (56), pp. A1, A14, A15; Jan. 31 (57), pp. A1, A16.

Frisch, R., Wyshak, G., Albright, N., Albright, T., & Schiff, I. (1989). Lower prevalence of nonreproductive system cancers among female former college athletes. *Medicine and Science in Sports and Exercise, 21*(3), 250–253.

Georgia Department of Human Resources. (1987, November). *State of Georgia five year plan on the acquired immune deficiency syndrome*. Submitted to Georgia General Assembly, Atlanta, GA.

Kolder, V., Gallagher, J., & Parasons, M. (1987). Court-ordered obstetrical interventions. *New England Journal of Medicine, 316*(19), 1192–1196.

Mulligan, J. (1976). *Three federal interventions on behalf of childbearing women: The Sheppard-Towner Act, Emergency MIC, the MCH: MRPA of 1963*. Unpublished doctoral dissertation, University of Michigan, Ann Arbor.

National Black Women's Health Project. (1990). Unpublished internal report, Atlanta, GA.

National Cancer Institute. (1989). *1991 budget estimate*. Bethesda, MD: Public Health Service.

National Center for Health Statistics. (1979). *Health United States*. (DHEW Publication No. HRA 80-1232). Hyattsville, MD: Public Health Service.

National Center for Health Statistics. (1990). *Health United States, 1989*. Hyattsville, MD: Public Health Service.

Ries, P. (1990). *Americans assess their health: United States, 1987* (Vol. 10, No. 174). National Center for Health Statistics. Hyattsville, MD: Public Health Service.

Robinson, J. (1984). Promiscuity isn't the cause. *New Statesman, 107*(2767), 14.

Society for Women's Health Research. (1991). *Women's health research: Prescription for change* [Annual report]. Washington, DC: Author.

Straus, M., Gelles, R., & Steinmetz, S. (1981). *Behind closed doors: Violence in the American family*. New York: Anchor Books.

Taking our bodies back [Film]. (1974). Cambridge Documentary Films.

Trussel, J. (1988). Teenage pregnancy in the United States. *Family Planning Perspectives, 20*(6), 262–272.

U.S. Department of Health and Human Services. (1985). *Report of the Secretary's Task Force on Black and Minority Health.* Washington, DC: U.S. Government Printing Office.

U.S. Department of Health and Human Services, Public Health Service. (1990). *Healthy people 2000: National health promotion and disease prevention objectives* (DHHS Publication No. PHS 91-50213). Washington, DC: U.S. Government Printing Office.

Wagner, M. (1989, February). Testimony from the World Health Organization's European office before the United Nations' Infant Mortality Commission, New York.

Wilson, W. J. (1987). *The truly disadvantaged: The inner city, the underclass and public policy.* Chicago: University of Chicago Press.

Women's Health Care Forum. (1991, March). Women's Health Care Forum sponsored by U.S. Public Health Service, Region I, Nashua, NH.

World Health Organization Regional Office for Europe. (1985). *Public health in Europe 26: Having a baby in Europe.* Copenhagen, Denmark: World Health Organization.

Worth, D. (1989). Sexual decision-making and AIDS: Why condom promotion among vulnerable women is likely to fail. *Studies in Family Planning, 20*(6), 297–307.

PART II

Critical
Health Topics

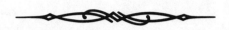

5

AIDS/HIV Epidemics
in the Black Community

Bill Jenkins

In June 1981, five previously healthy young white males with a history of having sex with other men were reported to the Centers for Disease Control (CDC) as having pneumocystic pneumonia. This was unusual because this disease was primarily observed among older patients with a severely impeded immune system secondary to treatment for another condition. This set of conditions, later to be called acquired immune deficiency syndrome (AIDS), became associated with being white, homosexual, and male (Centers for Disease Control [CDC], 1986).

AIDS is defined by a set of symptoms suggestive of the end stages of a human immunodeficiency virus (HIV) infection. It is characterized by a loss of immunity against otherwise nonthreatening diseases. The virus infects certain cells of the immune system and can also directly affect the brain. In fected persons remain in good health for many months to years before illness develops. Infected people who are in good health are classified as HIV positive but without illness. Once symptoms develop, the severity of illness varies from mild symptoms called AIDS-related complex (ARC) to life-threatening infections, classified as AIDS. Most infected persons eventually progress from a state of good health to severe disease (CDC, 1986).

The virus is spread by sexual contact, needle sharing, or less commonly through blood or blood products or organ donation. The virus may also be transmitted from an infected mother to an infant during pregnancy or birth or shortly after birth (possibly through breast milk). There have been few cases of transmission by an infected health care professional to patients; however, this represents an extremely rare event. Substantial discussion about this transmission speaks more to the fear of this disease than any reality of risk.

HIV was discovered to be the cause of AIDS by Luc Montagnier of the Pasteur Institute in 1986 (the discovery is also credited to Robert Gallo of the National Institutes of Health). With the discovery of HIV, a number of highly sensitive HIV antibody tests became available. For example, the Elisa is used for screening and is able to identify 99.7 percent of those infected (high sensitivity). The Western Blot, on the other hand, is used to confirm positive Elisa results, identifying 99.4 percent of those actually not having the disease (high specificity). The use of these two tests together has allowed the early identification of infected persons with a wider spectrum of disease manifestations. Early diagnosis has resulted in the use of "treatments" that may slow the spread of infection and retard the progression of infection to the more severe forms of disease. Research continues to develop even more specific tests that will detect disease earlier and more precisely.

The surveillance of severe disease associated with HIV infection (AIDS) remains an essential indicator of the course of the HIV epidemic. The active surveillance of AIDS cases began in 1981. The CDC is responsible for conducting national surveillance and developing criteria for the case definition of AIDS. The original surveillance case definition provided useful data on severe HIV disease (CDC, 1987). However, the national surveillance system does not include the full spectrum of diseases that we now know may be associated with being HIV positive. While this restrictive definition is good from an epidemiological point of view, its use as a criteria for entitlement of services and support has hampered the provision of resources to many HIV positive persons (Mitchell, 1988). This is especially true for women, whose spectrum of diseases may be different from the majority of male cases.

As early as January 1982, with about 250 reported cases, the CDC data suggested that blacks may be at higher risk for this disease. Although the ratio of AIDS cases per population among blacks was about 3.1 times higher than among whites, during that time the number of observations was small and the ratio fluctuated tremendously as new cases were documented. It was unclear that this association was "real."

By January 1983, with the documented number of cases exceeding 1,000, the higher risk of disease among blacks became more consistent. However, it was still unclear that this association was not due to other factors. For example, this observation may have been due to a specific subset of blacks, possibly Haitians immigrating to the United States. The supposition that Haitians were at a higher risk was the result of not being able to place them in any of the known categories of risk, such as homosexual men or intravenous drug users. It is now clear that the lack of response to questions regarding drug use or men having sex with other men was the result of language and cultural factors not then understood. However, U.S. blacks were still at a higher risk at that time, even when Haitians were removed from the analysis.

By January 1984, with over 3,000 cases analyzed, it was clear to some researchers that blacks were at a higher risk of AIDS. By 1984, the ratio of black to white cases stabilized above 2.1. A preliminary analysis was completed during the summer of 1984. However, in view of the public health and political implications of these observations, many questions arose as to their validity.

By January 1985 there was sufficient data—more than 8,000 cases—to substantiate an association. The black-to-white ratios of AIDS rates remained between 2.6 and 2.8 from January 1985 to January 1988. In 1988, the ratio of black to white rates of disease steadily increased to 3.0, and then it increased to 3.7 by 1990. Thus, in retrospect, blacks were clearly at a higher risk of disease as early as the second quarter of 1983. Figure 5.1 shows quarterly incidence rates of AIDS for black and white populations.

In 1985, a formal analysis of AIDS among blacks was initiated. During 1985, the first papers were completed (Bakeman, McCray, Lumb, Jackson, & Whitley, 1987) and recommendations were made to hold conferences on the subject. The CDC sponsored the first national conference on AIDS in minority communities in August 1987, an official acknowledgment that the HIV epidemic disproportionately affected blacks.

During this period, it also became clear that the AIDS epidemic was in fact several smaller epidemics at times interacting but generally independent of each other. They could generally be defined in terms of two variables, ethnicity and risk behavior groups.

Epidemiologists have developed estimates of the number of new AIDS cases expected in the black and Hispanic communities through 1994. Using the number of new cases diagnosed in each quarter since 1981, estimates were obtained on the number of new cases expected in the African-American and Hispanic communities to 1994. A relatively simple quadratic equation was assumed as the basic distribution. The model used in these projections is

Figure 5.1. Quarterly Incidence Rates of AIDS for Black, White, and Total United States, with Projections per Million.

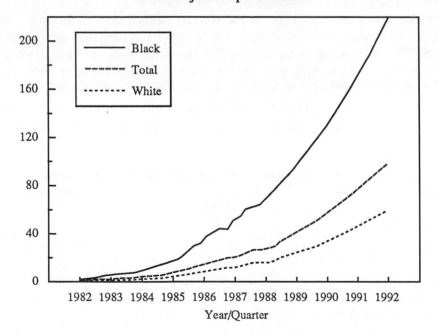

the following: number of cases/quarter = $2.86(T**2) + 61.76$, where $T**2$ is the square of the time unit in quarters beginning in 1980 and 61.76 is the number of cases at the beginning of the study in 1980. The model projected a total of 325,000 cases among blacks by 1993 and 600,000 by 1994. By 1995, the number of new cases among blacks may be expected to reach over one million. It is important to note that this model assumes that no major breakthrough will occur in the development of a vaccine or in substantially affecting the risk behaviors of African Americans.

We observe a substantial increase in the number of cases in these two populations and an even greater increase in the proportion of AIDS cases that are black. Thus, the number of new cases among blacks is expected to continue to increase at a substantial rate. Since some progress has been made in affecting the risk behavior of middle-class white homosexual males, and the recent data suggest a slowing of transmission in this group, the proportion of AIDS cases that are black is also expected to increase. The model suggests that the relative ratio of black-to-white rates of AIDS will exceed 4.0 after 1992.

As of July 1991, there were 182,834 cases of AIDS reported in the United States. Twenty-eight (28.6) percent of these cases were among blacks. Blacks are 3.5 times more likely to contract AIDS than whites. Black women are 13.8 times more likely to contract AIDS than white women. Black children are 12.8 times more likely to contract AIDS than white children. These rates are shown in Table 5.1.

Observation of surveillance data is also supported by population-based studies accessing HIV prevalence among military applicants, which indicated that blacks are four times more likely to have contracted an HIV infection than whites. More specifically, prevalence of HIV infections per 1,000 was found to be 3.5 for black military recruits, while 0.6 for white (Centers for Disease Control, 1990b). These data indicate a prevalence rate of 10.0 for black hospital patients and 7.0 for white patients. The disparity continues to be apparent in viewing job corps recruits with prevalence rates of 5.1 and 1.2 per 1,000 for blacks and whites, respectively (Centers for Disease Control, 1990a). Higher rates of HIV infections have also been found among black and white persons receiving care at public sexually transmitted

Table 5.1. AIDS Rates and Ratios for Blacks and Whites, U.S. 1991.

	Rates		
	Black	White	Ratios
Male	2.69	0.86	3.13
Female	0.55	0.04	13.75
Children	0.22	0.02	12.76

Source: Adapted from Centers for Disease Control, 1990a.

disease (STD) clinics and at drug treatment centers. Thus, the rate of disease among African Americans is not only a function of risk behaviors, but also of predisposing conditions such as sexually transmitted diseases, as well as of the social and economic factors of discrimination and alienation.

There is no evidence to suggest that blacks are biologically more susceptible to AIDS than whites. Differences in disease rates are likely due to differences in the distribution of risk behaviors, the existence of co-conditions (such as genital ulcer disease), and the lack of access to early diagnosis and treatment (National Research Council, 1989). Risk behaviors account for transmission of HIV infections, not membership in any particular ethnic group. However, some ethnic groups have a greater proportion of persons exhibiting certain risk behaviors. About 84 percent of whites with AIDS are men who have sex with other men, compared with only 44 percent of blacks with AIDS. Similarly, 45 percent of blacks with AIDS use intravenous (IV) drugs, while only 15 percent of white cases engage in this high-risk behavior. Thus, the higher proportion of blacks who use IV drugs in large measure determines the higher rate of disease among blacks, particularly among women and children.

Women and AIDS

The most obvious way in which the epidemiology of AIDS in blacks is different from that found among whites is the proportion of cases among women and children. Substantially, AIDS seen among black children is the result of higher rates of infection among their mothers. Higher rates of infection among black women is the result of higher rates of IV drug abuse and higher rates of infection among their drug-using sexual partners. Thus, women are at far greater risk of acquiring AIDS in the black community, both through their own risk behavior and through the risk behaviors of their sex and needle-sharing partners. They are also more likely to pass this infection on to their newborns.

The number of AIDS cases is growing faster among black women than any major race-gender group. It is now the eighth leading cause of death among women fifteen to forty-four years of age. Half of all AIDS cases among women are black (half are also IV drug abusers). Women are at increasing risk. Deaths from AIDS for black women in 1987 totaled 739 and had increased to 995 in 1988. Deaths for black men were 3,301 and 4,202 respectively for the same years.

Women who are HIV positive are more apt to develop conditions not now included in the official definition of AIDS and are thus less likely to receive entitlements of health services and support. Women are therefore also less likely to receive entitlements enabling them to receive early treatment. Six thousand infants are born to HIV-positive women each year, with 25 to 35 percent becoming HIV positive themselves (Ellerbrock, Bush, Chamberland, & Oxtoby, 1991). In addition to the increased risk of AIDS from infected parents, black children are far more likely to be orphaned at the death of both parents from AIDS (Rothenberg et al., 1987).

The incidence of IV drug abuse–related AIDS was 19.7 per million among whites and 188.9 per million among blacks in 1987. Thus, the rate of such cases is 9.6 times higher among blacks than whites. The relative risk of IV drug abuse–related AIDS has been consistently higher among blacks than among whites since 1982, when these data were first compiled (Selik et al., 1988). Thus, the greater proportion who abuse IV drugs in the black community accounts for many of the differences in the distribution of AIDS cases by race.

Black Men Who Have Sex with Other Men

It must also be noted that the increased rate of infection is not only due to risk behavior, but also to the capacity to change such behavior. Black men who have sex with other men are also more at risk for AIDS than their white counterparts. Black homosexual males are at a higher risk of transmission, 1.8 times higher than similarly situated whites (using the 10 percent estimate of homosexuality generally accepted in the literature). While white men who had sex with other men participated in risk behaviors in similar ways to their black counterparts, they were quite different in response to efforts toward organization and education. The white gay community has effectively organized around this issue and has moved away from high-risk behaviors to reduce transmission. Efforts of the black homosexual male community are less apparent. The black gay community remains harder to identify and reach.

Indeed, the sociology of AIDS is as complicated and intriguing as the epidemiology of AIDS. While the general population has known the factors associated with the transmission of this disease since 1983, behaviors that reduce the risks of HIV infections have not been readily adopted by many high-risk persons, especially blacks and Hispanics. From 1981 to 1986, the prime reason for this may have been the widespread self-righteous beliefs expressed by the phrase, "It's not my problem." Prior to the first conference on AIDS in minorities, many African-American leaders opposed any suggestion that blacks were at greater risk. However, after the conference many were concerned that it had not been held earlier. Within one week, the prevailing view went from not wanting to be involved in developing strategies to reduce the spread of HIV infection to demands for being actively involved. While many persons were frustrated by the conference, the goal was achieved: the African-American community was made aware that AIDS was a new threat that could no longer be ignored.

Concerns about blame remain a major problem for the African-American community. Even today, the issue of the origin of HIV occupies the thinking of many black Americans. These concerns are exhibited in two notions — that the virus originated in Africa, and that the AIDS epidemic was born out of a conspiracy to reduce the black population. It is important to understand that no group can be blamed for this epidemic. It is also enormously important that we not divert precious time and energy away from developing effective programs to prevent the spread of HIV in black communities. The inordinate amount of energy spent debating these issues in the African-American community speaks more to lingering alienation from American society than to any real importance of where this epidemic started or who started it. On the other hand, these issues demonstrate the need to develop culturally appropriate interventions that consider issues that may not appear to be relevant. Those responsible for ending this epidemic may be tempted to ignore issues that appear to be unfounded. However, like the concerns regarding transmission from health care workers, officials must respond not only to the "epidemic," but also to the "epidemic of fear" associated with this disease.

The history of public health programs in the African-American community has been less than positive. From the early 1930s to the early 1960s, these programs were often efforts to treat the African-American community. For example, programs attempted to reduce fertility among blacks, to study the effects of untreated syphilis, or to control the spread of infections. African Americans were treated as "subjects." In the 1960s, public health programs were developed to "improve" the African-American community. These programs provided maternal and child health services, comprehensive community health services, and community development efforts. However, they were generally managed from Washington or some other central authority. It was not until 1986 that a commitment was made to develop public health efforts with the African-American community. These programs provided funds to black and other minority communities and national organizations to develop HIV prevention messages and interventions. Since 1986, similar programs have provided support to minority organizations to develop activities aimed at the prevention of cancer, heart disease, drug abuse, and other conditions. This uneven history makes it clear why problems of implementation exist.

Public health officials find it difficult to include members of the community in decision making. They are often baffled by continued resistance to messages of prevention and do not appreciate the differences in perspective on roles. Some public health officials continue to find it difficult to work with African-American communities as "partners" and not as "clients" or "subjects." Responding to this need, the CDC funded fifteen minority community-based organizations in 1988 and twenty-four in 1990. On the other hand, minority organizations often do not have substantial experience in illness prevention programs. In 1987, the CDC funded three national minority organizations. Five were funded in 1988, seven in 1989, and ten in 1990. Historically, the better-known minority organizations have frequently been heavily sponsored by alcohol and tobacco companies, which do not encourage the development of public health prevention programs. Public

health agencies often lack understanding of how to gain minority participation and minority organizations often lack experience in the infrastructure
of public health.

While the five cases of HIV apparently contracted from a Florida
dentist named David Acer are highly unusual cases having little relevance to
the HIV epidemic in the United States, they have generated national attention from the news media and government. On the other hand, an earlier
case in Florida involving a very high rate of spread among residents of a small
town (Bel Glade) received little acknowledgment from the media or political
leaders. While the Bel Glade case occurred in a community that is poor and
black, the Acer case occurred among middle-class whites. The scientific
community generally acknowledges that the Acer case has little public health
importance. The number of such cases is expected to remain extremely
small. However, the Bel Glade case portends the coming tragedy of drug-
related heterosexually spread AIDS among poor minority communities.
Notable exceptions to this are more recent cases surrounding basketball star
Earvin (Magic) Johnson and retired tennis celebrity Arthur Ashe. These
examples show how the HIV epidemic is reaching all social echelons. Factors
of race and class continue to be apparent in the differences between the
populations affected, however.

Conclusion

While we can expect continued reductions in AIDS cases among whites,
indicators predict an increase of these disease rates among African Americans. Thus, treatment for those already infected will be the high priority for
white Americans, but the priority for black Americans must be prevention. In
view of the massive political forces on the far right and the far left backing
treatment over prevention, support for preventive measures will undoubtedly
face continued peril. We can also expect substantial difficulties in program
implementation as minority organizations learn to initiate prevention programs, and as public health officials learn to allow others to participate in the
management process.

References

Bakeman, R., McCray, E., Lumb, J., Jackson, R., & Whitley, P. (1987). The
    incidence of AIDS among blacks and Hispanics. *Journal of the National
    Medical Association, 79,* 921–928.
Centers for Disease Control. (1986). *CDC Reports on AIDS: June 1981–May
    1986.* Atlanta, GA: Department of Health and Human Services.
Centers for Disease Control. (1987). *Reports on AIDS: June–December 1986.*
    Atlanta, GA: Department of Health and Human Services.
Centers for Disease Control. (1990a). *AIDS public information data set.* Atlanta,
    GA: Department of Health and Human Services.

Centers for Disease Control. (1990b). *National HIV seroprevalence surveys: Summary of results, data from serosurveillance activities through 1989*. Atlanta, GA: Department of Health and Human Services.

Dewart, J. (1991), (Ed.). *The state of black America*. New York: National Urban League.

Ellerbrock, T., Bush, T., Chamberland, M., & Oxtoby, M. (1991). Epidemiology of women with AIDS in the U.S., 1981–1990. *Journal of the National Medical Association, 265*(22), 2971–2975.

Guinan, M. E., & Hardy, A. (1987). Epidemiology of AIDS in women in the U.S. *Journal of the National Medical Association, 257*, 2039–2044.

Mitchell, J. (1988). Women, AIDS, and public policy. *AIDS and Public Policy Journal, 3*, 50–52.

National Center for Health Statistics. (1991). *Health: United States, 1990*. Hyattsville, MD: Public Health Service.

National Research Council. (1989). *AIDS: The second decade*. Washington, DC: National Academy Press.

Panem, S. (1988). *The AIDS bureaucracy*. Cambridge, MA: Harvard University Press.

Rothenberg, R., Woefel, M., Stoneburner, R., Milberg, J., Parker, R., & Truman, B. (1987). Survival with the acquired immunodeficiency syndrome: Experience with 5833 cases in New York City. *New England Journal of Medicine, 317*, 1297–1302.

Selik, R., Castro, K., & Pappaioanou, M. (1988). Racial/ethnic differences in the risk of AIDS in the United States. *American Journal of Public Health, 78*(12), 1539–1545.

Valdiserri, R. (1989). *Preventing AIDS: The design of effective programs*. New Brunswick, NJ: Rutgers University Press.

6

Prevention, Intervention, and
Treatment of Chemical Dependency
in the Black Community

Donnie W. Watson

For a variety of reasons, some scientists, health professionals, and social psychologists describe alcohol and other drug addiction as a disease. Advocates of the disease model have suggested that some individuals have a genetic or hereditary susceptibility to drug dependency. Others perceive alcohol and other drug addiction as a disease because they view it as a manifestation of underlying psychological problems such as depression. It is also important to note that substance abuse may mask other medical and/or psychiatric problems. There are a significant number of patients who might present with a dual diagnosis of substance abuse and psychiatric disorder.

Other experts on the subject of addiction further assert that alcohol and other drug abuse actually alters brain chemistry, which makes future controlled use nearly impossible. Moreover, some minority researchers see substance abuse as a secondary problem resulting from the individual's response to primary problems of oppression, racism, economic deprivation, stress, and despair in society. Although there are a myriad of views on the nature of alcohol and other drug abuse, none of these views excludes the need for alcohol and other drug addiction treatment as a necessary component in the fight against addiction.

Most health care professionals do indeed view alcohol and other drug dependence as a disease process. In fact, the American Medical Association officially defines alcohol and drug addiction as diseases. Chemical dependency is a very complex primary disease process that has genetic, psychosocial, and environmental components. As with any disease, there is a recognizable set of symptoms that allows for accurate diagnosis.

The chemically dependent person may experience changes in tolerance, withdrawal symptoms, and blackouts. The disease of chemical dependency follows a predictable course that is characterized by the patients' compulsive and repeated use of mind-altering substances without regard to the serious impact of these substances on just about every aspect of their lives. This disease process affects the emotional, physical, spiritual, familial, social, psychological, and occupational aspects of the person's life. It cuts across gender, racial, ethnic, economic, and geographic lines and constitutes a progressive and ultimately fatal disease.

Understanding the psychological aspects of chemical dependency is an important dimension in examining this problem. Watson (1990) describes addiction as a "disease of feelings." That is, chemically dependent persons often use alcohol or other drugs to change their feeling state. A primary reason for the difficulty in weaning the patient from the substance is that the chemical produces a seemingly beneficial effect for the user at the early stages of the abuse. However, once the addiction process becomes activated, the desired effect of the chemical is no longer met.

Denial is the predominant defense mechanism in the treatment of people who are chemically dependent. Denial is characterized by patients' inability to accurately assess the devastation of the chemical dependency on their lives. They are the victims of a massive denial system that dictates that patients will not reach out for help (Talbott & Gallegos, 1990).

Other prominent characteristics are powerlessness and unmanageability. Chemically dependent people behave in erratic ways and are often hostile or abusive. Their behavior is out of control, and consequences have no meaning. Resentment, self-pity, and low self-esteem often occur. Shame and guilt are feelings that often paralyze addicts and decrease their ability to function appropriately. It should be noted that chemical dependency greatly affects families, since family members are impacted by the behavior of the addicts.

Adherents of the disease theory believe that chemically dependent people can never learn to responsibly use mind-altering chemicals. They point to the failed attempts of individuals to return to social drinking after treatment for chemical dependence (Bell, 1990).

Certain influences regarding chemical dependency affect both the black and white communities (Watson & Sobell, 1983). However, some authors in the community raise questions about the wisdom of the disease concept in the black community. In this regard, there is reasonable concern among blacks about viewing chemical dependency as a disease process. Genetic predisposition to addiction is an idea that is subject to close scrutiny by black and other minority communities. There is fear that the concept of a genetic predisposition invites racist notions of the superiority of one race over another (Bell, 1990). These concerns cannot and should not be taken lightly.

Some theorists, such as Nobles and Goddard (1989), would probably agree that black chemical dependency is greatly related to environmental influences. The devastating effects of oppression are readily recognized by taking a similar view of the problem. In fact, Nobles and Goddard (1989) assert that the primary factors leading to substance abuse in the African-American population include economic deprivation, racism, and stress. It is also postulated by some that blacks cannot wait for all social ills to be rectified before addressing chemical dependency in the community. Further, historically, blacks have demonstrated a strength of character in overcoming many hardships in the American culture.

Bell (1990) succinctly states that there is room in the disease theory to accommodate cultural differences. The problem is that many people in the field of chemical dependency treatment are only now becoming aware of the critical significance culture plays among racial minorities in recovery. Similarly, Bell and Evans (1981) note that addiction is a primary illness. They acknowledge the role of racism and oppression in substance abuse among blacks but clearly view chemical dependency as a primary process.

Scope of the Problem

The concept of prevention, intervention, and treatment for chemical dependency specifically targeted to the black community has received considerable and sustained attention in recent years. One has only to look at the increasing number of community, federal, state, and locally funded prevention and treatment programs as evidence of the importance of this concept. Likewise, one can observe the empirical evidence supporting the decrease of drug use within the black community. For example, results of the 1988 National Household Survey (National Institute on Drug Abuse, 1990) reveal a decrease in drug use among blacks in their lifetime (from 37.1 to 35.9 percent), a significant decrease in drug use among blacks in the past year (from 21.8 to 13.3 percent), and a significant decrease in drug use among blacks in the past month (from 15.7 to 7.8 percent). It should be noted that these statistics are collected only from those in households who respond to surveys. Howver, with the consistency of these results across surveys, one can be reasonably assured that they accurately reflect use patterns of blacks in the United States.

Results of the 1988 High School Survey (National Institute on Drug Abuse, 1990) report that over one-third of the eighteen- to nineteen-year-old blacks have dropped out of school, with drug use higher among the dropouts. Black students who stay in school are less likely than white students to use illicit drugs. Specifically, white seniors are twice as likely to report ever using cocaine than black seniors (13 percent versus 6 percent) and more likely to report ever using marijuana (50 percent versus 37 percent). Results from these surveys suggest that the prevalence of drug use within the black community is decreasing. Although promising, these results demonstrate that there is still a serious national chemical dependency problem within the black population in the United States.

The 1988 National Household Survey on Drug Abuse (NHSDA) revealed other significant facts about the black community. Defining illicit drug use as any nonmedical use of marijuana or hashish, cocaine (including crack), inhalants, hallucinogens (including PCP), heroin, or psycho-therapeutics (stimulants, tranquilizers, and sedatives), the National Household Survey revealed that nearly 8 million (36 percent) blacks have used illicit drugs at least once in their lifetimes, 3 million in the past year, and 1.7 million in the past month. Thus, although drug use within the black community is decreasing, there is still a significant number of drug users within the black population.

The NHSDA also revealed that within the population age thirty-five and older, blacks were more likely than whites or Hispanics to use an illicit drug currently (in the past month); blacks were more likely than whites or Hispanics to have used heroin once in their lifetime; blacks were more likely than Hispanics, but less likely than whites, to have used cigarettes; and black women were more likely than women in any other racial/ethnic group to have used crack cocaine.

Likewise, the black community is not immune to other problems resulting from chemical dependency. A 1989 report by the Centers for Disease Control (CDC) reveal that AIDS is a severe problem among blacks due to intravenous (IV) drug use. Of those living in households, blacks are twice as likely as whites to have used drugs intravenously. Even though blacks represent 12 percent of the population in the United States, they account for approximately 27 percent of all people with AIDS. Of those cases, 44 percent (12,609) reported injection of an illicit substance prior to diagnosis with AIDS (CDC, 1989). Blacks account for more than half of the AIDS cases who were heterosexual partners of IV drug users (CDC, 1989).

Furthermore, black patients accounted for 39 percent (63,002) of the 160,170 drug abuse–related emergency room cases reported to the Drug Abuse Warning Network of the National Institute on Drug Abuse (1988). Of the emergency room cases involving black patients, 62 percent were male, 40 percent were twenty to twenty-nine years old, and 57 percent involved cocaine — the most frequently mentioned drug in emergency room episodes (National Institute on Drug Abuse, 1988). Of the 6,756 drug abuse–related deaths reported by medical examiners to the Drug Abuse Warning Network, black decedents accounted for 30 percent (1,999) of those deaths. Over 74 percent of the black decedents were males, and 46 percent were thirty to thirty-nine years old (National Institute on Drug Abuse, 1988). Alcohol and drug abuse also play a significant role in black male–on–black male completed homicide (that is, either the victim, perpetrator, or both were under the influence at the time of the incident) (Office of National Drug Control Policy, 1989).

In spite of the devastating effects of chemical dependency, statistics show that the black community is receiving a certain measure of treatment. The 1987 National Drug and Alcoholism Treatment Survey reported that blacks represented about one-fourth of the drug abuse clients in treatment. The proportion of black clients was highest in the District of Columbia,

Georgia, Illinois, and Maryland. Thus, the black community is putting forth some effort to treat chemical dependency, but more needs to be done. As such, the topics of prevention, intervention, and treatment for the black community deserve considerable attention and resources. In this regard, the U.S. Department of Health and Human Services has concluded that black life expectancy is approximately six years shorter than that of whites—citing chemical dependency as one major reason (Gossett, 1988).

Prevention Methodology

According to the Office of National Drug Control Policy, "in the war against illegal drug use, the real heroes are not those who use drugs and quit; they are those who never use them in the first place. That is the primary goal of prevention: to see to it that Americans—especially school children—never start down a slippery slope of drug use that begins with experimentation, but can culminate in dependency" (1989, p. 47).

Prevention is a goal that this country must continuously strive to reach. The statistics reported by Ellis (1987) illustrate this point. Nearly half of all high school seniors have used an illegal drug at least once; almost 90 percent have used alcohol. In many ways, this behavior has become acceptable; for too many it has become a way of life. There are 5.3 million fourteen- to seventeen-year-old problem drinkers. Over half of the teenagers who have used drugs buy them at school. Increasingly, people accept the use of alcohol and marijuana, sexual intercourse, and teenage pregnancy as normal behavior for teenagers in this country (Ellis, 1987).

Prevention efforts are aimed at reducing the adverse effects of single bouts of drug use as well as the social and medical problems that arise as a result of persistent high-risk drug use. Prevention activities are undertaken by legislators, law enforcement officials, educators, health professionals, business leaders, and concerned citizens (Secretary of Health and Human Services, 1990). In recent years, a public health approach has emerged toward prevention of alcohol use (Secretary of Health and Human Services, 1990). A key element of this approach is the recognition that reducing alcohol-use problems requires strategies that affect the environment as well as individual behavior. These prevention efforts employ a variety of methods. These methods include changes in the social context of drinking, public information and education, and limitations on the availability of alcoholic beverages. The alcohol prevention research being undertaken also employs the public health model. The current emphasis is on studies concerning the host (for example, individual drinker) and the environment (for example, the immediate alcohol drinking context). Two types of prevention research are conducted (Secretary of Health and Human Services, 1990). Basic prevention research explores factors that influence the risk of developing alcohol and use problems. These factors include individual characteristics that may place one at risk (such as age, gender, and family history) and factors within the environment (including family interaction, workplace factors, characteristics of drinking establishments, and alcohol beverage prices). The other type of research, applied prevention research, evaluates the effectiveness of purposeful actions taken to reduce problems related to alcohol use. Such actions include measures to modify the drinking environment (for instance, legislation establishing minimum drinking age, laws regarding drinking and driving, and measures—such as educational programs—designed to change individual behavior). The findings of basic prevention research ideally contribute to the development and implementation of prevention strategies.

Drug prevention (which also includes alcohol) is similar to alcohol prevention. There are two approaches to influencing whether an individual decides to use drugs. One approach is to discourage use through information and moral persuasion. These factors obviously help shape an individual's preferences. The other approach is to make an individual fear the consequences and penalties that society will impose for drug use by making it clear that the costs will outweigh whatever temporary benefits drugs can provide. The "education/persuasion" approach has traditionally been thought of as demand reduction and the "consequences" approach as supply reduction. Both approaches reduce the demand, and both are critical to an effective prevention strategy (Office of National Drug Control Policy, 1989).

Knowledge of what works in preventing young people from using drugs has recently improved. For instance, much of the previous effort that focused on the passive approach was not successful. The passive approach, which consisted of presenting young people with information on the harmful effects of drugs, often in a context devoid of moral judgment, did little if anything to reduce the demand. In fact, according to the Office of National Drug Control Policy (1989), the problem may have even been fueled by stimulating young people's curiosity about drugs.

What does work is a more confrontational approach in which every facet of society clearly communicates that drug use is unacceptable. Schools have a major role to play in prevention, not only by presenting accurate drug information, but also by developing and enforcing firm and consistent policies that discourage the use and sale of drugs. However, there are other major influences in a young person's life that should also be dealt with without equivocation. Families (parents and siblings) must make it clear that drugs are unacceptable, and they must intervene at the first sign of drug use. Communities and neighborhoods must confront and not accept drug use, both potential and actual, at every turn. Employers and businesses must make it clear that drug use and employment are incompatible. Thus, young people and adults alike must be confronted on a consistent basis with the same message—that drugs are not only harmful but illegal and that their use will bring harmful consequences (Office of National Drug Control Policy, 1989).

According to Scott (1987), one of the developers of Oakland Parents in Action, the program that pioneered the phrase and strategy of "Just Say No," youngsters know what they want in a prevention program. They do not want information on alcohol and drug problems that is rife with scare tactics. They want factual information on how drugs affect them now, as opposed to how they will be affected twenty years from now.

Scott (1987) also points out several other factors that need to be included in prevention programs. One is that we must build skills in the areas of social competence by teaching such things as assertiveness and communication. Decision-making skills also play a critical role in prevention; these skills are not just effective relative to making a decision about whether to drink alcohol or take drugs, but they will assist individuals in making informed decisions throughout their lives. A third factor, as noted by Scott (1987) and Crayton (1987), is the improvement of self-esteem, which is particularly important for black youngsters. Many black youth in America have problems related to low self-esteem that can be a precipitating factor for substance abuse. A lack of self-esteem is largely related to identity confusion. Black youth need a greater sense of appreciation of their heritage. They need to know about the positive contributions of their African ancestry to world civilization as well as contributions of America's blacks to the development of the United States. Furthermore, a positive role model or mentor is also recommended by Scott (1987) and Carter (1987). According to Scott, the key to success for the Oakland Parents in Action program was to have willing teachers who wanted to volunteer their time.

Explicit group expectations of school and religious networks can interrupt young abusers' dependency as well as serve as deterrents. The New World Community of Islam in the West, Orthodox Jews, and the Amish experience very low addiction rates. The Nation of Islam has also been very successful in getting members off drugs while teaching more adaptive, healthier life-styles. These adaptive groups define the value and role of chemicals and establish clear ground rules that are incompatible with drug abuse (Gossett, 1988).

Community-based programs must involve the black church and other significant community and human service providers. Historically, the black church has been at the forefront of social change in the community. The church must play a significant role as change is implemented to "drug-proof" the community and empower it to make continual changes. One important way this can happen is by educating clergy on what chemical dependency is and how the churches can become involved in prevention, intervention, and treatment referral efforts.

Mayberry (1987) and Carter (1987) suggest that prevention programs be focused at the elementary school level. Mayberry contends that children need to focus on skills, particularly science and math, as well as reading and writing. An appropriate education is not only important, it is essential to a child's survival. Likewise, Carter (1987) suggests that elementary school children should participate in the process of creating a prevention program. Empowerment is increasingly becoming one of the necessary elements of success. According to Carter (1987), children can suggest activities they would like to engage in. Those activities should allow children (both younger and older) to work together on something that involves economics and determination. For instance, some of the activities of the Oakland Parents in Action program (Carter, 1987) include creating prevention messages that address the media and billboards that address the public. In other words, the key is a student component, because students have to actively participate to make it meaningful. The Office for Substance Abuse Prevention (1989) suggests that all prevention strategies should take on a systems approach, which is an approach that views the community and the environment as interconnected parts, each affected by the others and needing to work together. Since the individual parts have the potential either to support or to undermine each other's efforts, the goal of any community that is serious about drug prevention must be to make the parts work together through communitywide coalition efforts. Communities will move closer to creating environments for youth that consistently discourage involvement with alcohol and other drugs with support and cooperation.

Effective prevention strategies begin with an understanding of the various reasons why young people start to use alcohol and other drugs (Office for Substance Abuse Prevention, 1989). Those reasons appear in three main categories: individual influences, interpersonal and societal influences, and environmental influences. Individual influences include personality traits, genetics, attitudes and beliefs, and interpersonal and peer resistance skills. Interpersonal and societal influences include parents, the community, peers, school policy, local law enforcement, and personal situations. Environmental influences include the cost of alcohol and other drugs, federal laws concerning alcohol and illegal drugs, the minimum purchase age for alcohol, the marketing of alcohol, and the portrayal of alcohol, tobacco, and other drugs on television and in movies.

To implement these strategies successfully, it is important to have a planning guide (Office for Substance Abuse Prevention, 1989). Planning is important in that it helps communities concentrate on projects that will have the most impact on local alcohol and drug problems. Planning reduces the frustration and wasted effort that can occur when prevention efforts try to accomplish too much with too little. Furthermore, planning can assist communities in receiving financial support from the federal government as well as national organizations and private donors. The Office for Substance Abuse Prevention suggests nine steps to planning a successful prevention effort: (1) conduct a needs assessment, (2) develop prevention goals, (3) develop objectives, (4) identify resources, (5) identify funding resources, (6) assign leadership tasks, (7) implement the prevention program, (8) evaluate the prevention program, and (9) revise the program.

Efforts are successful when they relate to and build on the strengths and interests of the people involved in the prevention initiative (Office for Substance Abuse Prevention, 1989). Several types of strategies can be used to build on those strengths; these include strategies focused on the individual, strategies focused on the peer group, educational approaches targeting parents, prevention through school-based strategies such as student assistance programs, educational approaches for teachers, mass media approaches to prevention, and prevention through regulatory and legal actions. A comprehensive program will eventually need to incorporate all of these strategies.

Intervention for Those Who Are Chemically Dependent

Early intervention with substance abusers in the black community is essential since blacks suffer disproportionately from health problems related to substance abuse and tend to become involved much later in the treatment process.

Intervention, as defined by Johnson (1986), is a process by which the harmful, progressive, and destructive effects of chemical dependency are interrupted and the chemically dependent person is helped to stop using mind-altering chemicals and to develop new, healthier ways of coping with his or her needs. It implies that the person need not be an emotional or physical "wreck" before such help can be given. In past years, those in the substance abuse field have generally accepted that "hitting rock bottom" was the most effective way to get the chemically dependent person into treatment. Fortunately, those in the treatment field have come to discard this theory of "helping." It is particularly important that intervention efforts among blacks who are chemically dependent take place as soon as possible, given the oppression and hardship some blacks face under normal circumstances.

Intervention is not treatment; rather, it is part of the process to get the person into treatment. Intervention should occur early in the patient's chemical dependency. This maxim is particularly critical to black patients, since their successful recovery is impacted by preexisting oppressive societal conditions. Further, black patients sometimes lack the societal supports of their white counterparts. Take the example of the black employee in a predominantly white institution where there are strong undercurrents of prejudice. This worker is under closer scrutiny than white counterparts. As the chemical dependency problem becomes more severe and his or her job performance suffers, the worker has unwittingly given credence to prejudicial management. Support and encouragement are also less likely to be present among management for blacks' recovery process. Bell (1986) notes that the perception of racism in the majority of American society would make any mindful black health professional hesitant to step forward and admit an impairment, because it may put the impaired black health professional at the mercy of a system that means him or her ill will.

Johnson (1986, pp. 61–87) has summarized five principles of intervention:

1.   People who are important to the chemically dependent individual are involved.
2.   These people record specific information about the actions of the chemically dependent individual which validates their concern.
3.   These people should reveal to the dependent individual—in a nonjudgmental way—their feelings about how the individual is affecting his or her life and theirs.
4.   The chemically dependent individual is offered treatment options.
5.   When the chemically dependent individual consents to accept assistance, immediate help is made available.

Talbott and Gallegos (1990, p. 14) note other procedures that serve as the basis for interventions:

1.   Intervention "rehearsals" permit intervention team members to practice and refine their roles.
2.   All individuals on the intervention team should understand the intervention goals and objectives.
3.   The intervention team should anticipate denial defenses, and responses should be discussed beforehand.
4.   Time restraints should not be put on the intervention team; return visits should be anticipated and allowed.

Conversely, Talbott and Gallegos (1990, p. 15) identify reasons for intervention failure among health professionals that are applicable to general populations as well:

1.   Poor planning, preparation, choosing of intervention team members, information gathering, and failure to rehearse
2.   Failure to include professional(s) in intervention
3.   Support systems or meaningful individuals not adequately involved or excluded from intervention
4.   Insufficient time provided for the intervention and the intervention not repeated
5.   Intervention sabotaged by team members who become enablers
6.   Intervention team members who did not receive adequate disease education and therefore exhibit hostile and uncaring behavior
7.   Intervention site selection and time inappropriate and therefore not conducive to successful intervention

Ideally, the result of the intervention is to get the chemically dependent person in treatment. The reality is that the best efforts may result in the person not recovering. Nevertheless, even if the person continues to abuse chemicals and never enters treatment, Johnson (1986) argues that intervention properly done "works" every time because, at the very least, it offers a chance for recovery where none existed before.

Treatment for Chemically Dependent Blacks

There are social contexts of chemical dependency and recovery that are unique to the black chemically dependent person. Some authorities take it for granted that blacks have to contend with more race-related self-concept issues than whites. Basic identity problems seen normally are present in the recovering black, and so the healing process must deal with black identity and racial pain (McGee, Johnson & Bell, 1985).

Consider, for example, an African American who has worked hard to become successful in society, but the individual becomes chemically dependent. The disappointment and feelings of low self-worth are compounded by the realization that he or she was at a disadvantage to begin with; the person is now in a tenuous situation. There is pressure to succeed in treatment because this person feels he or she will not receive the same chances afforded whites.

Treatment centers sometimes make serious mistakes by discounting issues of race or self-esteem that black patients raise. Treatment based on the disease theory needs to develop a mechanism to allow chemically dependent individuals to talk about racial identity issues and cultural differences, while not allowing these differences to be used as an excuse to avoid treatment or to deviate from treatment goals.

One strategy is to allow blacks in recovery to express their feelings and concerns about being black and related self-esteem issues without automatically attributing it to an attempt to defocus. Ultimately, counselors and treatment management need education on cultural and group differences and how to discern their role in the treatment process.

Treatment for the chemically dependent black person can involve inpatient, outpatient, recovery residences, or self-help groups such as Alcoholics Anonymous or Narcotics Anonymous. Family treatment is also available in the form of Alanon, Naranon, and Adult Children of Alcoholics groups. Traditional psychological therapies involving the individual, family, marital unit and group can be used as well.

In addition to the self-help groups, behavior therapy, and/or other forms of psychotherapy, treatments using drugs to control the physiological impact on the individual are also available. For example, methadone maintenance treatment (usually provided on an outpatient basis) involves replacing heroin with methadone over a period of time, which allows the client to explore alternative ways of functioning. Detoxification (which can be inpatient or outpatient) employs similar techniques—but for a much shorter period of time—for those dependent on a wide range of drugs but who are not necessarily opiate dependent. However, because of the high rate of recidivism of detoxification programs, they are not recommended as a modality, but as a precursor to other — more effective — treatment modalities such as chemical dependency programs, therapeutic communities (for those with serious social handicaps, including a history of criminal behavior), or outpatient nonmethadone treatment programs. Because clients'/patients' drug use patterns in the latter two programs vary greatly from those in methadone treatment programs, treatment techniques are not geared toward any specific class of drugs, although like other treatment programs, they are now dominated by those who are cocaine dependent. Other treatment techniques for cocaine abuse involve medication to reverse some of the biochemical imbalances caused by the drug (National Institute on Drug Abuse, 1988, June; Gerstein & Harwood, 1990).

Although some view twelve-step programs based on the Alcoholics Anonymous self-help principles as primary, psychological therapies and twelve-step programs such as Alcoholics Anonymous can be closely aligned in the treatment of chemically addicted persons. In fact, Whitfield (1987) sees a clear connection between twelve-step self-help groups, recovery, and psychotherapy.

The role of spirituality is an important component of the twelve-step treatment approaches. Spirituality is the simple recognition of a higher power or divine presence underlying the totality of things in the universe. This is not to be confused with religion that deals with rules of belief and behavior toward that higher power (L., 1990). This author contends that a reliance on spirituality is especially important to the recovering black addict. It is essential, however, that persons be able to choose their own concept of spirituality in the recovery process.

Denial is a major obstacle to recovery in light of clients' inability to view themselves honestly. Group therapy confronts the denial system while providing honest, direct, and supportive feedback. Group therapy also offers a mechanism for addressing anger, resentment, and hurt. Individual therapy, on the other hand, is sometimes indicated to help clients deal with feelings of depression, despair, hopelessness, low self-esteem, and psychic pain that recovery often involves. Therapy can also aid the client in skills training, so that coping skills and problem-solving skills can be acquired to avoid relapse situations.

Treatment is only the beginning of the recovery process for the addicted black client. Health professionals as well as the larger community need to understand that addicts are "sick" people who need support toward becoming well, rather than "bad" people who are immoral.

Conclusion

Blacks face special challenges in dealing with recovery from chemical dependence because of (1) the basic recovery process and its nuances, (2) racism/oppression in society at large, (3) feelings of decreased self-esteem, which have been found to be exacerbated by chemical dependence, and (4) the difficulty of finding and maintaining "safe" places in the community to achieve sobriety. Blacks sometimes experience other special hardships in the recovery process, including a lack of family support and difficulty adjusting to predominantly white treatment systems that they perceive themselves as not belonging in (Richardson & Williams, 1990). Aftercare and continuing care treatment planning should address these issues and strive to develop solutions.

A continuum of services that impact chemical dependency in the black community must be offered. This effort should be made in the provision of prevention, intervention, and treatment services that work in unison and are culturally appropriate to the black community. The fact that the occurrence and maintenance of chemical dependency in the black community is a complex problem that involves political, economic, social, and cultural elements must not be ignored. However, waiting for optimal social conditions to attack this problem is not the answer. Rather, a proactive stance utilizing community, local, state, and federal resources is in order. Only then can the black community be empowered to reclaim the community in order to implement long-term changes and reverse the devastating impact of chemical dependency.

As Nobles and Goddard (1989) note, the solution to the substance abuse problem lies in the area of national interest and therefore in public policy. In this regard, black educators, clergy, health care professionals, laypersons, and grassroots planners must organize to implement education, prevention, research, and treatment efforts that are culturally appropriate to address the complexity of drug use in the community.

There are major barriers to treatment for chemical dependency in the black community. These include lack of funds to pay for treatment, long waiting lists for admission to affordable programs, and a lack of economic support to sustain clients or their families during inpatient treatment. Low-income single parents face particularly difficult barriers because of the lack of child-care options, possible loss of child custody, and threats to economic and family security posed by inpatient treatment. The black community can respond to these barriers by advocating for more treatment programs for low-income clients, supporting outpatient alternatives to hospital stays, advocating for more effective treatment of drug users in correctional facilities, and addressing the needs of the single parent. Although African Americans are faced with barriers to treatment, treatment does work when clients are treated by qualified professionals, are motivated, and have supportive families who understand the nature of the illness and have support systems in the environment to provide safe places for continuing care.

These efforts must also consider and address the sociocultural context of blacks living in America in order to make these efforts sensitive and viable to the communities served. The strengths rooted in cultural aspects of the black community must be utilized in this effort. This type of collaborative effort will lead to the development of models and policies that will improve the quality of efforts directed toward addressing chemical dependency in the black community, which will in turn strengthen the nation as a whole.

References

Bell, C. C. (1986). Impaired black health professionals: Vulnerabilities and treatment approaches. *Journal of the National Medical Association, 78*(10), 925–930.

Bell, P. B. (1990). *Chemical dependency and the African-American.* Center City, MN: Hazelden Foundation.

Bell, P. B., & Evans, J. (1981). *Counseling the black client.* Center City, MN: Hazelden Foundation.

Carter, A. (1987). [Summary of remarks.] *Proceedings of a national conference on preventing alcohol and drug abuse in black communities* (DHHS Publication No. ADM 89-1648, pp. 31–35). Rockville, MD: Office for Substance Abuse Prevention.

Centers for Disease Control. (1989, September). *HIV/AIDS surveillance.* Atlanta, GA: Department of Health and Human Services.

Crayton, B. (1987). [Summary of remarks.] *Proceedings of a national conference on preventing alcohol and drug abuse in black communities* (DHHS Publication No. ADM 89-1648, pp. 22–24). Rockville, MD: Office for Substance Abuse Prevention.

Ellis, K. (1987). [Summary of remarks.] *Proceedings of a national conference on preventing alcohol and drug abuse in black communities* (DHHS Publication No. ADM 89-1648, pp. 36–40). Rockville, MD: Office for Substance Abuse Prevention.

Gerstein, D., & Harwood, J. (Eds.). (1990). *Treating drug problems* (Vol. 1). Washington, DC: National Academy Press.

Gossett, V. R. (1988). Drug and alcohol abuse in black America. In D. Grant (Ed.), *A guide for community action.* New York: National Urban League.

Johnson, V. E. (1986). *Intervention: How to help someone who doesn't want help.* Minneapolis, MN: Johnson Institute.

L., Chris. (1990). *Step two: Becoming spiritual.* Minneapolis, MN: Johnson Institute

McGee, G., Johnson, L., & Bell, P. B. (1985). *Black, beautiful, and recovering.* Center City, MN: Hazelden Foundation.

Mayberry, C. (1987). [Summary of remarks.] *Proceedings of a national conference on preventing alcohol and drug abuse in black communities* (DHHS Publication No. ADM 89-1648, pp. 27–31). Rockville, MD: Office for Substance Abuse Prevention.

National Institute on Drug Abuse. (1988). *Drug abuse warning network.* Rockville, MD: NIDA Press Office.

National Institute on Drug Abuse. (1988, June). Drug abuse treatment. *National Institute on Drug Abuse Capsule.* Rockville, MD: NIDA Press Office.

National Institute on Drug Abuse. (1990). National Household Survey on

Drug Abuse: Main findings 1988 (DHHS Publication No. ADM 90-1682). Rockville, MD: Author.

Nobles, W. W., & Goddard, L. L. (1989). Drugs in the African American community: A clear and present danger. In J. Dewart (Ed.), *The state of black America* (pp. 161–182). New York: National Urban League.

Office for Substance Abuse Prevention. (1989). *Prevention plus II: Tools for creating and sustaining drug free communities* (DHHS Publication No. ADM 89-1649). Rockville, MD: Author.

Office of National Drug Control Policy, Executive Office of the President. (1989, September). *National drug control strategy* (S/N 040-000-00542-1). Washington, DC: U.S. Government Printing Office.

Richardson, T. M., & Williams, B. A. (1990). *African-Americans in treatment.* Center City, MN: Hazelden Foundation.

Scott, B. (1987). [Summary of remarks.] *Proceedings of a national conference on preventing alcohol and drug abuse in black communities* (DHHS Publication No. ADM 89-1648, pp. 24–27). Rockville, MD: Office for Substance Abuse Prevention.

Secretary of Health and Human Services. (1990, January). *Seventh special report to the U.S. Congress on alcohol and health* (DHHS Contract No. ADM 281-88-0002). Alexandria, VA: Editorial Experts, Inc.

Talbott, G. D., & Gallegos, K. V. (1990, September). Intervention with health professionals. *Addiction & Recovery*, 13–16.

Watson, D. W. (1990). *Psychological aspects of addiction.* Unpublished manuscript.

Watson, D. W., & Sobell, M. B. (1983). Social influences on alcohol consumption by black and white males. *Addictive Behaviors*, 7, 87–91.

Whitfield, C. L. (1987). *Healing the child within.* Deerfield Beach, FL: Health Communications.

7

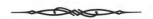

Alcoholism and
the African-American Community

Creigs C. Beverly

The U.S. Department of Health and Human Services reports that, overall, black life expectancy is 5.6 years less than that of whites and that chemical dependency stands out as a major reason (The Kerner Report Updated, 1988). For example, black men have excessive rates of alcohol-related illness. Prior to 1950, cirrhosis mortality rates among whites exceeded that of blacks. From 1951 to 1980, deaths due to cirrhosis more than tripled among black men, while they increased only slightly among white men. Esophageal cancer is also associated with alcohol consumption. During the 1980s, the rate of esophageal cancer among black men age twenty-five to thirty-four was ten times greater than among white men in the same age group (Marshall, 1989). If we add to these data the relationship between alcohol and crime and other ills (for example, domestic violence and family dissolution; fetal alcohol syndrome, which the National Urban League [1988] has labeled the single greatest preventable cause of mental retardation in the United States; automobile injuries and deaths; and loss of work and lack of productivity), it becomes clear why alcoholism in the black community is of grave concern.

An Imperfect Freedom

Alcoholism is of grave concern not only because of its negative effects, but also, and perhaps more important, because it adds one additional problem to the lives of people still engaged in a protracted struggle for political, economic, and social enfranchisement. A pertinent question often raised is whether alcohol abuse and misuse in the African-American community is one of the primary reasons the struggle for freedom and equality continues, or whether the imperfect freedom African Americans experience daily is one of the primary causes for use and abuse. The assumption underlying the first question is this: If alcoholism were not a problem at all, then African Americans would come closer to achieving social, political, and economic enfranchisement. This point deserves careful consideration. As far as it goes, however, an alcohol-free African-American community would still be confronted with the fallout from years of oppression, discrimination, educational inequities, economic underdevelopment, and to a great degree, societal beliefs and response patterns suggesting the social marginality and social insignificance of African Americans. Still, the goal of drastically reducing or eliminating alcoholism as a factor in the African-American community is not only worthwhile but also noble.

It would be naive to disregard the relationship between a lack of adequate social development and the tendency to compensate by using alcohol and other drugs. For this reason, any discussion of alcoholism and the African American creates a heavy burden on communities already beset by racism, poverty, and unequal access to resources. As The Kerner Report Updated (1988) proclaims, we must bring the problems of race, unemployment, and poverty back into the public consciousness and put them back on the public agenda.

Though socioeconomic and cultural realities are important in the understanding, treatment, and prevention of alcoholism in the African-American community, these issues should not preempt what Bell and Evans (1981) refer to as the "fundamental presenting problem." They suggest that addiction is primary and that though racism and oppression certainly contribute to alcohol abuse, abuse is not a secondary issue to psychological and emotional problems. They conclude, however, with the acknowledgment that alcoholism in the African-American community can be diagnosed, treated, and prevented most successfully when taking into account the cultural context in which the alcohol abuse developed.

A significant component of the cultural context in which alcohol abuse and addiction develop in the African-American community is the disproportionate accessibility of liquor and party stores. It is not unusual to see such stores on nearly every corner in some black neighborhoods across America; this is especially the case in low-income, inner-city neighborhoods. There is also a disproportionate number of billboards and other signs of every variety glorifying alcohol consumption. The same is true for cigarettes. The promotion of death-inducing behaviors in black America via target advertising, if not a conspiracy, represents, minimally, a level of corporate social irresponsibility that borders on criminality.

As dismal as the foregoing discussion is, there are some glimmers of hope, particularly in the area of drinking patterns among African-American youth. According to recent surveys (Office for Substance Abuse Prevention, 1990), African-American youth drink less than white, Hispanic, and Native American youth, and they are more likely to abstain from alcohol (see Table 7.1). However, the surveys are usually conducted on high school students, so that dropouts are excluded. Data show results that over one-third of the eighteen- to nineteen-year-old blacks have dropped out of school. Use of

**Table 7.1. Percent Reporting Alcohol Use in the Past Month
by Age Group and Demographic Characteristics, 1988.**

	Age Group (Years)		
Demographic Characteristics	12–17	18–25	Total
Total	25.2	65.3	53.4
Gender			
Male	26.8	74.5	60.6
Female	23.5	56.6	46.7
Race/ethnicity			
White	27.4	68.8	55.1
Black	15.9	50.0	44.3
Hispanic	25.4	61.4	49.2
Region			
Northwest	30.2	70.8	59.2
North central	27.9	73.0	55.7
South	21.2	53.2	45.1
West	24.7	74.7	60.3

Source: Compiled and abstracted from National Institute on Drug Abuse, 1989, Tables 13-A-B-C-D-E-F-G-H, p. 13.

substances, including alcohol, is generally higher among high school dropouts. This conclusion has major policy implications. Reducing the school dropout rates among African-American youth is a logical precursor to reducing their likelihood of engaging in alcohol and other drug abuse.

Beyond Description

Problem description is a precursor to problem prescription. Although fewer African-American youth use alcohol and other drugs than do other ethnic groups, the prevalence of this problem remains a cause for special concern within African-American families and communities (Office for Substance Abuse Prevention, 1990). Regarding alcoholism, several conclusions are compelling:

1. Alcoholism in America is a social problem of enormous proportions. Its devastating effects can be seen in the faces of the dispossessed and alienated who inhabit the skid rows of America as well as in those who have made it into the boardrooms of corporate America. Alcoholism destroys individuals and families, takes an alarming toll on youth, and directly contributes to massive absenteeism in the workplace. Moreover, it exacerbates medical problems and increases costs of medical treatment, correlates with personal, family, and institutional violence, and in general is a terrible cancer in American society (Beverly, 1989).

2. Alcoholism does not discriminate. Its victims are young and old, of all races and ethnic groups. It makes no distinction between rich and poor or

male and female; it assaults the dignity of all its victims. However, when the assault occurs among a cohort such as black Americans—a population already burdened with multilevel assaults in an inhospitable society—special care and attention are required for effective intervention.

3. Alcoholism is a multifaceted phenomenon in the African-American community. Therefore, its reduction or eradication will require an approach to the problem driven by wholes and quantum realities versus atomistic and mechanistic realities (King, 1987).

4. The African-American community is neither monolithic nor homogeneous. One can find ultraconservatives to left-wing radicals; congregational affiliations that span the theological spectrum; rugged individualists and communalists; the very rich and the very poor; the highly educated and the uneducated; and cultural values and practices that run the gamut from Eurocentrism to Afrocentrism. This reality must be factored into any formula designed to address alcoholism as it is manifest in and among African Americans.

Etiology

Before moving beyond description to problem-solving prescriptions, it is important to touch on the etiology or causes of alcoholism. In an insightful article titled "Alcohol Abuse and Dependence," Grinspoon and Bakalar (1990) explore the complex etiology of alcoholism: Alcohol abuse has touched as many as one-third of American families. It has often been eloquently described, not only in clinical case histories, but also by alcoholics themselves in confessions, memoirs, and imaginative literature. So there is some mystery about why it so easily eludes definition and identification. Even the symptoms are disputed. Almost everyone now understands that the image of alcoholism must not be oversimplified and exaggerated. Few alcoholics are on skid row, many do not have withdrawal symptoms, and most hold jobs and sustain family life for a long time. As the social stigma of alcoholism becomes milder, more and more people are defined as alcoholics or become willing to define themselves that way. But this has only heightened controversy, not only about the nature of the symptoms, but also about the kind of condition alcoholism is. Is it a behavior problem, a vice, a bad habit, a personality disorder, a progressive disease, or perhaps all of these? The answer often seems to depend on which alcoholic you are talking about and which moralist or expert you are listening to.

Current research, though still inconclusive, suggests that the causes of alcoholism are both psychosocial and biogenetic. Talbott (1986), among others, has studied chemically impaired physicians and has greatly contributed to our understanding of the biogenetic basis of addiction. The biogenetic approach to alcohol addiction holds that some individuals have a predisposition for addiction or a greater proclivity to be "at risk" for addiction due to genetic characteristics. The psychosocial view of addiction etiology rests on the premise that psychological and social development factors cause alcoholism. Family origin is a critical factor in both biogenetic and psychosocial theories (Grinspoon & Bakalar, 1990). From this standpoint, it is possible for a person to become addicted to alcohol at any point along the biogenetic-psychosocial continuum, depending on the operable mix of factors. Understanding the etiology of alcohol addiction is crucial to framing prevention programs as well as to providing focus and direction for clinical intervention once addiction has occurred.

Prescription/Intervention

It has been established that alcoholism in the African-American community is only one of a myriad of problems facing African Americans. Given this reality, the issue of alcoholism cannot be addressed in isolation from other social and economic conditions. Prescriptions for the problem must be forged in a comprehensive program of actions designed to raise the quality of life of African Americans at all levels. It is also important that within the overall action plan, attention be paid to specific treatment issues for persons already addicted to alcohol. The systems designed to assist them with recovery and hopefully prevent a relapse into dysfunctional behavior (secondary prevention) should not be neglected, either.

Treatment

To treat an affliction, we must have some familiarity with it. First, what is addiction? Second, what is alcoholism? Shaef and Fassel (1988) define addiction as any substance or process that takes over people's lives and over which they are powerless. It may not be a physiological addiction, though the idea that alcoholism has a physiological grounding is widely held. This is the basis for classifying alcoholism as a disease. An addiction is any process or substance that begins to have control over us in such a way that we feel we must be dishonest with ourselves or others about it. Addictions lead us into increasing compulsiveness in our behavior. Shaef and Fassel (1988) also note that an addiction is anything we feel we have to lie about. If there is something we are not willing to give up in order to make our lives fuller and healthier, it probably can be classified as an addiction.

Regarding a precise definition of alcoholism, Grinspoon and Bakalar (1990) argue that it is not surprising that authorities do not agree on what weight to give various symptoms or how numerous and severe the symptoms must be to justify a diagnosis of alcoholism. No single symptom is decisive, not even high alcohol consumption. The problems take different forms in different people. Grinspoon and Bakalar (1990) do agree, however, that alcoholism is usually defined by patterns of alcohol use (drunken binges, morning drinking, need to drink daily, repeated unsuccessful efforts to cut

down, continued drinking despite an illness exacerbated by alcohol), consequences (blackouts, violence and accidents, drunk driving, loss of job, arguments with family and friends, mental and physical illness), and feelings
about drinking. It is, therefore, important to think about alcoholism in terms
of a constellation of symptoms rather than a single symptom. This is necessary because a single symptom may be applicable to a whole range of
physical and psychological conditions. The more symptoms that can be
observed within an individual that correlate with what we know about
alcoholism, the more likely the diagnosis is to be accurate.

     Within the field of alcoholism, there are various modalities of treat-
ment intervention. These modalities range from what may be considered the
most traditional, Alcoholics Anonymous and the other highly respected
twelve-step programs, to programs deeply steeped in cultural and religious
transformation—as evident in the Nation of Islam model. Grinspoon and
Bakalar (1990) identify and define the prevailing modalities of treatment
independent of ethnicity.

Behavior Therapy

Behavior therapists assume that alcohol abuse is a learned habit that can be
unlearned by altering contingencies (that is, the factors in a given situation
that determine whether or not a person takes a drink). Early behavior
therapists thought that alcoholics had become conditioned to use drinking
as a way to relieve anxiety. To break this supposed conditioning, they experi-
mented with techniques such as chemical and electrical aversion—giving
electric shocks or injecting a nauseating drug while the alcoholic drank.
These treatments have not been very successful, and most experts now think
that conditioned anxiety is not the main cause of alcohol abuse.

Cognitive Behavior Therapy

More recently, behavior therapists have emphasized cognitive behavioral
therapy. Alcoholics are encouraged to identify and record the situations and
feelings that cause them to drink. Then they are trained to avoid these
situations and feelings and to substitute other responses. They may be taught
how to refuse drinks politely and how to monitor the level of alcohol in their
blood by paying close attention to physical sensations. Therapists also encourage better diet and exercise. The aim is to learn a skill, the social skill of
controlled drinking. Abstinence is not regarded as the ultimate goal but as
one way, which may or may not be the best, to exercise self-control.

Detoxification

Although a few experimental drugs offer promise, there is no established
sobering agent—nothing that counteracts the effects of alcohol or speeds its

breakdown and passage out of the body. Stimulants reverse some of alcohol's effects on thinking and motor coordination, but they are unreliable and have dangers of their own. Opiate antagonists do not affect alcohol intoxication or alcohol withdrawal.

Many alcoholics can withdraw on their own, but some are so severely dependent that they have to be detoxified—supervised as they go through a gradual withdrawal. The most common withdrawal symptoms are tremors, nausea, dry mouth, sweating, weakness, and depression. These symptoms begin six to eight hours after sudden withdrawal, reach their greatest intensity after ten to thirty hours, and subside in a few days.

Drug Treatment

Drugs are generally not very useful for sober alcoholics, and some drugs create a serious danger of dependence. A few alcoholics suffering from severe depression will be helped by antidepressants, but more often the depression results from alcohol abuse and clears up a week to two weeks after withdrawal. Recent studies suggest that lithium is usually prescribed for mood disorders; it helps alcoholics who are not depressed as much as those who are.

Alcoholics Anonymous (Group Therapy)

Group therapy allows alcoholics to rebuild the personal relationships they have lost through drinking. The results are more hope, new skills, and a new sense of community or family. Patients gain a sense of social effectiveness and power over their circumstances by finding a place in the group and helping others while helping themselves. Some varieties are couples therapy, psychodrama, and group therapy with a professional leader. By far the most popular form of group treatment is Alcoholics Anonymous, one of the oldest and most respected mutual aid organizations.

The Twelve Steps

The basic strategy of Alcoholics Anonymous is known as the twelve steps. Recovering alcoholics must admit their powerlessness over alcohol and seek help from a higher power, which can be understood in any way a member chooses. Members are urged to pray or meditate to get in touch with that power. They are asked to make a "moral inventory," confess the wrongs they have done, beg forgiveness, make amends, and carry the message to other alcoholics. Alcoholics Anonymous takes the position that anyone who has once been an alcoholic is always an alcoholic; the disease can be arrested, but vulnerability is permanent.

There are also a wide range of support groups for alcoholics and those people whose lives have been affected by an alcoholic. The recognition of the codependency syndrome has contributed greatly to the development of such groups for families, teens, and even workers in business and industry whose lives have been touched by alcoholism in the workplace. The idea of codependency reflects the belief that though the alcoholic is dependent on the drug, the behaviors that emanate from the addiction affect everyone else in the addict's social environment. A very recent development consistent with this support-group phenomenon is the establishment of the National Association of Children of Alcoholics–Adult Children of Alcoholics.

Within the African-American community proper, beyond the attention being given to the problem by long-standing organizations such as the NAACP and the Urban League, there has been a significant increase in issue-specific groups. Some examples include the Institute on Black Chemical Abuse, Cork Institute on Alcohol and Other Substance Abuse of the Morehouse School of Medicine, the National Black Alcoholism Council, and the Institute for the Advanced Study of Black Family Life and Culture. The efforts of these groups, in combination with an ever-increasing body of literature generated by black scholars, have helped to focus specific attention on treatment issues felt to be of primary importance in intervention with black alcoholics (Nobles, 1989; Womble & Brisbane, 1985; Beverly, 1989; Marshall, 1989).

The scope of this chapter does not allow for a detailed articulation of all the current thinking and practice-based research available on treating black alcoholics. Readers are therefore encouraged to pursue the primary sources. It is, however, rather instructive to provide a sample of the range of topics available for in-depth study. For example, in the reader *Treatment of Black Alcoholics*, edited by Womble and Brisbane (1985), one will find detailed discussions of (1) how Alcoholics Anonymous functions for blacks, (2) spirituality: the treatment of black alcoholics, (3) misdiagnosis of alcohol-related organic brain syndrome, (4) inpatient rehabilitation, (5) designing employee assistance programs to meet the needs of black clients, (6) treatment needs of black alcoholic women, and (7) alcohol users in an emergency room setting, as well as other discussions of treatment.

Another very instructive way to approach the treatment of black alcoholism is to reconstruct the characteristics, attitudes, and achievements of blacks who do not become substance addicts or self-destructive individuals. Primm (1988) describes these attributes as follows:

> Some characteristics, attitudes, and achievements of blacks who do not become substance addicts or self-destructive individuals are: (a) a realistic perception of the "American dream"—material possessions alone do not insure happiness; (b) the ability to solve problems rather than trying to forget them; (c) feelings of self-worth emanating from a positive acceptance of oneself as a black person; (d) models of physical, emotional, and career fulfillment; (e) experience of success or mastery which develops

confidence to overcome environmental handicaps; (f) a sense of identification with a larger group in whose accomplishments one can take pride; (g) achievable short-range goals; (h) sources of help; (i) unglamorized picture of drug effects and drug life-styles; (j) a perception of self by standards other than normative.

Constructing rather than reconstructing these attributes could also provide a foundation for developing strong alcohol prevention programs in African-American communities.

From Treatment to Social Development

Though undeniably necessary, treatment of alcoholism in the African-American community will inevitably reflect the prevailing national cliché of "too little and too late." It is much like trying to rescue dying and dead fish, rather than seeking out the causes of the destruction and eradicating them. A much more effective strategy is what might be called the *social development approach*. The social development approach recognizes and takes into account the interrelatedness of all quality-of-life factors in human behavior. According to the social development model, alcoholism and related devastating effects are merely symptomatic of broader issues of human underdevelopment, including personal and communal impotence.

Just as some people attempt to overcome feelings of impotence through the use of force—with a gun, a knife, or a strong arm—the use and abuse of alcohol is every bit as much a behavior designed to compensate for impotence. Thus, the community development model seeks to ensure that the institutions that serve the African-American community, both indigenous and exogenous, are organized, structured, and operate in such a way as to eliminate or markedly reduce the need for people to engage in destructive behaviors to themselves, to others, and to society in general. Indeed, these institutions need to operate to promote the optimal capacity of all individuals to realize their fullest potential and forever remove from the social fabric of the African-American community the need for people to "take revenge on life for negating itself to them." The model just mentioned operates on the assumption that social development occurs best in communities that hold human values paramount, that regard the maintenance of life and improvement of the quality of life as ultimate goals, and that view people as capable of acting on and changing the world and in the process, contributing to the betterment of humankind.

Some readers will be skeptical of the social development approach and say "impossible." They will say that even when America is experiencing great economic expansion, the African-American community receives a disproportionately small share of the fruits of the expansion. It is therefore important to understand that goals represent ideals. They represent what is most desirable, and as such, they provide a sound basis for rational decision making and the formation of specific objectives. Even more important is the need—perhaps the absolute imperative—for African Americans to organize, mobilize, and activate their own resources, human and material, to address factors of community underdevelopment. In spite of the treacherous terrain most African Americans have had to traverse, thousands have done exceptionally well in every field applicable to the development of the African-American community. All must give back to those left behind. There is no reason not to do so. Alcoholism, among other debilitating conditions that beset the African-American community, will not be eradicated until and unless this community takes its destiny into its own hands.

Conclusion

Social policy issues that bear on the eradication of the effects of alcohol on the African-American community are not separate from other factors that bear on the overall quality of American life. Among the policies that need immediate attention are the following:

1. A comprehensive educational program specifically targeted to the African-American community on the causes and consequences of excessive abuse of alcohol
2. Massive and comprehensive programs designed to keep American youth in school, since the high correlation between school dropout and the use and abuse of substances is well established
3. A national commitment to dedicated research designed to more clearly define life stressors peculiar to or exacerbated by the social and racial status that can be correlated with substance abuse
4. More research on the effectiveness of generic alcoholism intervention methodologies overlayed with Afrocentric understandings in the treatment of black alcoholics
5. Continued local, state, and national efforts to reduce the number of liquor stores in African-American communities and to reduce targeted advertisements glorifying alcohol consumption in African-American communities
6. Promotion at every level of those personal attributes of African Americans known to reduce their vulnerability index to substance abuse
7. The creation of a third-wave movement capable of mobilizing African Americans of all persuasions to reclaim their humanity by committing themselves to reclaiming the greatness of a people whom "they could not kill!"

Systematic efforts are needed toward the development of effective social policy. The will of black people in overcoming the problem of alcoholism, as with other maladies, deserves such support.

References

Bell, P., & Evans, J. (1981). *Counseling the black client: Alcohol use and abuse in black America*. Minneapolis, MN: Hazelden Foundation.

Beverly, C. (1989). *Treatment issues for black alcoholic clients*. *Social Casework, 70*(6), 370–374.

Grinspoon, L., & Bakalar, J. (Eds.). (1990). Alcohol abuse and dependence [Special issue]. *Harvard Medical School–Mental Health Review, 2*.

The Kerner Report Updated. (1988). *Report of the 1988 Commission of the Cities: Race and poverty in the United States today*. Racine, WI: Johnson Foundation.

King, L. (1987). Comparative paradigms in mental health research. (Monograph No. 2) Los Angeles, CA: Fanon Center, Drew Medical School.

Marshall, O. M. (1989). *Substance abuse prevention in the minority community*. Unpublished manuscript. Resource for Public Health Policy, School of Public Health Regional Think Tank, University of Michigan, Ann Arbor.

National Urban League and the Institute on Black Chemical Abuse. (1988). *Alcohol and drug abuse in black America: A guide for community action*. New York: National Urban league.

Nobles, W. (1989). *Afrocentric deep structure: Toward an understanding of the cultural foundation of African American substance prevention*. Office for Substance Abuse Prevention Advisory Roundtable, Morehouse School of Medicine, Cork Institute, Atlanta, GA.

Office for Substance Abuse Prevention (1990, August). *Alcohol and other drug use is a special concern for African American families and communities*. Rockville, MD: Author.

Primm, B. (1988). The alcohol/opiod abuser: A brief review of history and treatment. *Bulletin of the New York State Chapter of the National Black Alcoholism Council*.

Shaef, A. W., & Fassel, D. (1988). *The addictive organization*. New York: Harper & Row.

Talbott, G. D. (1986). Alcoholism and other drug addictions: A primary disease entity. *Journal of the Medical Association of Georgia, 75*, 490–494.

U.S. Department of Health and Human Services. (1985). *Report of the Secretary's Tash Force on Black and Minority Health*. Washington, DC: U.S. Government Printing Office.

Womble, M., & Brisbane, F. (1985). *Treatment of black alcoholics*. New York: Hawthorn Press.

8

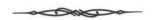

Heart Disease, Stroke, and Hypertension in Blacks

Carolyn J. Hildreth
Elijah Saunders

Blacks experience excess mortality compared with whites from hypertension and from related conditions including heart (cardiovascular) disease and stroke (cerebrovascular) disease. While this chapter focuses primarily on hypertension, it is important to acknowledge the interrelatedness of these three disease entities. Certain adverse effects of hypertension on cardiovascular and cerebrovascular disease are clearly established. For example, the principal cause of stroke in blacks is hypertension. It is the third leading cause of death in blacks and in the United States, generally. It is estimated that the rate of mortality from strokes among blacks is approximately 66 percent higher than among whites (Hypertension Detection and Follow-up Program Cooperative Research Group, 1982). Little doubt exists that stroke is potentially preventable by controlling blood pressure. However, poor control rates continue to be a major factor in the high prevalence of stroke in the black community despite a steady decline among black females.

Although historical gains in the treatment of hypertension occurred largely from the reduction of mortality and morbidity from stroke (Veterans Administration Cooperative Study Group on Antihypertensive Agents, 1970), continued improvements in mortality and morbidity are typically in the cardiac effects of hypertension. Thus, an understanding of both the indirect and direct contribution of hypertension as an antecedent to the development and expression of atherosclerotic coronary heart disease is of primary importance. Mortality from heart failure is 50 percent higher in blacks than in whites. The 1987 age-adjusted death rate for heart disease is 27 percent higher in black men than white men, and 55 percent higher in black women than white women (Saunders, 1991). While the 1987 age-adjusted death rate represents a marked decrease since 1962 for the overall U.S. population, it remains excessively high.

There are an estimated sixty million people with hypertension living in the United States. Approximately 28 percent are black Americans (Saunders, 1985). This is disproportionately higher than their representation in the population as a whole. Hypertension in black Americans tends to appear at an earlier age than in white Americans and frequently is not treated either early or aggressively enough. Consequently, there is a higher prevalence of more severe hypertension among black patients. Hypertension in blacks is also more frequently accompanied by target organ damage. Furthermore, effective treatment of hypertension in this population is hampered by limited access to medical care, occasionally prohibitive cost of treatment, and lack of education about the disease, all of which affect compliance.

The treatment of hypertension, along with the morbidity from related diseases, is generally improving in this country. Unfortunately, this is not occurring for black people at the same rate as among white Americans. In addition to the factors just mentioned, others that are not entirely clear account for this phenomenon.

Incidence and Epidemiology

The first studies to demonstrate clear differences in blood pressure between blacks and whites in this country were reported by Adams (1932) in New Orleans. He documented that mean systolic and diastolic blood pressures were higher in blacks at all ages. Since that time, practically every study done in the United States in which prevalence and incidence were examined for blacks and whites showed clearly higher rates among blacks.

Most studies have found that hypertension differences in children of the two races were not significant until approximately age ten; however, the Bogalusa Heart Study found differences in children between the ages of five and fourteen (Voors, Foster, Frerichs, Webber & Berenson, 1976). Other studies conducted in communities in the United States do not show racial differences in blood pressure before the teenage or prepubertal years. A more recent survey of black and white children age six to ten years showed minor differences for same-age, same-gender groups, but such differences disappear after adjustment for weight or other indices of body size (Prineas, Gillum, Horibe, 1980). It appears that the statistically significant racial differences in blood pressure occur sometime after age seventeen.

The 1971–1974 Health and Nutrition Examination Survey (Roberts & Maurer, 1977) estimated that 17 percent of white Americans had mild to moderate high blood pressure (defined as systolic blood pressure > 160mmHg or diastolic > 95mmHg), whereas the estimate for black populations was 28.2 percent. Similarly, the Maryland Statewide Household Survey of 6,425 adults age eighteen and older showed a prevalence among blacks of 26.8 percent, compared with 20.1 percent for whites (Saunders, 1985) (see Table 8.1). In the Maryland surveys, when the patient population was broken down into age groups eighteen to forty-nine years and fifty years and over, blacks had higher prevalence rates for all categories (see Table 8.2). The rates of hypertension are extremely high in blacks over fifty and are higher in females than in males (see Table 8.3).

A 1973–1974 study indicated that the three-year incident rate of hypertension for blacks was approximately two to three times higher (Saunders, 1985) (see Table 8.4). The Hypertension Detection and Follow-up Program Cooperative Research Group (1977) found that not only was hypertension one and one-half to two times more common in blacks than in white

Table 8.1. Prevalence of Hypertension[a] in Maryland Adults, 1982.

Age, Race, and Gender	%
All blacks	26.8
All whites[b]	20.1
All males	23.2
All females	19.9
All 18–29 years	4.1
All 30–49 years	17.2
All 50+ years	41.7

[a] Diastolic BP ≥ 90, or < 90 on medication.
[b] Includes all nonblacks.

Table 8.2. Prevalence of Elevated Blood Presure in Maryland Adults by Age, Race, and Gender, 1982.

Age, Race, and Gender	DBP ≥ 90 (%)	BP > 150/90 (%)
18–49 black male	12.2	12.6
18–49 black female	9.6	10.0
18–49 white male	12.0	12.5
18–49 white female	3.7	3.8
≥ 50 black male	40.5	45.5
≥ 50 black female	19.1	26.7
≥ 50 white male	21.0	27.2
≥ 50 white female	10.9	19.7
Total	11.4	14.0

Table 8.3. Prevalence of Hypertension[a] in Maryland Adults, 1982.

Age, Race, and Gender	%
18–49 black males	16.0
≥ 50 black males	56.2
18–49 white males[b]	15.1
≥ 50 white males[b]	38.8
18–49 black females	16.9
≥ 50 black females	59.7
18–49 white females[b]	6.0
≥ 50 white females[b]	38.3
All groups	21.5

[a] Diastolic BP ≥ 90, or < 90 on medication.
[b] Includes all nonblacks.

Table 8.4. HDFP Three-Year Incidence of Hypertension.[a]

Race and Gender	Incidence (%)	Estimated Incidence After Two-Stage Screen
Black men	28.6	20.5
Black women	23.3	16.4
White men	8.2	6.2
White women	9.6	7.8

[a] Among persons not on antihypertensive medication in 1973–1974.

Americans between the ages of thirty and sixty-nine, but severe hypertension (diastolic BP > 115mmHg) was five times more common in black than white men and approximately seven times more common in black women than their white counterparts. Several major studies have shown that marked black-white differences in hypertension prevalence occur with increasing age, being extremely common in older blacks (Meyer, et al., 1981).

Genetic Research and Hypertension in Blacks

No validated research findings have yet determined any genetic differences between black and white hypertensives. However, familial aggregation of essential hypertension has been documented (Meyer et al., 1981; Woods, Beevers, & West, 1981). Gillum (1979) found that estimates of the heritability of blood pressure are statistically significant within black populations and are very similar to those in whites. Unquestionably, both black and white hypertensives frequently give histories of elevated blood pressure in blood relatives. It is rare to encounter a hypertensive person who does not know of family members with hypertension or with hypertension-related morbidity or mortality. Findings by Grim and colleagues (1980) suggest that genetics plays a major role in hypertension etiology in both blacks and whites. Their ongoing studies are with black monozygotic and dizygotic twins.

It remains controversial whether genetic markers such as skin color can be related to hypertension prevalence. A population-based study of blacks in Charleston, South Carolina, showed a significant association between blood pressure and skin darkness among black men and women (Boyle, 1970). The effect was independent of age but was minimized by consideration of socioeconomic status. Later, a different study from the same area showed that skin color, measured by photoelectric reflection meter on the medial aspect of the upper arm, was not significantly associated (independent of socioeconomic status) with the fifteen-year incidence of hypertension in a cohort of black women over the age of thirty-five (Keil, 1981). These studies, however, differ from a Detroit, Michigan, study of black men, which found a significant relationship between high blood pressure and skin color (measured by subjective coding of skin color of the forehead, between the eyes). Once again, other studies failed to confirm this, and, according to Tyroler and James (1978), socioeconomic and psychosocial factors may be responsible for what was thought to be a correlation between skin darkness and blood pressure elevation.

Hormonal and Physiological Factors in Hypertensive Blacks

Hormonal and physiological differences may be associated with the ethnic disparity in prevalence of hypertension. For example, Voors, Foster, Frerichs, Webber, & Berenson (1976) showed that in children between the ages of five and thirteen (63 percent white) the renin levels were higher in whites over all blood pressure strata compared to the renin levels in blacks. Table 8.5 shows plasma renin measurements in normotensive blacks and whites reported by several investigators. Many determinations were done on ad lib sodium intake. In each of these studies, the renin levels were lower in blacks with and without renin stimulation.

Table 8.5. Plasma Renin Measurements in Normotensive Black and White Americans.

		Ad Lib Sodium Intake		Renin Stimulation	
		White	Black	White	Black
Adults					
Helmer		1.32 ± 0.24 [a] (8)	0.84 ± 0.1 (6)		
Kaplan	Males	2.0 ± 1.4 [a] (29)	1.4 ± 0.8 (27)	4.6 ± 2.6 [a] (29)	3.2 ± 2.2 (27)
	Females	1.5 ± 1.0 [a] (47)	1.2 ± 1.0 (24)	3.2 ± 2.2 [a] (47)	2.2 ± 1.5 (24)
Grim	Males	2.82 ± 0.23 (105)	2.49 ± 0.20 (36)		
	Females	2.47 ± 0.15 [a] (121)	2.03 ± 0.14 (53)		
Luft		7.2 ± 0.43 [a] (94)	5.7 ± 0.5 (94)	29.4 ± 1.9 [a] (94)	19.7 ± 2.4 (94)
Luft	Males	5.2 ± 0.8 (19)	4.4 ± 0.9 (19)	27.7 ± 4.0 [a] (19)	14.3 ± 2.0 (19)
	Females	5.6 ± 0.9 (15)	4.4 ± 0.9 (15)	18.0 ± 4.0 (15)	21.6 ± 5.0 (15)
Children					
Berenson		7.1 ± 2.5 [a] (128)	5.3 ± 3.7 (130)		
Hohn	FH + [b]	4.8 ± 2.8 [a] (33)	2.4 ± 1.7 (36)	12.7 ± 5.5 [a] (32)	7.8 ± 5.1 (34)
	FH − [c]	4.6 ± 3.5 [a] (41)	2.0 ± 1.5 (18)	13.0 ± 7.9 [a] (42)	5.1 ± 3.1 (19)

[a] $P < 0.05$ between groups. Numbers in parentheses indicate subjects studied.
[b] Family history positive.
[c] Family history negative.

The findings of suppressed renin in many black hypertensives could be due to alterations of the blood supply to the juxtaglomerular apparatus. This could lead to a disruption in the normal homeostatic response to renin release, to changes in plasma volume, and to renal blood flow. This occurs in diabetic nephropathy, in which early onset of afferent and efferent arteriolar sclerosis results in low renin states. A second mechanism for the low renin status in blacks could be primary volume expansion due to other intrarenal factors that promote sodium and water retention or prohibit sodium excretion.

Other hormonal and physiological aberrations found in black hypertensives may have some genetic basis. For example:

1. Many blacks show lower values for some indices of sympathetic nervous function such as lower levels of dopamine beta hydroxylase (DPH). This seems to correlate with the diminished role of the sympathetic nervous system in the pathogenesis of hypertension in blacks (Voors, 1979; Voors, Foster, Frerichs, Weber, & Berenson, 1976). Studies by psychologists at Duke University (Anderson, 1989) suggest that blacks may be more reactive to alpha adrenergic stimulation, which results in vasoconstriction and therefore in a rise in blood pressure. Although these responses were elicited in the laboratory by cold pressor testing, the investigators suggested that such reactivity might be comparable to that seen in response to chronically stressful life-styles and life circumstances.

2. Deficiency in the natriuretic vasodilatory renal kallikrein-kinin system has been postulated by Warren and O'Connor (1980) to form the basis for the pathophysiological profiles in many black hypertensives.

3. The kidneys of hypertensive blacks excrete significantly less sodium and potassium when the patient is challenged with a sodium load (Lilley, Hsu, & Stone, 1976).

4. The frequency of hypertension in blacks may correlate with the increased sodium-potassium ratio found in the urine of many black hypertensives. This could be related to low dietary intake of potassium in blacks, which itself may be due either to economic factors or to food preferences that exclude potassium-rich foods.

5. Cellular transport mechanisms recently have received considerable attention as potential mechanisms for development of hypertension. Sodium-potassium cotransport and sodium-lithium counter transport have been found to be abnormal in black persons with essential hypertension (Canessa, Adragna & Solomon, 1980). Numerous other transport systems are currently under investigation. These include circulation material that may decrease the activity of sodium-potassium ATPase and thereby account for the volume-expanded form of hypertension frequently found in blacks, particularly the elderly. Conceivably, this might lead to a diminished capacity to extrude sodium from smooth muscle cells, thereby promoting an increase in intracellular calcium, which in turn increases vasoactivity (Blaustein & Hamlyn, 1983). In this study, these authors explore the role that calcium and

magnesium may play in hypertensive blacks. They suggest that the presence of a circulation hormone (natriuretic hormone) may facilitate the increased calcium in vascular smooth muscle cells, increasing tone and therefore propensity to development of hypertension.

6. Recent data linking insulin resistance to hypertension prevalence may have special applicability to the black population, in which type II diabetes mellitus and obesity (especially in black women) represent special problems.

Environmental Theory

The environmental theory suggests that an interaction of the environment with genetics is necessary for the development of hypertension. Proponents of the environmental theory contend that blacks are more frequently exposed to conditions of poverty, low education, low occupational status, and high stress. They propose that these environmental factors can cause stress-inducing transient blood pressure elevation, and they postulate that this stress when repeated frequently can lead to permanently elevated blood pressure. Studies conducted in Detroit involving blacks and whites in high-stress areas (characterized by high rates of poverty, crime, density of housing, residential mobility, and marital breakup) and low-stress areas (characterized by low rates of the same stress indicators) revealed blood pressure to be highest among black men from high-stress areas (Harburg, Erfurt, & Hauenstein, 1973). Suppressed hostility, measured by structured interviews, was related to high blood pressure levels of black men in these high-stress areas.

Barriers to Control of Hypertension in Blacks

There has been a decline in stroke and other cardiovascular morbid and mortal events since the 1940s. Since 1968, there has been a steeper decline attributed to improved hypertension awareness, treatment, and control (Ouellet, Apostolides, Entwisle, & Hebel, 1979; Tyroler, Heyden, & Hames, 1975). However, despite this encouraging trend from the population in general, surveys from the 1970s and the most recent survey from the Maryland Hypertension Program indicate that hypertension control among blacks remains unacceptably poor, particularly in view of the high prevalence. Of particular concern are black men, who have the highest prevalence of any group and the poorest control rate (see Tables 8.1 to 8.4).

According to Gillum and Gillum (1984), high rates of noncompliance with follow-up and drug therapy seriously compromise the efforts of communitywide programs. These researchers indicate that noncompliance with treatment and preventive health counseling is now the major barrier, nationally, to effective hypertensive control. Impediments to ideal hypertension control and compliance in the black community can further be divided into three categories: (1) severity of hypertension in blacks (2) barriers related to the medical care system, including inadequate financial resources, inconveniently located health care facilities, long waiting times, and inaccessibility to health education, specifically as it relates to hypertension in black people, and (3) barriers related to the social, psychosocial, and sociopolitical environment, which include problems of unemployment, underemployment, and strained racial relationships. In spite of generally improved hypertension control in the United States, the group that has the worse problems (blacks, especially males) is not benefiting as much as the general population.

Treatment Considerations

In any treatment initiation for hypertension in black patients, considerations must be made for the social, psychosocial, political, and environmental factors previously discussed. The medical cause of the patient's hypertension will most likely be classified as "essential" hypertension (meaning the cause is unknown). However, for compliant patients who present with hypertension that is refractory to aggressive, treatment must be considered for possible secondary hypertension—secondary to renal, renal vascular, or adrenal hormonal disease. Appropriate laboratory and radiographic studies must be carried out to evaluate each of these possibilities if the circumstances suggest them. One should expect this to be a rare occurrence; however, consideration of secondary hypertension in blacks should not be excluded.

For the average patient with essential hypertension, full control can be achieved with a well-adhered-to treatment plan. This plan should begin with a consideration of factors that likely contribute to the individual patient's hypertension or that can exacerbate otherwise well-controlled hypertension. These include diet and other life-style and personal habits such as activity level, smoking, and alcohol intake. The sedentary person—whether young or old, slim or obese, or with degenerative joint disease and diabetes mellitus— must be encouraged to initiate a program of mild to moderate exercise for improved cardiovascular fitness. Patients should be encouraged to begin simply by walking more. Taking a short walk to start, then walking at a moderate (three to four miles an hour) pace for thirty minutes, three to four times a week, can be a tremendous help in developing cardiovascular fitness. All patients, but particularly those with diabetes mellitus or peripheral vascular disease, should be encouraged and assisted in obtaining properly fitted, comfortable shoes. Referral to a podiatrist should be made if necessary. Patients who additionally have osteoarthritis of the knees or hips must be reassured that this type of exercise will be dually beneficial in maintaining strength and flexibility in their lower extremities as well as in building the cardiovascular fitness that they need. Patients should be encouraged to seek out partners and to use their neighborhood parks or shopping mall. Such facilities often have structured programs for people who wish to walk, and if indoors, are convenient in inclement weather. Throughout the year, various fruits and vegetables that are seasonal should be suggested to substitute for other high-calorie choices.

Cigarette smoking is extremely prevalent among persons of lower socioeconomic and educational status. Many blacks are affected. Cigarette smoking adds to cardiovascular morbidity and can affect the treatment of hypertension (Materson, Reda, Freis, & Henderson, 1988). While there has been a nationwide decline in smoking in the United States, this decline has been less for both black men and women. Young black women in particular have a high rate of continued cigarette smoking (Fielding, 1987; Willet, Green, & Stamfer, 1987). The overall impact this has on the black community is manifest in the increased rates of cancer and cardiovascular disease morbidity and mortality for blacks and the documented lower life expectancy for both black men and women compared to their nonblack counterparts in the United States. The National Center for Health Statistics (1989) reported that in 1985 the life expectancy for blacks was 5.8 years less than for whites. In 1986 the age-adjusted death rates from all causes were 51 percent greater in black men than in white men, and 52 percent greater in black women than in white women. The 1987 age-adjusted death rates from heart disease were 27 percent greater in black men than in white men, and a remarkable 55 percent greater in black women than in white women. Hypertensive heart disease undoubtedly accounted for a significant percentage of these deaths.

Frequent excessive alcohol intake also contributes to elevated blood pressure, and patients need to be counseled on exactly what amount is too much. While there is a great deal of controversy over the cardiac benefits of some daily alcohol ingestion (Jackson, Scragg, & Beaglehole, 1991; Rimm et al., 1991), there has been no disputing the adverse effect on systolic and diastolic blood pressure of ethanol intake greater than 30 ml per day (Mac-Mahon & Norton, 1986; Joint National Committee, 1988). This is equivalent to one ounce of 100 proof whiskey, eight ounces of wine, or two 12-ounce cans of beer. Patients with hypertension should be discouraged from drinking alcohol in amounts exceeding these intakes.

Patients' dietary habits should be addressed as personally as their activity level and other personal behavior. Patients may benefit from referral to a registered dietician who is sensitive to both personal and cultural differences in food preferences. They need specific guidelines to allow them to make appropriate choices for achieving the best compromise on what they should eat and what they may be more accustomed to eating. Patients also need to be made aware of the appropriate quantities from each food group that contribute to a nutritionally balanced diet with adequate caloric intake. Often, overall changes will need to be drastic, but made gradually, these should be incorporated into an entire package of life-style changes that a patient with commitment can make.

Eventually, and in some patients concurrently with nonmedical modalities, drug therapy may be necessary. Several factors should be remembered in considering when and whether to initiate drug therapy and in deciding which to choose. Many blacks have limited access to the health care system. Often the first elevated blood pressure recorded may be indicative of need for evaluation of cardiovascular and renal disease that has existed for some time. Laboratory analysis of renal function will be necessary along with an electrocardiogram to begin to assess the effect the hypertension has had on the heart. Echocardiographic evaluation for left ventricular hypertrophy (LVH) and left ventricular function is prudent in evaluating blacks with hypertension (Dunn et al., 1983). This is particularly true with those with known cardiovascular risk factors and a family history of hypertension involving family members who themselves have not had regular medical follow-up care previous to documentation of an elevated blood pressure.

Hypertensive patients with LVH documented by echocardiograph should seriously be considered for medical treatment if they have other cardiovascular risk factors, even if they have mild hypertension (diastolic BP 90–104mmHg). In the recently reported Systolic Hypertension in the Elderly Program (SHEP) study of the effectiveness of treating isolated systolic hypertension (systolic BP greater than or equal to 160mmHg), both cardiovascular and cerebrovascular morbidity were reduced with treatment of the hypertension. The Hypertension Detection and Follow-up Program (HDFP) (1984) had previously documented a reduction in cerebrovascular morbidity and mortality from treating even mild hypertension. The lesser reduction in cardiovascular morbidity in many of the earlier studies is felt to be possibly related to the frequent use of non-potassium-sparing diuretics as first-line and often as the only treatment. There is evidence that particularly in patients with LVH, the propensity for the development of life-threatening arrhythmias is enhanced by loss of potassium and possibly magnesium while using these diuretics (Hollifield, 1986).

Drugs should be chosen that have been documented to have a beneficial effect on LVH, particularly calcium channel blockers, beta blockers, and angiotensin converting enzyme (ACE) inhibitors. The latter two may need the addition of a diuretic in some patients. It is known that blacks may respond less well to beta blockers and ACE inhibitors used without diuretics than to calcium channel blockers used alone (Cubbeddu, Aranda, & Singh, 1986; Freis, Materson, & Flamenbaum, 1983). When used appropriately, each of these drug classes can be quite effective.

Consideration must be made for other medical problems, particularly diabetes mellitus, peripheral vascular disease, hypercholesterolemia, and arthritis, as well as for advanced age (Flamenbaum, 1987). Care must be taken to avoid untoward interactions with drugs being prescribed concurrently for these and other maladies. The guidelines set forth by the Joint National Committee (1988) can be helpful when initiating drug therapy in patients

with mild to moderate hypertension with or without other medical problems, keeping in mind the patients' other individual characteristics.

A major concern for many patients is their financial inability to
acquire prescription medication that may be required for the rest of their
lives. This limits access to care and unfortunately will also limit the choice of
medications for many physicians prescribing for these patients. Despite this,
each physician must decide whether the long-term benefits any drug choice
will have for the patient (reduction in morbidity, mortality, hospital admissions, and thus long-term expenses) outweigh the immediate financial burden. All mechanisms for assisting patients in their efforts to acquire appropriate medications must be supported by medical providers. This also
reinforces the need for complete and continued compliance with nonmedicinal modalities.

As previously established, black patients have severe hypertension
more frequently than whites do. These patients need aggressive drug therapy
and often will be first encountered in a crisis situation with a hypertension
urgency or emergency. They must be treated appropriately in a hospital
setting. In many cases, these patients do not have primary care providers and
have accessed the health care system for crisis intervention only. Adequate
counseling must be done during the hospitalization to convince the patient
of the absolute need for long-term outpatient follow-up care and to make
clear the inevitable consequences of failure to seek out and receive this care.
Access to this care must be available in a timely manner.

Promoting Compliance

The issue of compliance is complex. It involves understanding by the health
care provider of all factors that could limit the patients' willingness or ability
to comply with the care plan as it becomes established. In one model, the
patients' likelihood of being compliant has been analyzed based on their
readiness to undertake recommended behavior changes and the modifying
and enabling factors that contribute to or deter them from this behavior
(Becker, 1976). This model lists factors that lead to patients' compliance,
including personal motivation and perception of the value of treatment and
the likelihood that treatment will reduce threat of further illness. The acknowledgment of these factors by providers and the impact of their own
attitude toward the patient should help to support efforts toward increasing
compliance.

Efforts to increase compliance must be ongoing. An open discussion
must be held with each patient at the beginning of therapy about the need for
long-term treatment and the benefit of well-controlled (normal) blood pressure in preventing cardiovascular problems. Most patients have some idea of
the consequences of hypertension. It is helpful to clarify their understanding
of how sustained or poorly controlled hypertension can affect the "target

organs." Specifically, patients need to know that treatment is aimed at preventing morbid sequelae in the heart, brain, and kidneys. Furthermore,
patients need to have reassurances that their continued nonmedicinal efforts
toward blood pressure control will continue to be important. These efforts
need to be acknowledged and reinforced at all visits, even after medication
has been initiated.

Patients need to be given the fullest understanding possible of all
drugs being used to treat their blood pressure. It is important that they
understand exactly how to take each medication and what side effects to
expect. Many patients will inquire into this aspect of their care, and it is
important to acknowledge their concerns and attempt to eliminate ap-
prehension about side effects. Patients need to be allowed to ask questions
about all aspects of their care and the complete therapeutic program that
they have been advised to follow. Receiving thoughtful and honest answers to
these inquiries helps to further promote compliance with the total health
care plan.

Community Projects to Increase Education and Compliance

Because of the general societal awareness of the high prevalence of and risks
from undetected and untreated hypertension, there has been excellent cooperation and collaboration between black community groups (churches, bar-
ber shops, and so on) and community health providers and organizations.
This has led to greater access of community members to health education
provided in a familiar and comforting setting. For example, Saunders (1985)
was instrumental in piloting the concept of this type of collaboration into a
structured format within churches in Baltimore, Maryland. Church-based
blood pressure control centers were established. Members of the community
were trained to take blood pressure and give basic layperson's advice on
appropriate follow-up needs. These "church nurses" received an eight-hour
standardized training program directed by the local heart association or
state health department.

The impact and the availability of this type of voluntary community-
based screening program has yet to be critically evaluated. It can be specu-
lated, however, that this type of community involvement can be instrumental
in patient education and ultimately in patient compliance. It is important
that the medical community continue to initiate and support these types of
community programs.

Conclusion

Hypertension, stroke, and heart disease in blacks are community health
issues that medical providers must address from the social, environmental,
and medical perspective. Blacks must first be empowered to manage those

factors in their lives that they can control and that contribute to cardiovascular morbidity and mortality. Their confidence must be developed in health care providers and the medical system such that they appropriately seek advice and medical attention when needed. This advice must be directed to each person individually; his or her uniqueness should be recognized. Medical providers must be committed to taking the extra time that this will require to establish good and lasting provider-patient relationships. The long-term benefit to the overall health of the community and the gratitude received from individual patients will be well worth the time and effort.

All medical providers treating black patients with hypertension and related diseases must be cognizant of the issues discussed in this chapter. The tendency to use a particular protocol approach to this disease entity complicates the problem, because the "disease" is only one aspect of the overall problem. The social and environmental components of this health problem are equally important and must be addressed and treated by the health delivery system with care and sensitivity.

References

Adams, J. M. (1932). Some racial differences in blood pressures and morbidity in groups of white and colored workmen. *American Journal of Medical Science, 184,* 342–350.

Anderson, N. B. (1989). Racial differences in stress induced cardiovascular reactivity and hypertension: Current status and substantive issues. *Psychological Bulletin, 105,* 89–105.

Becker, M. (1976). Sociobehavioral determinants of compliance. In D. Sackett and R. Haynes (Eds.), *Compliance with therapeutic regimens* (pp. 40–50). Baltimore: Johns Hopkins University Press.

Blaustein, M. P., & Hamlyn, J. M. (1983). Role of a natriuretic factor in essential hypertension: An hypothesis. *Annals of Internal Medicine, 98* (Suppl.), 785–792.

Boyle, E., Jr. (1970). Biological patterns in hypertension by race, sex, body height, and skin color. *Journal of the American Medical Association, 213,* 1637–1643.

Canessa, M., Adragna, N., & Solomon, H. S. (1980). Increased sodium-lithium countertransport in red cells of patients with essential hypertension. *New England Journal of Medicine, 302,* 772–776.

Cubbeddu, L. X., Aranda, J., & Singh, B. (1986). A comparison of verapamil and propranolol for the initial treatment of hypertension: Racial differences in response. *Journal of the American Medical Association, 256,* 2214–2221.

Dunn, F. G., Oigman, W., Sungaard-Riise, K., Masserli, F., Ventura, H., Reisin, E., & Frohlich, E. D. (1983). Racial differences in cardiac adaptation to essential hypertension determined by echographic indexes. *Journal of the American College of Cardiology, 5,* 1348–1351.

Fielding, J. E. (1987). Smoking and women: Tragedy of the majority [Editorial]. *New England Journal of Medicine, 317*(21), 1343.

Flamenbaum, W. (1987). Management of unique hypertensive situations: A focus on difficult, problematic, elderly black patients. *Journal of the National Medical Association, 79* (Suppl.), 31.

Freis, E. D., Materson, B. J., & Flamenbaum, W. (1983). Comparison of propranolol or hydrochlorothiazide alone for treatment of hypertension: III. Evaluation of the renin-angiotensin system. *American Journal of Medicine, 74,* 1029–1041.

Gillum, R. F. (1979). Pathophysiology of hypertension in blacks and whites: A review of the basis of racial blood pressure differences. *Hypertension, 1,* 468–475.

Gillum, R. F., & Gillum, B. S. (1984). Potential for control and prevention of essential hypertension in the black community. In J. D. Matarazzo & N. Miller (Eds.), *Behavioral health: A handbook of health enhancement and disease prevention,* 825–835. New York: Wiley.

Grim, C. E., Luft, F. C., Miller, J. Z., Meneely, G. R., Battarbee, H. D., Hames, C. G., & Dahl, L. K. (1980). Racial differences in blood pressure in Evans County, Georgia: Relationship to sodium and potassium intake and plasma renin activity. *Journal of Chronic Disease, 33,* 87–94.

Harburg, E., Erfurt, J. C., & Hauenstein, L. S. (1973). Socioecological stress, suppressed hostility, skin color, and black-white male blood pressure in Detroit. *Psychosomatic Medicine, 35,* 276–296.

Hollifield, J. W. (1986). Thiazide treatment of hypertension: Effect of thiazide diuretics on serum potassium, magnesium, and ventricular ectopy. *American Journal of Medicine, 80* (Suppl. 4A), 8–12.

Hypertension Detection and Follow-Up Program Cooperative Research Group. (1977). Race, education, and prevalence of hypertension. *American Journal of Epidemiology, 106,* 351–361.

Hypertension Detection and Follow-Up Program Cooperative Research Group. (1982). Reduction in stroke incidence among persons with high blood pressure: Five-year findings of the Hypertension Detection and Follow-Up Program III. *Journal of the American Medical Association, 247*(5), 633–638.

Hypertension Detection and Follow-Up Program Cooperative Research Group. (1984). The effect of antihypertensive drug treatment on mortality in the presence of resting electrocardiographic abnormalities at baseline: The HDFP experience. *Circulation, 70*(6), 996–1003.

Jackson, R., Scragg, R., & Beaglehole, R. (1991). Alcohol consumption and risks of coronary heart disease. *British Medical Journal, 303,* 211–216.

Joint National Committee. (1988). The 1988 report of the Joint National Committee on Detection, Evaluation, and Treatment of High Blood Pressure. *Archives of Internal Medicine, 148,* 1023–1038.

Keil, J. E. (1981). Skin color and education effects on blood pressure. *American Journal of Public Health, 71,* 532–534.

Lilley, J. L., Hsu, L., & Stone, R. A. (1976). Racial disparity of plasma volume in hypertensive man [Letter to the editor]. *Annals of Internal Medicine, 84,* 707–708.

MacMahon, S. W., & Norton, R. N. (1986). Alcohol and hypertension: Implications for prevention and treatment. *Annals of Internal Medicine, 105,* 124–125.

Materson, B., Reda, D., Freis, E. D., & Henderson, W. G. (1988). Cigarette smoking interferes with treatment of hypertension. *Archives of Internal Medicine, 148*(10), 2116–2119.

Meyer, P., Garay, R. P., Nazaret, C., Dagher, G., Bellet, M., Broyer, M., & Feingold, J. (1981). Inheritance of abnormal erythrocyte cation transport in essential hypertension. *British Medical Journal, 282,* 1114–1117.

National Center for Health Statistics. (1989). *Health, United States, 1988* (DHHS Publication No. PHS 89-1232). Hyattsville, MD: Public Health Service.

Ouellet, R. P., Apostolides, A. Y., Entwisle, G., & Hebel, J. R. (1979). Estimated community impact of hypertension control in a high-risk population. *American Journal of Epidemiology, 109,* 531–538.

Prineas, R. J., Gillum, R. F., & Horibe, H. (1980). The Minneapolis Children's Blood Pressure Study: Standards of measurement for children's blood pressure. *Hypertension, 2* (Suppl. 1), 18–24.

Rimm, E. B., Giovannuci, E. L., Willett, W., Colditz, G., Ascherio, A., Rosner, B., & Stampfer, M. J. (1991). Prospective study of alcohol consumption and risk of coronary disease in men. *Lancet, 338,* 464–468.

Roberts, J., & Maurer, K. (1977). Blood pressure levels of persons 6–74 years, United States, 1971–1974 (DHEW Publication No. HRA 78-1648). *Vital and Health Statistics* (Series 11, No. 203). Washington, DC: National Center for Health Statistics.

Saunders, E. (1985). Special techniques for management of hypertension in blacks. In W. D. Hall, E. Saunders, & N. B. Shulman (Eds.), *Hypertension in blacks: Epidemiology, pathophysiology, and treatment* (pp. 209–236). Chicago: Year Book.

Saunders, E. (1991). *Cardiovascular disease in blacks.* Philadelphia, PA: F. A. Davis.

State of Maryland Demonstration of Statewide Coordination for the Control of High Blood Pressure (NHLBI Contract No. 1-HV-2986). (October 1977–September 1983).

Systolic Hypertension in the Elderly Program Cooperative Research Group. (1991). Prevention of stroke by antihypertensive drug treatment in older persons with isolated hypertension: Final results of the systolic hypertension in the elderly program (SHEP). *Journal of the American Medical Association, 265*(24), 3255–3264.

Tyroler, H. A., Heyden, S., & Hames, C. G. (1975). Weight and hypertension: Evans County studies of blacks and whites. In O. Paul (Ed.), *Epi-*

demiology and control of hypertension (pp. 177–204). New York: Stratton Intercontinental.

Tyroler, H. A., & James, S. A. (1978). Blood pressure and skin color. *American Journal of Public Health, 68,* 1170–1172.

Veterans Administration Cooperative Study Group on Antihypertensive Agents. (1970). Effects of treatment of morbidity in hypertension: II. Results in patients with diastolic blood pressures averaging 90 through 114 mm Hg. *Journal of the American Medical Association, 213*(7), 1143–1152.

Voors, A. W. (1979). Racial differences in blood pressure control. *Science, 204,* 1093.

Voors, A. W., Foster, T. A., Frerichs, R. R., Webber, L. S., & Berenson, G. S. (1976). Studies of blood pressure in children, ages 5–14 years, in a total biracial community: The Bogalusa Heart Study. *Circulation, 54,* 319–327.

Warren, S. E., & O'Connor, D. J. (1980). Does a renal vasodilator system mediate racial differences in essential hypertension? *American Journal of Medicine, 69,* 425–429.

Willet, W. C., Green, A., & Stamfer, M. J. (1987). Relative and absolute risk of coronary heart disease among women who smoke cigarettes. *New England Journal of Medicine, 317*(21), 1303–1309.

Woods, K. L., Beevers, D. G., & West, M. (1981). Familial abnormalities of erythrocyte cation transport in essential hypertension. *British Medical Journal, 282,* 1186–1188.

9

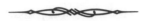

Cancer and
Black Americans

Claudia R. Baquet
Tyson Gibbs

Cancer is the second leading cause of death in the United States and is a significant burden to many Americans in terms of morbidity, years of life lost, and economic and emotional costs. This burden is borne disproportionately by black Americans, who have the highest overall age-adjusted cancer incidence and mortality rates of any population group in the United States. For many cancers, mortality rates among blacks are increasing in contrast to decreasing rates among whites. Trends in cancer incidence, mortality, and survival point to increasing disparities between blacks and whites (Baquet, Horm, Gibbs, & Greenwald, 1991).

Research indicates that the potential for reducing cancer incidence and mortality through targeted prevention and intervention is high. The Department of Health and Human Services (DHHS) has established an overall objective of reducing cancer mortality by achieving a rate of no more than 130 deaths per 100,000 persons by the year 2000 (the age-adjusted baseline is 133 deaths per 100,000 persons in 1987) (U.S. Department of Health and Human Services, 1991). DHHS has delineated sixteen cancer-related objectives for the year 2000 that address health status, risk reduction, services, and protection. Achieving these goals depends in large measure on the development and implementation of prevention messages and culturally appropriate intervention strategies directed at specific populations. These are the populations at elevated risk because of various risk factors and exposures and underserved by quality cancer prevention, early detection, treatment, and rehabilitation services. Blacks are both at high risk for cancer and are underserved.

Methods, Data Sources, and Data Deficiencies

Surveillance and assessment of the impact of cancer on the general population and on subsets of the population require measurement of incidence rates (the number of new cases per year per 100,000 persons) and mortality rates (the number of deaths per 100,000 persons) and a determination of the proportion of persons alive at some point (usually five years) following a diagnosis of cancer (observed survival rate). The relative survival rate, calculated by adjusting the observed survival rate for the normal life expectancy of the general population of the same age, is an estimate of the chance of surviving the effects of cancer.

The National Cancer Act of 1971 mandated the collection, analysis, and distribution of data useful in the prevention, diagnosis, and treatment of cancer. Consequently, the National Cancer Institute (NCI) established the Surveillance, Epidemiology, and End Results (SEER) Program to collect data on cancer incidence and survival in the United States. Through the SEER program, NCI collects data from nine population-based tumor registries on all newly diagnosed patients with cancer and follow-up information on persons previously diagnosed. Some SEER registries provide data on selected racial and ethnic groups. The geographic areas that make up the SEER program's database represent approximately 9.6 percent of the U.S. population and cover approximately 8.3 percent of U.S. blacks. Cancer incidence, mortality, and survival rates and trends are derived from this database, which is the primary source of cancer incidence and relative survival data in this chapter.

National mortality data are obtained annually from the National Center for Health Statistics (NCHS). Information on each death occurring in the United States includes cause of death, age at death, gender, and geographic area of residence. SEER also presents mortality data for the SEER areas. The Bureau of the Census provides population data by racial/ethnic group, age, and gender. Data related to socioeconomic status (for example, income, education, and population density) are also available from the Bureau of the Census. Population counts supply the denominators for cancer rate calculation.

Each year since 1957, NCHS has conducted the National Health Interview Survey (NHIS). The data collected are a principal source of information on the health, illness, and disability status of the noninstitutionalized population. Interviews are conducted in approximately 50,000 representative households. In 1987, the Cancer Control Supplement of the NHIS collected information on cancer risk factors, knowledge, and use of cancer screening services. Some data from the Cancer Control Supplement are provided later in this chapter.

Despite a wealth of available data, deficiencies in the quality of certain cancer data do exist. These problems include inaccurate coding of race/ethnicity, errors in validity of cause-of-death data, differences in methods of data collection and reporting (which limits the comparability of data), and population undercounts. In addition, the heterogeneity of the black population mandates specific studies of different segments of the population (urban/rural; northern, western) to truly understand the cancer control needs of the black community in varying geographic and socioeconomic settings. One's ability to understand the health status of any population and to plan effective intervention programs will be enhanced by improvement in surveillance and data systems.

Cancer Statistics

Blacks have significantly higher age-adjusted cancer incidence rates than whites for all cancer sites combined—approximately 6 to 10 percent higher, depending on the time period and geographic area (Baquet, Horm, Gibbs, & Greenwald, 1991; Ries, Hankey, & Edwards, 1990). The specific cancers for which blacks have higher incidence than whites include oral cavity, esophagus, lung (males), breast (females under age forty), cervix uteri, prostate, stomach, and pancreas (Table 9.1). Trends in age-adjusted cancer incidence from 1976–78 to 1985–87 indicate that blacks experienced higher increases in incidence than whites for most sites and lower decreases in incidence for those sites where decreases occurred (National Cancer Institute, 1989). The one exception to this trend is cancer of the cervix, for which black women experienced a greater decrease in incidence than white women, although the incidence rate remained more than twice as high in blacks as in whites.

The disparity between blacks and whites is most striking for cancer mortality (Table 9.2). Blacks have mortality rates 20 to 40 percent higher than the general population (National Cancer Institute, 1989). Further, for sites where mortality rates for whites are decreasing—for example, colon and rectum, pancreas, and stomach—the rates for blacks are either increasing (colon and rectum and pancreas) or not decreasing as fast (stomach) as they

Table 9.1. Black/White Ratios[a] in Cancer Incidence, Four SEER Areas,[b]
1975–76 to 1987–88.

Site	1975–76	1979–80	1987–88	Trend
Oral cavity	1.1	1.4	1.3	Increasing
Esophagus	2.7	3.2	2.8	No change
Colon and rectum	0.9	1.0	1.0	No change
Lung	1.2	1.3	1.2	No change
Male	1.3	1.4	1.4	No change
Female	0.9	1.0	0.9	No change
Breast (female)	0.8	0.8	0.8	No change
Cervix uteri	2.5	2.5	2.2	Decreasing
Prostate	1.7	1.7	1.5	Decreasing

[a] Ratio is black cancer incidence rate divided by white cancer incidence rate. A black/white ratio greater than 1.0 indicates that blacks have an excessively high incidence of cancer compared with whites.

[b] The four areas are the metropolitan areas of San Francisco–Oakland, Detroit, Atlanta, and the state of Connecticut.

Source: National Cancer Institute.

Table 9.2. Black/White Ratios[a] in Cancer Mortality, United States, 1969–70 to 1987–88.

Site	1969–70	1979–80	1987–88	Trend
Oral cavity	1.2	1.8	1.8	Increasing
Esophagus	2.9	3.5	2.9	No change
Colon and rectum	0.9	1.0	1.2	Increasing
Lung	1.1	1.2	1.2	Increasing
Male	1.2	1.3	1.3	Increasing
Female	1.0	1.0	0.9	Decreasing
Breast (female)	0.9	1.0	1.1	Increasing
Cervix uteri	2.7	2.8	2.6	Decreasing
Prostate	1.9	2.1	2.1	Increasing

[a] Ratio is black cancer mortality rate divided by white cancer mortality rate. A black/white ratio greater than 1.0 indicates that blacks have an excessively high cancer mortality rate compared with whites.

Source: U.S. Mortality (NCHS; Bureau of Census).

are in whites. Blacks experience excess mortality for esophageal cancer, cancers of the cervix, breast, and uterus, multiple myeloma, and prostate cancer (Ries, Hankey, & Edwards, 1990).

Blacks also experience poorer five-year relative survival for all sites combined. For the period 1981 to 1986, five-year relative survival rates are 38.2 percent for blacks (both genders) and 52.0 percent for whites, or about 30 percent lower for blacks (Ries et al., 1990). Poorer survival for blacks is particularly marked for cancers of the rectum, larynx, breast (females), corpus uteri, prostate, and bladder. Improvements in survival that have occurred over the past thirty years have not been shared equally by blacks (Table 9.3). If survival rates are analyzed by proxy measures of socio-economic status (that is, income), within various income strata blacks have poorer survival than whites. Blacks are also slightly less likely than non-minorities to receive cancer treatment. The reasons for these differences have not been delineated.

Contributing Factors

Factors that contribute to the cancer experience of black Americans are numerous, complex, and often not well understood. Major categories of contributing factors include (1) exposures to tobacco and ethanol, occupation, and diet/nutrition, (2) knowledge, attitudes, and practices, and (3) health and medical resources and other variables, including biological factors and socioeconomic status. These factors have been identified through analytical epidemiological studies (mainly case-control), cross-sectional surveys, and health services research. A discussion of these factors follows.

Tobacco use, particularly in the form of cigarette smoking, is the best-documented cause of early cancer morbidity and mortality. Tobacco use contributes to over 35 percent of all cancer deaths (Shopland, Eyre, &

Table 9.3. Black/White Ratios[a] in Cancer Five-Year Relative Survival, SEER, 1974–76 to 1981–86.

Site	1974–76	1977–80	1981–86	Trend
Oral cavity	0.6	0.6	0.6	No change
Esophagus	0.8	0.6	0.7	No change
Colon and rectum	0.9	0.9	0.8	Decreasing
Lung	0.9	0.9	0.8	Decreasing
Male	1.0	0.8	0.8	Decreasing
Female	0.8	1.0	0.8	No change
Breast (female)	0.8	0.9	1.0	Increasing
Cervix uteri	0.9	0.9	0.8	Decreasing
Prostate	0.9	0.9	0.8	No change

[a] Ratio is black five-year relative survival rate divided by the white five-year relative survival rate. A black/white ratio less than 1.0 indicates that blacks have a poorer five-year survival rate compared with whites.

Source: National Cancer Institute.

Pechacek, 1991), including nearly 45 percent of all male cancer deaths and 22 percent of all female cancer deaths. The vast majority of excess tobacco-related cancer mortality is due to lung cancer as a result of cigarette smoking.

Cigarette smoking is also an established cause of several other sites of cancer, including the larynx, oral cavity, esophagus, and bladder, and it contributes to an elevation in the death rates for cancer of the kidney and pancreas in men and women, cervical cancer in women, and to some additional cases and deaths from stomach cancer in both men and women (U.S. Department of Health and Human Services, 1989). Use of smokeless tobacco is an established cause of increased cancer morbidity and mortality. Users of pipes and cigars have substantially elevated risks for cancer of the larynx, oral cavity, pharynx, and esophagus—risks that often equal and sometimes exceed those of regular cigarette smokers.

Smoking prevalence is higher in blacks than whites; 34 percent of blacks smoked in 1987 compared to 28.8 percent of whites. The higher prevalence rates observed among black Americans is due almost exclusively to the higher rates among black males; no difference in smoking prevalence exists between black and white females (Shopland & Massey, 1990). Documented trends in smoking prevalence over the past thirty years have shown higher rates among black males compared to their white counterparts, while no difference has been observed between white and black females. While overall rates are high among black males, they initiate smoking somewhat later than whites and, on average, smoke fewer cigarettes per day (National Cancer Institute, in press). However, compared to whites, blacks tend to smoke cigarette brands with higher tar and nicotine levels (Wagenknecht et al., 1990).

Certain chemicals and other agents in the environment are carcinogenic. Some of these carcinogens, including some solvents and dyes, heavy metals, organic and inorganic dusts, and pesticides and herbicides, can be found in the workplace. Historically, blacks have been more likely than whites to be employed in less skilled jobs, where exposures to hazardous substances tend to be greater. Blacks have also been placed in more hazardous jobs than whites in work settings that have included the steel (Lloyd, 1971), rubber (Monson & Nakano, 1976), and chemical industries (Schulte et al., 1985), where hazardous substances tend to be greater. The higher representation of blacks among blue-collar workers who have higher smoking rates also increases the cancer risk for these individuals. Tobacco use plus workplace carcinogen exposure likely act synergistically to put a worker at even greater risk of developing certain cancers. This fact may in part explain the elevated lung cancer rates among black males who smoke infrequently.

Estimates of the proportion of cancer deaths in the United States that are associated with diet range from 10 to 70 pecent (U.S. Department of Health and Human Services, 1988). Obesity and high-fat, low-fiber diets have been reported to be associated with various cancers, particularly colon, breast, and prostate cancers. Although information on dietary patterns among black Americans is limited, anecdotal and some survey data suggest that blacks consume diets high in fat (Hargreaves, Baquet, & Gamshadzahi, 1989). The consumption of meats that have a high fat content or are smoked or salt cured and that are less expensive (in contrast to fruits and vegetables) may contribute to cancer risk. Methods of cooking, including frying, barbecuing, and overcooking of vegetables with fat (salt pork or fatback) are also risks. Additionally, the high rate of obesity in black women over age forty-five (61 percent, compared with 32 percent of white women of the same ages) may contribute to breast, colon, and corpus uteri cancers (Baquet, Clayton, & Robinson, 1989).

Knowledge, Attitudes, and Pratices

In general, blacks have less knowledge of health promotion/disease prevention measures, including cancer prevention and control strategies, than the general population (Cardwell & Collier, 1981). Lack of knowledge may result in nonparticipation in cancer screening programs, failure to recognize early warning signs of cancer, and delays in seeking cancer diagnosis or treatment. For example, among women age forty and older, 29.4 percent of black women stated they had never heard of mammography, compared with 12.2 percent of white women; however, 40.9 percent of black women had heard of mammography but never had it, compared with 48.9 percent of white women (National Center for Health Statistics, 1987).

Certain surveys suggest that fatalistic or pessimistic attitudes about cancer—lack of belief that early detection is likely to be successful in inhibiting disease progression and that treatment can be effective—are prevalent in the black community (EVAXX, Inc., 1981). Similar attitudes among blacks were reported by researchers in Buffalo, New York, where three- to six-month delays in seeking diagnosis and treatment were found to occur (Natarajan, Nemoto, Mettlin, & Murphy, 1985).

Health and Medical Resources

Access, availability, continuity, and compliance with cancer control services are affected by social class, employment status, type and extent of medical coverage, and utilization patterns of health services. Blacks do not access the health care system as frequently as whites, irrespective of income level (Blendon, Aiken, Freeman, & Corey, 1989), and use hospital emergency rooms or hospital outpatient departments as their principal sources of health care, in contrast to higher use of private physicians' offices by whites (Sparer & Simpson, 1985). Blacks also are much more likely than whites to be under-insured or without health insurance—factors that restrict access to quality health care, including cancer screening, early detection, treatment, and rehabilitation. According to the National Center for Health Statistics (1987), among those under sixty-five with no health insurance coverage, blacks constituted 22.6 percent and whites 14 percent. Thirty-seven percent were families with income under $10,000 annually and 3 percent were families with income over $35,000. Poorer survival for blacks is thought to be related in part to the fact that blacks generally have more advanced disease than whites at the time of diagnosis. Poverty as a risk factor for cancer mortality also contributes to poorer survival.

Due to high rates of comorbidity or poorer overall health status of black Americans, cancer treatment may be more difficult. For example, blacks have high prevalence rates of cardiovascular, pulmonary, and renal diseases, which may preclude the administration of optimal doses of cancer chemotherapeutic agents such as adriamycin, bleomycin, and cisplatin.

Other Factors

Biological factors also contribute to higher cancer incidence and mortality rates among blacks. For certain cancers such as bladder and uterine (corpus uteri), blacks have more aggressive histological tumor patterns than whites, which may contribute in part to poorer survival of blacks (Baquet & Ringen, 1986). More research is needed on the relationship of histological tumor patterns and other aspects of tumor biology and differentials in survival, as well as on the role of genetics in cancer incidence and survival.

Many of the factors already discussed that contribute to the higher cancer incidence among blacks than among whites are related in some way to the generally lower socioeconomic status of black Americans. Nearly four times as many blacks as whites are considered to live below the poverty level, and more than 40 percent of black children live in poverty. Just over 50 percent of blacks are high school graduates, compared with nearly 70 percent of whites. Additionally, nearly 60 percent of blacks live in central cities, where overcrowding and poverty are commonly found.

When socioeconomic status is described in terms of income, education, and occupational category, the relationship to blacks' cancer experience can be generalized as follows: lower income restricts access to health care and medical resources and may affect dietary intake, because limited food purchasing power may lead to the selection of lower-cost, higher-fat items; lower educational attainment may result in lack of knowledge about the importance of early cancer detection; persons holding low-paying jobs are more likely to be exposed to hazardous substances in the workplace and to smoke cigarettes.

Using income, educational level, and population density as surrogates for socioeconomic status, a recent study found a statistically significant relationship between both cervical cancer and lung cancer and socioeconomic status (Baquet et al., 1991). For blacks and whites, incidence of lung cancer increased as population density increased. After adjustment for population density and education, the incidence of lung cancer in blacks was significantly lower than for whites. Only cancer of the colon, of the seven cancer sites studied, was not found to be significantly associated with race. This growing evidence of linkages between race, socioeconomic status, and cancer incidence affords opportunities to develop more in-depth studies of socioeconomic status to develop targeted cancer prevention and control programs. Because the exact nature of the relationship of socioeconomic status and cancer incidence or survival is not known, more investigation in the following areas is critically important: risk factors and exposures; knowledge, attitudes, and practices; aspects of cancer care; health and medical resources; and other factors, such as biological behavior of cancer and socioeconomic status. Only to the extent that we can better understand the factors that contribute to cancer among specific populations will we be able to improve our prevention and intervention strategies.

National Cancer Intervention Plans

National cancer intervention plans have been in progress since the mid 1980s via aggressive cancer prevention and control research and outreach activities. Cancer control encompasses both primary prevention (incidence rate reduction) and secondary prevention (screening, diagnosis, treatment, and interventions) to improve survival and mortality rates (Greenwald & Cullen, 1985). The cancer control research process is a continuum that proceeds through four phases: (1) systematic review of existing data from etiological research and randomized clinical trials, (2) methods development, (3) trials of primary and secondary prevention methods and diffusion of state-of-the-science treatment, and (4) studies of effective interventions in defined populations. Numerous developmental, controlled trials and phase IV activities in the black population are in various stages of implementation.

The Healthy People 2000 (U.S. Department of Health and Human Services, 1991) objectives for cancer focus on those areas with the greatest potential for reducing cancer incidence, morbidity, and mortality and provide a framework for expanding and coordinating efforts to apply current knowledge of cancer detection, prevention, and control strategies. Some of the objectives have special population targets, including blacks, persons with lower levels of educational attainment, blue-collar workers, and low-income groups. These objectives are preventing health, disability, and health status disparities and enhancing quality of life.

National Cancer Institute

In the United States, NCI is the lead federal agency responsible for meeting the challenge of cancer. It is committed to ensuring that advances emanating from research reach all Americans, including racial and ethnic minorities. NCI's Special Populations Studies Branch, a component of the Cancer Control Science Program within the Division of Cancer Prevention and Control, is charged with developing targeted cancer control intervention research among groups that experience higher cancer rates or are underserved by the lack of culturally appropriate cancer prevention and control programs. NCI supports a wide range of programs targeted to minority populations and is involved in activities such as establishing research networks and other collaborative efforts, conducting intervention research including population-based studies and clinical trials, supporting basic laboratory research that emphasizes minority cancer issues, promoting minority participation in research through special training opportunities (for example, the Minority Oncology Leadership Award), and developing and making educational materials available via services such as the toll-free 1-800-4-CANCER Cancer Information Service.

Networks and Other Collaborative Efforts

Recognizing the need for local participation in cancer control interventions, NCI has supported the development of a national outreach structure through the establishment of six operational regional offices. The National Black Leadership Initiative on Cancer (NBLIC), established by the National Cancer Advisory Board and NCI in 1987, is a network of concerned and active black leaders who organize, implement, and support cancer prevention programs at the national and local levels. By identifying and mobilizing local black leaders, establishing community cancer coalitions, and developing networking relationships with many national, state, local, grassroots, and special interest organizations across the country, the NBLIC has directly or indirectly reached fifteen to twenty million black Americans. Examples of local coalition activities demonstrate the potential of the NBLIC model. In collaboration with the Department of Health and Human Services, one NBLIC coalition (the Philadelphia NBLIC) was instrumental in deterring the marketing of a brand of cigarettes to the black community. Through local networking activities to identify and enlist the cooperation of health service organizations, other coalitions have been able to offer no-cost or low-cost mammograms and provide information on breast self-examinations. Along with the American Cancer Society, another coalition in Los Angeles County helped coordinate Black Cancer Awareness Sunday, in which more than 250 churches participated by providing cancer prevention messages to their congregations. Another phase of NBLIC activities involves further coalition building and addresses cancer control barriers, including risk factors and service utilization in black communities.

The National Cancer Control Research Network (NCCRN) is another national collaborative effort initiated by NCI to reduce cancer incidence and mortality among black Americans by increasing research that addresses the causes, prevention, and treatment of cancer in that population. This national network of cancer researchers (individuals and institutions) with a special commitment to the black community intends to achieve its objectives through a variety of approaches, including sponsorship of scientific symposia, funding of developmental research projects, maintenance of information resources such as a database and bibliography, facilitation of collaborative, multiinstitution research projects, and support of faculty development programs. The NCCRN, which is incorporated and seeking tax-exempt status, has been supported in its developmental stages by NCI, the Office of Minority Health in the Public Health Service (PHS), and the contributions of member institutions.

The D.C./NCI Cancer Initiative in Washington, D.C., was developed in response to the high cancer mortality rates among blacks in the nation's capital. In collaboration with the D.C. Commission on Public Health, the D.C. Cancer Control Consortium, and the Howard University Cancer Center, NCI is undertaking efforts to promote primary prevention, early detection, and prompt treatment for cancers of the breast, cervix, lung, and head and neck, which have especially high mortality rates in the District of Columbia. Planned activities, all specifically targeted to the black community, include inservice training for primary health care providers on cancer detection and screening, school-based smoking prevention and healthy eating behavior programs, and adult educational programs tied to screening and follow-up.

Other collaborative efforts aimed at the problem of cancer among black Americans involve the National Medical Association program to address cancer prevention awareness at the state level and the Links, Inc. (an organization of professional black women) program to incorporate cancer prevention as a priority in local projects.

Intervention Networks

To identify and remedy key factors that contribute to the excess cancer experience of blacks, NCI supports specially designed intervention research and clinical trials. One group of projects addresses avoidable mortality from cancers in black populations. Institutions funded under this initiative are examining several approaches to reducing mortality from breast and cervical cancers among blacks. For example, a clinic-based intervention is being tested as a way of increasing the availability, accessibility, and use of breast cancer screening services in three institutional settings that serve low-income black residents. Another project is examining the effectiveness of a comprehensive community education program to increase the rate of participation by black women in cervical cancer screening programs. Other interventions are aimed at increasing the participation of black women in screenings for cervical and breast cancers through a nurse-delivered educational program and a culturally appropriate home education program.

Cigarette smoking is the targeted risk factor in NCI's Primary Prevention of Cancer in Black Populations initiative. Funded institutions are developing innovative smoking prevention or cessation interventions and evaluating their long-term effectiveness in black populations. Interventions being tested include a skills-based prevention approach for black youth in grades seven through nine, a community-based effort to reduce smoking among low- and middle-income blacks in both urban and rural settings, a smoking cessation and motivational education program for mothers of children in Head Start, and a primary care physician counseling program to stop smoking among black patients in a large inner-city hospital.

The National Cancer Institute hopes to stimulate the development of culturally sensitive intervention methods and assessment instruments through its intiative on Developmental Research in Special Populations. Research studies that are funded seek to identify barriers to cancer control, test intervention methods that can be used or adapted for special populations, and validate assessment instruments. One currently funded project includes studies on dietary modification opportunities in rural, low-income blacks.

Population-Based Studies and Clinical Trials

NCI conducts a number of case-controlled and epidemiological studies on minority and medically underserved groups and seeks to increase the participation of minority patients and health care providers in clinical trials. A large population-based case-control study of pancreatic, esophageal, and prostatic cancers and mutliple myeloma is in progress to assess reasons for the excess risk of these cancers among black Americans. Information on risk factors is being collected from laboratory and genetic studies as well. A study of the etiology of uterine cervix cancer is focused on human papillomavirus (HPV) infection and differential incidence rates in minority women, including blacks, and nonminorities. This study also will examine whether black American women have a higher prevalence of HPV infection and whether HPV proliferates more rapidly in blacks, thus leading to a more rapid progression of cervical lesions to cancer.

Cancer centers that serve large or predominantly minority populations are focusing on ways to increase accrual and participation of minority patients in clinical trial programs, expand research on cancers affecting minority populations, promote cancer prevention and control measures in communities, and extend the benefits of clinical research and improved oncology practice to populations who reside outside of major medical and urban centers. NCI also funds a number of minority Community Clinical Oncology Programs, which involve community physicians in clinical trials, thereby expanding access of minority populations to state-of-the-art therapies.

The Cancer Prevention and Clinical Research in The Underserved Populations initiative is intended to stimulate the establishment and implementation of a research program that will integrate and deliver comprehensive cancer prevention screening and early detection as well as quality treatment services to underserved low-income, high-risk populations. The initiative emphasizes applying mechanisms that will facilitate the rapid spread of state-of-the-art cancer prevention and control technology and increase the participation of these populations in clinical trials.

Basic Research

Several ongoing basic laboratory research projects have a special emphasis on cancers that disproportionately affect blacks. An internal NCI breast cancer work group was formed to study the aggressiveness of breast cancer in black American women and will analyze potential molecular markers. A novel therapeutic agent is being evaluated for treatment of multiple myeloma, which is rising in incidence among blacks. Basic research on prostate cancer, which has an unexplained disproportionately higher incidence and mortality in black men, has provided new information about the influence of growth factors that is being used in the development of new treatments. Studies are also in progress to develop treatment and vaccine for adult T-cell leukemia, a disease that primarily affects black Americans and is caused by a human retrovirus (National Cancer Institute, 1989).

Training and Related Programs

NCI has recognized the need to rapidly increase the pool of minority scientists to prevent potential shortages of scientists in the future. Culturally sensitive investigators are needed to address the problem of excess cancer rates among special populations. Therefore, blacks (and other minorities) need to have more opportunities to pursue careers in science, other areas of research, and health care. NCI provides grants for the support of minority undergradutes, graduate research assistants, and faculty members, and it co-funds other programs aimed at increasing minority participation in research. It is also exploring ways of encouraging minority students to consider research careers at an early stage in their education. For example, the Science Enrichment Program is a pilot program that recruits underrepresented minority high school students, including black students, who are interested in science, mathematics, or computer science to participate in a summer program that includes hands-on academic instruction, special seminars and speakers, specialized laboratory exposure, and educational and cultural field trips. This five- to six-week residential program has a rigorous evaluation and tracking component.

Educational Materials and Services

To meet its responsibilities to distribute cancer-related information, NCI has developed educational materials and services for special populations as well as for the general public. The Cancer Prevention Awareness Program for black Americans was developed to provide information through the mass media and intermediary organizations. By focusing on the "good news" about cancer control and ways to decrease personal risk, the program has attempted to alleviate pessimistic attitudes about cancer among blacks. A new theme of information targeted to black Americans is "do the right thing . . . get a new attitude about cancer." This theme was applied to information about nutrition, smoking, and screening for breast and cervical cancers and distributed as part of Minority Cancer Awareness month.

The Cancer Information Service is a nationwide program that offers free, current information about cancer prevention and treatment. By calling the toll-free telephone number 1-800-4-CANCER, consumers, cancer patients, and health professionals can speak to skilled information specialists about a variety of cancer topics. Information on state-of-the-art cancer treatments, names of organizations and physicians that provide care to cancer patients, and detailed summaries of clinical protocols for treating cancer can be obtained from the Physician Data Query (PDQ) system.

Conclusion

Data continue to indicate that black Americans bear a disproportionate burden of cancer. Compared with whites, blacks experience a higher incidence, increasing mortality rates for many sites, and shorter survival after a diagnosis of cancer. The reasons for these disparities are complex and difficult to decipher but are related to exposures and risk factors, including smoking, diet, and occupational exposures; knowledge, attitudes, and practices; health and medical resources distribution; and other factors, such as cancer biology, genetics, and socioeconomic status. One of the three major goals of the Year 2000 Objectives for the Nation is to reduce health disparities among Americans. NCI is leading a national effort to implement cancer prevention and control initiatives specifically targeted to the black population. Activities encompassed by these initiatives include network building and collaborations, intervention studies, population-based studies and clinical trials, basic research, training opportunities, and education and information distribution. Realization of the national goal of reducing the cancer mortality rate requires redoubling our efforts to ensure that all Americans share equally in the benefits derived from cancer prevention and control research. Through the aggressive and consistent mobilization of all parts of the black community—adults, children, clergy, grassroots organizations, health professionals, policy makers, and private-public groups—a substantial reduction in the cancer burden in the black community can be achieved.

References

Baquet, C. R., Clayton, L. A., & Robinson, R. G. (1989). Cancer prevention and control. In L. Jones (Ed.), *Minorities and cancer* (pp. 67–76). New York Springer-Verlag.

Baquet, C. R., Horm, J. W., Gibbs, T., & Greenwald, P. (1991). Socioeconomic factors and cancer incidence among blacks and whites. *Journal of the National Cancer Institute, 83*(8), 551–557.

Baquet, C. R., & Ringen, K. (1986). In *Advances in cancer control: Health care financing and research*. New York: Liss.

Blendon, R. J., Aiken, L. H., Freeman, H. E., & Corey, C. R. (1989). Access to medical care for black and white Americans. *Journal of the American Medical Association, 261*, 278–281.

Cardwell, J., & Collier, W. (1981, October). Racial differences in cancer awareness: What black Americans need to know about cancer. *Urban Health*, 29–32.

EVAXX, Inc. (1981). Black Americans' attitudes toward cancer and cancer tests: Highlights of a study. *CA—A Cancer Journal for Clinicians, 31*, 211–218.

Greenwald, P., & Cullen, J. (1985). The new emphasis in cancer control. *Journal of the National Cancer Institute, 74*, 543–551.

Hargreaves, M., Baquet, C. R., & Gamshadzahi, A. (1989). Diet, nutritional status, and cancer risk in American blacks. *Nutrition and Cancer, 12*, 1–28.

Lloyd, J. (1971). Long-term mortality of steel workers: V. Respiratory cancer in coke plant workers. *Journal of Occupational Medicine, 13*, 53–68.

Monson, R., & Nakano, K. (1976). Mortality among rubber workers: II. Other employees. *American Journal of Epidemiology, 103*, 297–303.

Natarajan, N., Nemoto, T., Mettlin, C., & Murphy, G. P. (1985). Race-related differences in breast cancer patients. *Cancer, 7*(56), 1704–1709.

National Cancer Institute. (1989). *1991 budget estimate*. Bethesda, MD: Public Health Service.

National Cancer Institute. (In press). *Comprehensive approaches to community based smoking control* (STCP Monograph Series, No. 1). Bethesda, MD: Author.

National Center for Health Statistics. (1987). *National health interview survey.* Hyattsville, MD: Public Health Survice.

National Center for Health Statistics. (1990). *Health, United States, 1989.* Hyattsville, MD: Public Health Service.

Ries, L.A.G., Hankey, B. F., & Edwards, B. K. (Eds.). (1990). *Cancer statistics review, 1973–87* (NIH Publication No. 90-2789). Bethesda, MD: National Cancer Institute.

Schulte, P., Ringen, K., Hemstreet, G., Altekruse, E., Gullen, W., & Patton, M. (1985). Risk assessment of a cohort exposed to aromatic amines: Initial results. *Journal of Occupational Medicine, 27,* 115–121.

Shopland, D. R., Eyre, H. J., & Pechacek, T. F. (1991). Smoking attributable cancer mortality in 1991. Is lung cancer now the leading cause of death among smokers in our society? *Journal of the National Cancer Institute, 83*(16), 1142–1148.

Shopland, D. R., & Massey, M. (Eds.). (1990). *Smoking, Tobacco, and Cancer Program: 1985–1989 status report* (NIH Publication No. 90-3107). Bethesda, MD: National Cancer Institute.

Sparer, G., & Simpson, N. (1985). *Health services patterns in U.S. black and minority patients* (Report prepared for the Division of Cancer Prevention and Control, NCI). Bethesda, MD: National Cancer Institute.

U.S. Department of Health and Human Services. (1988). *The Surgeon General's report on nutrition and health* (DHHS Publication No. PHS 88-50210). Washington, DC: U.S. Government Printing Office.

U.S. Department of Health and Human Services, Office on Smoking and Health. (1989). *Reducing the health consequences of smoking: 25 years of progress* (DHHS Publication No. CDC 89-8411). Washington, DC: U.S. Government Printing Office.

U.S. Department of Health and Human Services. (1991). *Healthy People 2000: National health promotion and disease prevention objectives* (DHHS Publication No. PHS 91-50212). Washington, DC: U.S. Government Printing Office.

Wagenknecht, L., Cutter, G., Haley, N., Sidney, S., Manolio, T., Hughes, G., & Jacob, D. (1990). Racial differences in serum cotinine levels among smokers in the Coronary Artery Risk Development in (Young) Adults Study. *American Journal of Public Health, 80,* 1053–1056.

10

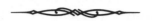

Diabetes and
the Black Community

Frederick G. Murphy
M. Joycelyn Elders

The United States has made positive gains toward improving the health status of its citizens over the past generation. However, not all segments of the population have fully benefitted from these improvements. The country's poor and ethnic minority populations continue to be plagued by disproportionately high rates of death and disability. In 1984, the secretary of the Department of Health and Human Services formed the Task Force on Black and Minority Health to analyze the disparities in health status. The Task Force identified six health areas that account for more than 80 percent of excess deaths among U.S. minorities; diabetes mellitus was cited as one of the six. Relatively uncommon among black Americans at the beginning of this century, diabetes is now the third leading cause of death from disease in this population. According to the U.S. Bureau of the Census, black Americans comprised 12.2 percent of the U.S. population in 1988. Some 29.3 million Americans are black—a 14 percent increase since 1980. Census figures also document that blacks have higher rates of poverty and unemployment than do their white counterparts (Public Health Service, 1988).

Defining Diabetes

For the purposes of this chapter, it is important to first define diabetes in the most practical terms possible. Diabetes mellitus is a common, chronic, systemic disease characterized by glucose intolerance or the inability of the body to properly use glucose. People develop diabetes because their pancreas does not make enough insulin or stops making insulin entirely, or because the cells in the body do not receive the insulin properly. As a result, too much sugar begins to build up in the blood and another source of energy has to be sought. Any of these conditions leads to problems that seriously threaten the body's health. Some of the clinical manifestations of diabetes often include unusual thirst, frequent urination, eating excessively, weight loss, fatigue, and a constant feeling of being ill.

Diabetes mellitus generally can be divided into two major forms. One results from damage or destruction of the beta cells of the pancreas, leading to partial or complete insulin deficiency; the other is a consequence of insulin resistance occurring at the tissue level, with little or no impairment of insulin synthesis or release. These forms of diabetes differ in their age of onset, occurrence in the population, clinical manifestations, inheritance, and treatment. In 1979, the National Diabetes Data Group revised the previous names and classification of diabetes mellitus and established criteria for its diagnosis.

Insulin-dependent diabetes mellitus (IDDM), also known as type I diabetes, may occur at any age but typically develops in children or young adults. IDDM accounts for approximately 5 to 10 percent of the diabetic population in the United States. In this country, it is less common in blacks than in whites. Some clinical manifestations of IDDM are characterized by modest hyperglycemia for several days, weeks, or even months before hyperglycemia becomes severe. IDDM is characterized by low levels or a total absence of insulin; individuals with this kind of diabetes must inject insulin in order to live. Other complications may manifest gradually during the course of the disease and are often associated with control of the disease. Examples include limited joint mobility, growth failure, delayed puberty, and cataracts. Chronic complications include retinopathy, nephropathy, neuropathy, and coronary disease.

Non-insulin dependent diabetes mellitus (NIDDM) is the most common type of diabetes, accounting for 90 to 95 percent of all cases. It most often affects adults, usually over age forty, seems to run in families, and is more common in women than in men. NIDDM is more common among blacks than whites, with many studies suggesting a ratio of 2 to 1 or less. The black to white ratio is higher for women than for men. The prevalence of diabetes among black men and women increases with age, as it does among whites, but the age of peak onset among blacks appears to be lower. People with the disease are often obese. They may have high, normal, or low levels of insulin, but their ability to use it effectively is impaired. Individuals with NIDDM often can manage the disease through diet, weight control, and exercise, although some may require treatment with oral hypoglycemic agents or insulin. The most distressing difficulties with NIDDM are related to the chronic complications of cardiovascular disease, retinopathy, neuropathy, and nephropathy.

Impaired glucose tolerance constitutes a heterogeneous grouping of patients who fit into neither the IDDM nor NIDDM category. These patients have abnormal glucose metabolism, which may be demonstrated by the impaired ability to dispose of a glucose load or fasting hyperglycemia; however, inadequate insulin secretion or action is not the primary pathogenic abnormality.

Maturity-onset diabetes mellitus of youth (MODY), a very specific genetic form of carbohydrate intolerance, has an autosomal dominant mode of inheritance and has been shown to be due to an abnormality of the insulin molecule. Gestational diabetes is a mild form of diabetes that affects women only during pregnancy. The prevalence of gestational diabetes has been stated to range between 1 and 14 percent, depending on the type of patients selected for study. In select patient populations, the incidence rate is 2 to 7 percent of pregnant women, with no significant differences between black, white, and Hispanic populations. Women who have had this form of diabetes are more likely to develop NIDDM when they are older.

Pregnant women with diabetes are usually seen by a physician or nurse more often during their pregnancy than other women who are pregnant. The National Diabetes Advisory Board and Centers for Disease Control (CDC) recommend that pregnant women with diabetes be cared for jointly by an obstetrician, a pediatrician, a health educator, and a primary care practitioner or an internist familiar with diabetes. With the new knowledge, skills, and equipment available today, the probability of delivering a healthy baby even when the mother or baby has developed a medical problem is much greater than in previous years (CDC, 1991).

Overview of the Problem

In 1986, diabetes mellitus was the seventh leading cause of death in the United States, and the thirteenth leading cause of years of potential life lost before age 65 (Centers for Disease Control, 1991). Other studies have shown that diabetes is identified as the underlying cause of death in approximately 25 percent of the death certificates on which it appears and is recorded on only 50 percent of the certificates for persons who have the disease at the time of death. Moreover, diabetes contributes to a much larger number of deaths than is apparent from death certificates. The *Diabetes Surveillance Report* (1991) from the Division of Diabetes Translation at the Centers for Disease Control describes the number of deaths resulting from diabetes and the associated death rates for the period 1980 through 1986. It examines the number and rates of deaths from diabetes by age, gender, calendar year, and state. Death rates for the general U.S. population, as well as for persons with diabetes (PWD), are discussed.

From 1980 to 1987, the number of PWD in the United States increased by more than one million, so that by 1987 nearly seven million people knew that they had the disease. This increase was related to both growth in the U.S. population and in the prevalence rate of diabetes.

The National Center for Health Statistics (NCHS) reported in 1987 that, in just two decades, the prevalence of diagnosed diabetes in black Americans increased fourfold, from 228,000 in 1963 to approximately one million in 1985. Another one million blacks are estimated to have undiagnosed diabetes. During the period 1980–1987, diabetes prevalence rates were significantly higher among blacks than whites. Black males had a rate four times higher than white males, and black females had a rate approximately two times higher than white females (CDC, 1991).

The National Diabetes Data Group (NDDG) of the National Institutes of Health reported that the rate of non-insulin-dependent diabetes among Black Americans is 50 to 60 percent higher than it is among white non-Hispanic Americans. In the sixty-five- to seventy-four-year-old age group, one in four has diabetes. Among black women, diabetes can almost be termed epidemic; one in four black women age fifty-five and older has diabetes — double the rate for white women of the same age. Black Americans experience high rates of the serious complications of diabetes: blindness, amputation, and end-stage renal disease (ESRD) (NIH, 1990). The rates of severe visual impairment are 40 percent higher in blacks with diabetes than in whites. Black patients evidence twice as many amputations as do whites. A Michigan study found that the rate of ESRD was four times higher among blacks with diabetes than whites (NIH, 1990).

The annual number of deaths attributed to diabetes as an underlying cause steadily increased from 1980 through 1986, reaching 37,184 in 1986. In each year, the number of deaths from diabetes as any listed cause was about four times greater than the number of deaths from diabetes as an underlying cause. Among the entire diabetic population, both minority and nonminority, the age-standardized mortality rate for diabetes as an underlying cause of death declined by 14.5 percent between 1980 and 1986. This trend, however, was somewhat erratic, with small rate increases noted during the periods 1981–1983 and 1984–1985. Black females — the group with the highest mortality rates — had annual mortality rates that were two times higher than those for white females. Mortality rates for black males were 20 to 40 percent higher than those for white males (CDC, 1991).

Two national conferences have been held to define issues and priority areas for activities to reduce the impact of diabetes on black Americans. Both conferences were chaired by Louis W. Sullivan, secretary of the Department of Health and Human Services. Sponsors of the conference included the National Institute of Diabetes and Digestive and Kidney Diseases (NIDDK), the Office of Minority Health (OMH), the Centers for Disease Control (CDC), the American Diabetes Association (ADA), and the National Black Nurses Association. The first conference was held in September 1988 and focused on epidemiologic research findings relevant to diabetes and its complications among blacks. The second conference focused on how to increase diabetes awareness within the professional and black lay communities. Some of the conference's major findings included the following:

- Black Americans have a higher prevalence of obesity, a strong risk factor for non-insulin-dependent diabetes mellitus (NIDDM). Among people with diagnosed diabetes, 82 percent of adult black women are obese compared with 62 percent of white women; among men, 45 percent of blacks are obese compared with 39 percent of whites.

- Black Americans are known to have a higher prevalence of hypertension, which is associated with retinopathy and renal and cardiovascular complications—major complications in black patients. Studies are needed to elucidate the disease processes involved in these conditions and to develop better methods of prevention and treatment.
- Studies of dietary habits of black Americans indicate that they consume less fiber and more cholesterol-rich foods than whites, although their total calorie consumption and fat intake are lower.
- Black people tend to have less access to financial, social, health, and educational resources that would help improve their health status and health awareness. Educational resources—including materials and programs—are needed to take into account life-styles, interests, and cultural and economic considerations of the black population (CDC, 1990).

A higher incidence of diabetes in minority populations contributes to the higher death rate from cardiovascular disease, the leading cause of death among people with diabetes in the United States. Heart disease is two to four times more likely to affect PWD than the general population. Not all the connections are clear, but it is apparent that the higher incidence of PWD with coronary risk factors, such as hypertension, cigarette smoking, increased fat, and elevated cholesterol in the blood, contributes to their chances of developing heart disease. Over half of all deaths among people with diabetes are attributable to heart disease. Coronary artery disease alone claims 38,000 diabetics annually, and it is estimated that preventive (risk reduction) measures could reduce this mortality rate by 45 percent (PHS, 1988).

Studies have found that a history of stroke is four times more common among PWD than in those without the disease. In addition, cerebrovascular disease has been found to be listed on 25 percent of the death certificates in which diabetes is the underlying cause of death. Since high blood pressure is a major risk factor for stroke, the correlation between stroke and diabetes may be largely due to the increased prevalence of hypertension, especially in black PWD. Controlling high blood pressure might prevent a vast majority of strokes from occurring among PWD.

Kidney diseases occur among PWD when high blood sugar forces the kidneys to filter more blood than is actually needed in an effort to keep wastes in the blood low. This overwork may lead to gradual degeneration of the kidneys' vital cleaning system. Known as *diabetic nephropathy*, this condition develops with diabetes. ESRD, which is the most severe form of kidney disease, requires dialysis or transplantation for survival. It is a leading complication for diabetics. The number of ESRD cases steadily increased over the period 1980–1986, with the age-adjusted incidence rate of ESRD increasing from 9.6 to 36.7 per million. The rate of increase was similar among gender and race groups. For males, the age-adjusted incidence among blacks was 2.9 times the incidence among whites. For females, the black rate was 4.3 times that of whites.

Diabetes is the leading cause of blindness in persons between the ages of twenty and seventy-four, with the highest rates of blindness due to diabetes occurring in nonwhite, minority populations. The primary vision disorder affecting diabetics is retinopathy, a condition in which enlarged and damaged capillaries lead to swelling and hemorrhaging within the retina, often impairing the portion of the eye specializing in detail vision. As capillaries become closed off, new blood vessels form, breaking through and leaking into the inner surface of the retina and seriously interfering with vision. Retinopathy can be detected before damage is evident, and a variety of treatments, including laser therapy and surgery, can improve vision and slow retinal damage.

However, many blacks cannot obtain or afford such care. Consequently, a disproportionate number of blacks may lose their vision as a result of this barrier to eye care. The number of persons who lose their vision because of diabetes is estimated to be between 12,000 to 24,000 annually (Will, Geiss, & Wetterhall, 1990). These numbers could be substantially reduced by an increase in accessibility to care for PWD.

Forty-five percent of amputations not caused by injury occur as complications of diabetes. Most often these amputations — usually of the foot or lower leg — are necessitated by gangrene and ulceration or from peripheral arterial disease. This condition, which is four times more common in PWD than in those without the disease, involves both hardening of the normally elastic arterial walls and deposit of plaque within the artery. Among diabetics, 60 percent of the 24,000 new cases of peripheral arterial disease per year are estimated to be preventable. From 1980 to 1987, blacks accounted for 13 to 25 percent of all hospital discharges for lower-extremity amputations (LEA) related to diabetes. Hospital discharge rates for blacks with diabetes were consistently higher than those for whites with diabetes, particularly for the time periods 1980–1981 and 1984–1987, when rates were 1.5 to 2 times higher (CDC, 1991).

Building a Research Agenda

During a 1988 national conference, James R. Gavin III of the Howard Hughes Medical Institute cited the need for a variety of scientific, behavioral, and social investigations to address the diabetes problem, which he indicated is "ravaging the black population." He called for studies to define the genetic pedigree of diabetes in blacks, studies to determine the nature and role of fat distribution in blacks and its relationship to diabetes, research to assess the influence of socioeconomic and psychosocial factors in the black population, research to develop optimum treatment strategies for the complications of diabetes and for hypertension in blacks, behavioral studies on dietary and cultural influences in the black community, and development of educational resources that are relevant to black concerns and life-styles (NIH, 1990).

Concrete recommendations such as Gavin's must be brought to the forefront through the utilization of innovative, yet appropriate, strategies and methodologies. The importance of cultural and linguistic variables cannot be overemphasized when health interventions and medical research initiatives are being planned for minority communities. Particularly in the black community, special considerations must be taken into account when attempting to introduce concepts or programs such as primary and secondary prevention, risk reduction, community empowerment, community ownership, and infrastructure building. Without such attention, research efforts will prove irrelevant and preventive interventions will be short-lived, with little or no substantive impact or outcomes. Prevention and primary care strategies and methodologies for the black community must above all be designed with effectiveness and longevity in mind. This is not an easy task, especially considering the socioeconomic, psychosocial, ecological, environmental, political, and religious determinants that dynamically coexist within the black community today. Such a constellation of critical determinants could make the development and implementation of appropriate methodologies a lifelong task for the dedicated health professional.

Chronic diseases such as diabetes mellitus must be battled forthrightly in black communities. Health professionals have to begin to spend more time on the identification and/or development of appropriate health intervention strategies to reduce risk factors, morbidity, and mortality associated with diabetes. These interventions must prove effective, translatable, and replicable. Reputable institutions, both private and public, must continually develop and publish research findings and develop policies focusing on diabetes and other chronic diseases. This, however, must be done with the assurance that these policies have been formulated based on sound research principles and designed with cultural sensitivity. Only then will they be feasible, acceptable, and usable by professionals and/or agencies involved in the delivery of community-level primary, secondary, and tertiary health care. Any attempt to do otherwise will prove futile, wasting dollars at a time when our country can ill afford missappropriations.

The Year 2000 Health Objectives for the Nation can serve as a blueprint for health professionals at all levels in establishing milestones, including goals, objectives, and recommendations for improving our nation's health. This document draws attention to diabetes and correlates of morbidity and mortality as well as risk reduction. It lists some specific yet comprehensive programmatic and evaluation issues that must be addressed. These include the following:

Personnel

- Establish the number and types of health professionals, including allied/associated public health fields needed to accomplish the practice, educational, and research aspects of diabetes.

- Provide an appropriate curriculum on diabetes and chronic disabling conditions in all schools and programs that prepares students for careers in the health professions, including allied/associated public health fields, and ensure that all graduates of such schools and programs demonstrate knowlege of these subjects.
- Increase the provision of continuing education on chronic and disabling conditions by national professional associations whose members have roles in this area.

Data Collection

- Establish national and state surveillance systems that can be used to monitor prevalence, complications, mortality, and major risk factors associated with diabetes.
- Establish racial and ethnic identifiers in national databases and statistically reliable samples of high-risk minority populations in national surveys.
- Collect more detailed information on race and ethnicity recorded on hospital discharge abstracts and ESRD treatment forms.
- Improve diabetes reporting on birth certificates to monitor reproductive and birth outcomes among women with diabetes.
- Establish mechanisms for tracking blindness in general and due to diabetes specifically.

Research

- Conduct basic and clinical research to better understand the etiology and pathogenesis of diabetes and its complications.
- Conduct research to develop optimal capabilities for the diagnosis, treatment, cure, and prevention of diabetes and its complications.

Community and Prevention Infrastructures

As essential as the preceding recommendations may be, it should be recognized that given a "hands-on" approach, community residents, both PWD and those without the disease, tend to give priority to other concerns not traditionally characterized as health or medical in nature (such as employment, housing, transportation, and so on). This is not to say, from a holistic viewpoint, that socioeconomic variables are not intricately interwoven into the fabric of public health, just as they are into the overall concept of "quality of life." In fact, when one begins to analyze existing socioeconomic problems or other public health problems impacting on residents of the black community (for example, poverty, racism, AIDS, substance abuse, teen pregnancy, violence, and environmental problems), it is not reasonable to expect diabetes or other chronic diseases to be considered priorities. Individuals in the black community are more apt to give priority to diabetes, and other chronic diseases, when primary preventive measures are no longer appropriate and treatment regimens are required (Anderson, et al., 1991).

Community Infrastructures

Attitudes and behaviors toward preventive health in the black community will require significant change to combat the diabetes epidemic. Community leaders must begin to come together and address chronic, infectious, and environmental health issues that negatively affect their community. Community "infrastructures" must be built where individuals representing public health, medicine, religion, business, education, politics, public safety, and other entities come together with residents of the community to form working coalitions, boards, and task forces. These working groups must develop strategies on how they can effectively work together to reduce risk factors, morbidity, and mortality plaguing their neighborhoods. Community ownership, not reticence, must become the order of the day. Through the establishment of creditable infrastructures, communities can be mobilized to begin transforming the attitude of their residents into one of education and commitment to changing their health profile and overall quality of life.

Central to this process is participation by community members in solving their own health problems. Community leaders must begin to work together to assess their circumstances, identify and prioritize their needs, and formulate and implement action plans to meet such needs. They must begin to embrace the fact that appropriate prevention and treatment interventions must not only be established but must become a way of life for the entire community. Key members in the community must become proactive toward all strategies focusing on the design and implementation of public health intervention programs in their target area. They must serve as diplomatic linkages, culture brokers, and translators who facilitate dialogue and negotiations with various institutions located both in and outside the community. They must work to ensure that resources and technical assistance are funneled to the neediest areas within their community.

Empowerment of community members has been cited by Paulo Freire and others as an effective prevention model that can promote health in all personal and social arenas. The model suggests that participation of people in group action and dialogue efforts enhances control and belief in the ability of people to change their own lives (Freire, 1968). Empowerment is intended to result in increased self-efficacy and an enhanced ability on the part of PWD to achieve their own self-care goals (Funnell, Anderson, & Arnold, 1991). Health and illness behaviors are culture bound, and primary prevention efforts to address preventable disease and illness must emerge from a knowledge of and respect for the culture of the target community. Community organization and development, community-oriented primary care, and other innovative approaches must begin to take place as intricate parts of health-related intervention strategies (Braithwaite, Murphy, Lythcott,

& Blumenthal, 1989; Katz, 1984). Involvement of this nature will help guarantee that cultural sensitivity is thoroughly incorporated into intervention planning and design (Randall-David, 1989).

Various institutions or "anchor agencies" (public health, medical, social work, and education sectors) are accessible to almost every community throughout the United States. These institutions can be valuable in enabling and reinforcing effective intervention programs and strategies over extended periods of time. Many of these agencies were conceived with the intent that they would provide resources and technical assistance to minority, low-income, and inner-city communities. An important step that can be taken by anchor agencies is to train and employ more health professionals from diverse racial and ethnic populations. The need is great as evidenced in the fact that African Americans comprise only 3 percent of all physicians, 4.5 percent of all registered nurses, and 3.2 percent of all registered dieticians (Public Health Service, 1990).

Traditionally, programs such as community health promotion and disease prevention have focused almost exclusively on the content of program development (for example, identifying program models or developing public information materials or curriculum). The process for translating programs has received much less attention. This lack of attention to the "translation" aspect of the process has led to failures even in the best-conceived and highly funded community-based programs. What has resulted has been difficulty in maintaining sponsoring organizations, difficulty reaching high-risk target populations, and difficulty integrating program objectives into the mission of indigenous community institutions or mediating structures.

Conclusion

The fight against diabetes in black Americans must incorporate cultural sensitivity, community organization and development, infrastructure building, and community empowerment. Such structuring will enable linkages to be formed between providers and recipients and will create an atmosphere conducive to reciprocity, where vertical (communities to institutions and institutions to communities) and horizontal (community member to community member), diabetes translation activities can more efficiently and effectively occur. Without the creation of appropriate forums where these translation activities can take place, interventions will have only a minimal chance of success, and risk factors and morbidity and mortality rates will continue to rise throughout the twenty-first century.

References

Anderson, R. M., Herman, W. H., Davis, J. M., Freedman, R. P., Funnell, M. M., & Neighbors, H. W. (1991). Barriers to improving diabetes care for blacks. *Diabetes Care*, *14*(7), 605–609.

Braithwaite, R. L., Murphy, F., Lythcott, N., & Blumenthal, D. S. (1989). Community organization and development for health promotion within an urban black community: A conceptual model. *Health Education, 20*(5), 56–60.

Centers for Disease Control, Division of Diabetes Translation. (1991). *Diabetes surveillance report* (pp. 4–11). Atlanta, GA: Author.

Centers for Disease Control, International Diabetes Center. (1983). *The prevention and treatment of five complications of diabetes: A guide for patients with an introduction to day-to-day management of diabetes.* Atlanta, GA: Author.

Centers for Disease Control, Division of Diabetes Translation. (1991). *The prevention and treatment of complications of diabetes: A guide for primary care with a practitioner.* Atlanta, GA: Author.

Freire, P. (1968). *Pedagogy of the oppressed.* New York: Scarbury Press.

Funnel, M. M., Anderson, R. M., & Arnold, M. S. (1991). Empowerment: A winning model for diabetes care. *Practical Diabetoloty, 10,* 15–18.

Katz, R. (1984). *Empowerment and synergy: Expanding the community's healing resources: Studies in empowerment.* New York: Hawthorne Press.

Murphy, F. G., Satterfield, L. D., Anderson, R. M., & Lyons, A. E. (1992). Diabetes educators as cultural translators. *Diabetes Education* (In Press).

National Institutes of Health, National Institute of Diabetes and Digestive and Kidney Diseases, National Diabetes Information Clearinghouse. (1989). *Diabetes: Related programs for black Americans: A resource guide* (pp. 5–7). Washington, DC: Author

Public Health Service, Bureau of Health Professions. (1990). Minorities and women in the health fields. HRSA-P-DV 90-3, p. 17. Washington, DC: Author.

Public Health Service, Office of Minority Health Resource Center. (1986). *Closing the gap* (1st ed.). Washington, DC: Author.

Public Health Service, Office of Minority Health Resource Center. (1988). *Closing the gap* (3rd ed.). Washington, DC: Author.

Randall-David, E. (1989). Strategies for working with culturally diverse communities and clients. In *Association for the care of children's health.* Washington, DC: U.S. Department of Health and Human Services, Bureau of Maternal and Child Health and Resources Development, Office of Maternal and Child Health.

Will, J. C., Geiss, L. S., & Wetterhall, S. F. (1990). Diabetic retinopathy. *New England Journal of Medicine, 323*(9), 613.

11

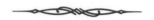

Homicide and Violence: Contemporary Health Problems for America's Black Community

Deborah Prothrow-Stith
Howard Spivak

Violence in America is a health problem that takes its greatest toll on young black men. The United States consistently has a very high homicide rate when compared to other industrialized countries. The 1980 rate of approximately 10 per 100,000 is five times that of Canada and twenty times that of the Netherlands (Wolfgang, 1986). Those who are most affected are poor, young, and male. Young black men are overrepresented among the poor and are overrepresented among the homicide victims. Homicide is the leading cause of death for black men age fifteen to forty-four at a rate several times higher than the rates for any other age/gender/race category (Centers for Disease Control, 1983; Alcohol, Drug Abuse, and Mental Health Administration, 1980).

Homicide is only the tip of the iceberg. The national rate of nonfatal interpersonal violence is significantly higher than the homicide rate, whether police, emergency room, or school data are used. There are less adequate data on nonfatal interpersonal violence because assaults are not mandatorily reported and because the emergency and school data are not routinely collected. When these data are collected, they consistently demonstrate the greater magnitude of the base of the iceberg of violence in America.

The Northeastern Ohio Trauma Study measured the incidence of cause-specific trauma by collecting emergency room data for the year 1977. The study reported an assault rate of 862 per 100,000 population, which was 100 times the homicide rate for that year (Barancik, 1983). This study also showed that the number of assaults reported to the emergency room was four times the number reported to the police. Police assault rates consistently underestimated the problem of nonfatal violence, when compared to emergency room rates or rates calculated from victimization surveys.

Schools do not consistently and reliably report the occurrence of violence. Suspension rates are often subject to collection, interpretation, and political biases. Some school-based data are available and reveal an even broader base to the iceberg. During the 1969–70 school year, Seattle Public

Schools had four assaultive injuries per 1,000 students (Johnson, Carter, Harlin, & Zoller, 1974). In the United States generally, there are approximately 75,000 assaultive injuries to teachers a year, at a rate of 35 per 1,000 (Baker & Dietz, 1979). A school-based victimization survey was conducted by the Boston Commission for Safe Schools (Boston Commission on Safe Public Schools, 1983). The commission's 1983 report revealed that 50 percent of the teachers and 38 percent of the students in the four schools surveyed reported being victims of a school-based crime during the previous school year. Weapon-carrying behavior was reported in this Boston survey, with 17 percent of the girls and 37 percent of the boys carrying a weapon at one time during the previous school year.

Many urban centers reported their most violent year in 1990, with homicide rates that were higher than any of the previous years. Violence in America is an increasing and devastating problem that takes its greatest toll on black Americans. Urban blacks are overrepresented among all the indicators of violence, emergency room rates, arrest rates, school suspension rates, and homicide rates. Poverty appears to account for this. In a study of domestic homicide in Atlanta, data that were corrected for socioeconomic status using the number of people per square foot of housing no longer showed a racial bias (Centerwall, 1984). Urban blacks are overrepresented among the poor and are overrepresented among the victims of fatal and nonfatal violence (Joint Center for Policy Studies, 1985).

The magnitude of violence in America and the contact health professionals have with the outcomes of violence have created impetus for a movement to address violence as a health problem. Additional motivation comes from knowledge of the characteristics of the violence and from the apparent applicability of prevention and intervention public health strategies used for other health problems.

Family and Friend Violence

The characteristics of homicides indicate a clear and consistently present pattern of friend and family violence. Half of the yearly 23,000 homicide victims in the United States die at the hands of someone they knew. Family members are responsible 20 percent of the time and friends or acquaintances are responsible for 30 percent. As illustrated in Figure 11.1, the leading precipitating cause of the homicides is an argument, which accounts for 47 percent. Significantly smaller percentages (15 percent) are caused by the commission of another felony (burglary, robbery, selling drugs), and an even smaller percent (1 percent) is due to gang activity. The news media report stranger, gang, and racial violence preferentially, yet these are not the dominant types of violence. Other correlates of violence include use of alcohol, cocaine, or other drugs and handgun availability (Prothrow-Stith & Weissman, 1991).

Figure 11.1. Homicide by Precipitant (United States Data).

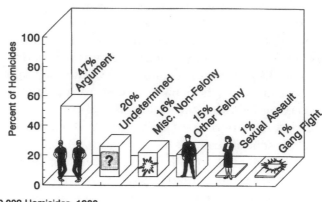

20,000 Homicides, 1986

Source: Reprinted with permission from Prothrow-Stith, *Violence Prevention Curriculum for Adolescents*, Educational Development Center, Inc., 55 Chapel Street, Newton, Massachusetts 02160, 1987, p. 26.

America's response to violence has been traditionally based in criminal justice, with law enforcement (punishment) and rehabilitation as the major strategies. Public health strategies are applicable to the problem of violence. Such strategies add prevention to the current responses to violence. Current criminal justice responses are triggered by a violent episode and are focused on establishing blame and instituting punishment. More recently, victim protection and retribution have become major concerns as well. Prevention is not a major concern, except through the deterrence yielded with punishment. There is considerable controversy as to whether current methods of punishment are deterrents of future violence at all. Even if they are, they are certainly not means of primary prevention, which is a strength within public health. Incarceration is not associated with a decline in violent crime. The 1990 report on incarceration rates in the United States reveals the impact of the "get tough" era of the last ten years. In addition to having incarceration rates for black men that are four times those of South Africa, the United States has doubled its prison population, which now numbers one million. The yearly costs are $16 billion (Bureau of Alcohol, Tobacco and Firearms, 1991).

Public Health Strategies

Public health prevention strategies are applicable to violence and offer unique opportunities for prevention. The movement within public health to address violence as a health problem is illustrated in the words of ex–Surgeon General Koop (1986, p. 35): "Violence is as much a public health issue for me and my successors in this country as smallpox, tuberculosis, and syphilis were for my predecessors in the last two centuries."

Public health strategies include the application of a multi-institutional and multidisciplinary model to change knowledge, attitudes, and behavior. This model has been applied with notable successes to other public health problems. The national campaign to reduce smoking is an example. Public health professionals, motivated by the first *Surgeon General's Report* on the health hazards of smoking, initiated a national effort to change the public's attitude from one that views smoking as glamorous and desirable to one that labels it offensive and unhealthy. The media, health care institutions, public schools, job sites, health fairs, and county fairs became the source of education and information. Advertisements were banned from television, and cigarettes were labeled with a warning. Once public attitudes changed, laws were enacted that banned smoking in public places. Each of these strategies contributed to the success of the smoking prevention efforts, though it is impossible to determine which strategy was responsible for what proportion of the success.

Today, a glamorous view of violence prevails. It is greatly enhanced by the television and movie heroes, who choose violence as a first response, are always successful, are always rewarded, and are never hurt badly. In addition, adults often encourage children to fight or feel that a certain child was justified in fighting. Parents do not want children who are wimps. Also of great concern is the fact that some parents use violence to solve their spousal conflicts or as the primary disciplinary technique. Children in those violence-plagued homes appear to be at higher risk for violence when they are adolescents and young adults. Alternatives to violence have to be taught, particularly to those children whose adult role models use violence.

A national public health campaign to prevent violence would utilize primary, secondary, and tertiary prevention strategies. Figure 11.2 illustrates a possible relationship between criminal justice and public health in each of these categories. Primary prevention strategies would focus on youth who do not fight as a rule, but who nevertheless participate in the "egging-on" of fights and who are exposed constantly to the glorified view of violence. The *Violence Prevention Curriculum for Adolescents* (Prothrow-Stith, 1987) and the Violence Prevention Project (Prothrow-Stith, Spivak, & Hausman, 1987) of the Boston Department of Health and Hospitals are examples of primary prevention.

The Violence Prevention Curriculum

The *Violence Prevention Curriculum for Adolescents* is designed to do the following:

1. Provide statistical information on adolescent violence and homicide
2. Present anger as a normal, potentially constructive emotion

Figure 11.2. An Ideal Relationship Between Public Health and Criminal Justice in Preventing Violence.

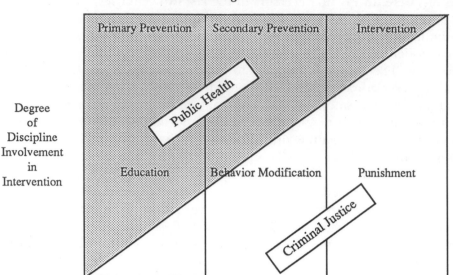

Type of Intervention

Source: Reprinted with permission from Prothrow-Stith, *Violence Prevention Curriculum for Adolescents*, Education Development Center, Inc., 55 Chapel Street, Newton, Massachusetts 02160, 1987.

3. Create an awareness in students of alternatives to fighting by discussing the potential gains and losses from fighting
4. Have students analyze situations preceding a fight and practice avoiding fights by using role play and videotape
5. Create a classroom ethos that is nonviolent and values violence-prevention behavior

The curriculum is specifically aimed at raising the individual's threshold for violence, by creating a nonviolent ethos within the classroom and by extending the student's repertoire of responses to anger. It acknowledges the existence of societal and institutional violence and the existence of institutional racism. Students are not taught to become passive agents, but are expected to claim anger and become intentional and creative about their responses to it. Anger is presented as a normal, essential, and potentially constructive emotion. Creative alternatives to fighting are stressed. The classroom discussion during the pivotal session focuses on the good and bad results of fighting. The students list the results. The list of bad results is invariably longer than the good list—hence the need for alternatives. This exercise illustrates the fact that violence rarely solves problems and often causes a person to lose more than he or she gains. There is emphasis on fighting or not fighting as a choice with potential consequences that are important to consider when making the choice.

In addition to providing education on handling anger, the schools (at all levels) are appropriate for mediation activities. Such activities involve the use of peer mediators and teachers who are trained to recognize the signs of an escalating conflict and to interject mediation techniques. These programs have been successfully implemented at elementary school (using fourth and fifth graders), high school, and college levels.

The Violence Prevention Project

The Violence Prevention Project of the Boston Department of Health and Hospitals is a health education and information campaign to reduce the incidence of adolescent violent behavior through adult and peer training. Through outreach and education, this community-based primary prevention effort is endeavoring to change individual behavior and community attitudes about violence. A supportive network of secondary therapeutic services and a hospital-based secondary prevention service project directed toward patients with intentional injuries supplement the primary prevention activities to provide a comprehensive program. The project is modeled after other prevention initiatives that have focused on individual behavior modification through risk communication and education. This community-based model has been successfully used in the prevention of heart disease and hypertension (Farquhar, 1978).

Peer violence, family and domestic violence, and to some extent stranger violence are promoted by society's glamorous portrayal of violence. Some are more at risk, particularly those who have been victimized by or witnessed violence as children. This learned violent behavior can be changed, and public health, including health care providers, has a role to play.

Individual clinicians have many opportunities to incorporate violence prevention in their medical care. One such opportunity involves raising the issue of violence prevention as part of anticipatory guidance (Stringham & Weitzman, 1988). Because we know that violence is a learned behavior, parents can be enlisted to help prevent violent behavior in their children. Parents have daily opportunities to teach their children how to handle anger, such as by encouraging verbal rather than physical expression of angry feelings. With some guidance, parents, can play an active, conscious role in teaching their children positive, nonviolent strategies in directing and resolving their anger. Pediatric health providers can facilitate this process. Issues such as styles of discipline, regulating television viewing, and negotiating conflicts between siblings also can be addressed during pediatric encounters.

Designing violence prevention strategies that are effective with adolescents requires an understanding of adolescence and knowledge of the impact of race and poverty on development.

Adolescence

In the United States, adolescence is not only the period of dynamic physical maturation, but it is also a turbulent period of psychosocial maturation. The transition from childhood to adulthood includes many ambiguities and cultural dilemmas. The physical changes occur without mishap in a large majority of adolescents, yet the psychosocial ones frequently create problems. The psychosocial changes include both cognitive maturation from concrete to abstract thinking and the mastering of specific developmental tasks. The major developmental tasks are the following:

1. Individuation from family, with the development of same-sex and opposite-sex relationships outside the family
2. Adjustment to the physical changes of puberty, with the development of a healthy sexual identity
3. Development of a moral character and a personal value system
4. Preparation for future work and responsibility

These tasks are accomplished simultaneously, and their successful completion is a major requisite for healthy adulthood. The experience of poverty and of racism can significantly hinder the accomplishment of these essential tasks. The development of a healthy self-identity requires a sense of self-esteem and a healthy racial identity, both of which can be undermined by poverty and racism. Preparing for future work and responsibility is a meaningless enterprise when unemployment rates are astonishingly high. Developing a sense of moral character and a functional personal value system is also not easy, when television and the street are the main sources of values.

It is often difficult to determine what is normal behavior for adolescents. In the developmental assessment of children, there is a clear set of tasks and an age range for accomplishment. Children should sit up by a certain age and walk and talk before certain ages. Normal behavior for adolescents includes a variety of experimental behaviors that at other developmental stages would be abnormal. Defining what is normal is even more difficult in cases where there is a subcultural experience. In his book *Manchild in the Promised Land*, Brown (1965, p. 263) describes such an experience: "Throughout my childhood in Harlem, nothing was more strongly impressed upon me than the fact that you had to fight and that you should fight. Everybody would accept it if a person was scared to fight, but not if he was so scared that he didn't fight."

The example clearly illustrates the dilemma. How much fighting is too much? When is it problematic? Many would agree that violence in self-defense is appropriate, yet if a homicide results, would running not have been a better response? On the other hand, in a violent world, is it not healthier to defend oneself rather than be beaten or harassed?

There are several characteristics of adolescence that make a teenager more prone to violence. One such characteristic is narcissism. Narcissism helps the adolescent make the transition from family to the outside world. Yet this narcissism is also responsible for the extreme self-conscious feelings of adolescents that make them highly vulnerable to embarrassment. They feel that they are always in the limelight and on center stage. Adolescents are particularly sensitive to verbal attack, and it is nearly impossible for them to minimize or ignore embarrassing phenomena.

Peer pressure is the single most important determinant of adolescent behavior (Jessor & Jessor, 1977). This vulnerability to peer pressure is a normal part of adolescence. It is a necessary product of the separation from family and the development of a self-identity. Yet it is a characteristic of adolescence that increases the potential for violence. If fighting is the expectation of peers, as illustrated in the quotation from Brown (1965), then an adolescent is most unable to disregard those expectations.

Race and Poverty

Erikson (1968) describes a social moratorium from responsibility that is necessary during adolescence to allow the requisite experimental behavior to occur without compromise of future options. Thus, the adolescent is able to experiment with a variety of roles without making a commitment. There is debate as to whether this moratorium occurs at all, yet many agree that in the situation of poverty, it does not. The poor adolescent struggles with developmental tasks without the protection of a social moratorium.

The black adolescent has to develop a healthy racial identity in addition to the developmental tasks just mentioned. Contact with racism results in anger that appears to contribute to the overrepresentation of black youth in interpersonal violence. According to Akbar (1980), psychologist Lewis Ramey used "free floating anger" to describe anger not generated by a specific individual or event but stemming from global factors such as racism and limited employment options. This anger is the excess baggage that an individual brings to an encounter that lowers his threshold for directed anger and violence. This concept is helpful in that it attempts to account for the environmental and socioeconomic factors and does not blame the victim by labeling the individual as deficient. The anger is normal and appropriate. Violence prevention is therefore designed to achieve a healthier response to anger, not to eliminate the anger itself.

Violence prevention programs that are appropriate for adolescents developmentally and that have a realistic cultural context can be expected to be effective. Developmentally appropriate programs utilize peers in education and counseling and reflect an understanding of the stages of adolescent development. The cultural context has to acknowledge the violence, racism, and classism that many adolescents experience.

The problem of interpersonal violence has been long appreciated by front-line health providers, school administrators, teachers, and counselors.

Despite an incomplete understanding of the causal factors, prevention and intervention programs have been developed with moderate success. The majority of these prevention programs are either based in a school or linked to a school because teens are a captive audience. Most are interdisciplinary and multi-institutional.

Beyond the level of primary prevention, clinicians have the opportunity to play an important role in the early identification of youth at high risk for violent behavior. Work that has focused on identifying characteristics of persons who are victims or perpetrators of violence can be used to recognize potentially violent youth. School, community, and health care screening of children and youth for a history of family or peer violence, substance abuse, depression, and low self-esteem or carrying of weapons can lead to the identification of youth at risk. These youth may be helped through referral to early intervention programs.

This effort of primary care health providers must, of course, be linked to the increased development and availability of intervention services directed toward violent behavior. Merely identifying high-risk youth without appropriate referral resources would lead to considerable frustration on the part of clinicians. Educational, mental health, and support services for adolescents need to be enhanced, and intervention strategies addressing the underlying emotional and behavioral components of violence behavior must be developed.

Of equal importance is the need to modify the response of health care professionals to youth with intentional injuries. Health care institutions, particularly emergency departments, are the major site of contact with persons with violence-related problems. Diagnostic and intervention services for such events as rape, child and sexual abuse, and suicide attempts are well established in the medical setting, as are support services for children and families with these categories of problems. On the other hand, peer violence is generally managed by treating the injury itself without investigating or responding to the circumstances of the injury or the underlying issues and behaviors that may have led to the injury. It is a "stitch them up and send them out" approach to violence, which will not reduce the risk for future injury. Some patients who present as victims may be assailants in the future, because many intentional injury victims often explicitly express their intent to seek revenge (Dennis, 1980). In addition, there is evidence that victims are not necessarily passive in creating the violent encounter and may in fact display provocative behaviors that led to the injury-related event (Wolfgang, 1958).

The labeling of those involved in violence is arbitrary and inaccurate for many situations. Often the more injured person is labeled the victim and the other, the perpetrator. Because public health is not designed for blame and punishment, it can be free of the victim-perpetrator labels. Rather than responding to an event, public health professionals can determine associated risk factors and try to engage in prevention. Routine and adequate assessment of intentional injury victims is of extreme importance. This assessment should include efforts to understand the risk of subsequent violence as well as the individual patient's lifelong risk. Detailed information on the precipitating event, including information on the relationship between victim and perpetrator and causal factors, must be obtained. Minimal information includes the following (see Spivak, Prothrow-Stith, & Hausman, 1988, for further discussion):

1. Circumstances of the injury event
2. Victim's relationship to the assailant
3. Use of drugs or alcohol
4. Presence of underlying emotional or psychosocial risk factors (especially violence in the family)
5. History of intentional injuries or violent behaviors
6. Predisposing biological risk factors
7. Intent to seek revenge

In many cases, this information can help to identify a need for referral to appropriate intervention and support services that may reduce the risk of further problems.

Conclusion

Violence and homicide remain largely unaddressed by the current health care system. Yet it has become increasingly obvious that the health care system will need to play a larger role in society's efforts to prevent violence, for the following reasons:

1. Current criminal justice strategies are inapplicable to the acquaintance and family violence that accounts for half of the American homicides.
2. Current criminal justice strategies are not prevention strategies. Instead they are limited to responding to a violence episode once it occurs. The focus of this response is blame and punishment.
3. Health care providers have a tremendous amount of contact with those involved in violence.
4. The "stitch them up and send them out" response to violence is woefully inadequate; it is unlike the medical response to any other situation and possibly exacerbates the problem.
5. Prevention efforts used in health care for other problems related to behavior (heart disease, obesity, drunk driving, teen pregnancy) are models for similar efforts to prevent violence.

Understanding American violence as a health problem has tremendous policy implications for the health care system and other related service systems (schools, juvenile justice, social service). Increased awareness, understanding, and attention to violence by health care providers will contribute significantly to society's efforts to address this problem.

References

Akbar, N. (1980). Homicide among black males: Causal factors. *Public Health Reports*, *95*(6), 549

Alcohol, Drug Abuse, and Mental Health Administration. (1980). Symposium on homicide among black males. *Public Health Reports*, *95*(6), 549.

Baker, S. P., & Dietz, P. E. (1979). Injury prevention — interpersonal violence. In *Healthy people — The Surgeon General's Report on Health Promotion and Death Prevention Background papers* (DHEW Publication No. 79-55071A, pp. 71–74). Washington, DC.: U.S. Government Printing Office.

Barancik, J. I. (1983). Northeastern Ohio trauma study: I. Magnitude of the problem. *American Journal of Public Health*, *73*(7), 746–751.

Boston Commission on Safe Public Schools. (1983, November). *Making our schools safe for learning*. Boston: Boston Commission on Safe Public Schools.

Brown, C. (1965). *Manchild in the promised land*. New York: Macmillan.

Bureau of Alcohol, Tobacco and Firearms. (1991). *Firearm Census Report*. Washington, DC: U.S. Treasury Department.

Centers for Disease Control. (1983). Violent deaths among persons 15–24 years of age — United States, 1970–78. *Morbidity and Mortality Weekly Report*, *32*(35), 453–457.

Centerwall, B. (1984). Race, socioeconomic status, and domestic homicide, Atlanta 1971–72. *American Journal of Public Health*, *74*, 1813–1815.

Dennis, R. E. (1980). Homicide among black males: Social costs to families and communities. *Public Health Reports*, *95*, 556

Erikson, E. (1968). *Identity, youth, and crisis*. New York: Norton.

Farquhar, J. (1978). The community-based model of life style interventions. *American Journal of Epidemiology*, *108*, 103–111.

Jessor, R., & Jessor, S. L. (1977). *Problem behavior and psychosocial development: A longitudinal study of youth*. New York: Academic Press.

Johnson, C. J., Carter, A., Harlin, V., & Zoller, G. (1974). Student injuries due to aggressive behavior in the Seattle public schools during the school year 1969–70. *American Journal of Public Health*, *64*, 904.

Joint Center for Policy Studies. (1985). A fighting chance for black youth. *Focus*, *13*(9), 4.

Koop, C. E. (1986). *Surgeon General's workshop on violence and public health* (DHHS Publication No. HRS-D-MC 86-1, pp. 35–43). Washington, DC: U.S. Government Printing Office.

Prothrow-Stith, D. (1986). Interdisciplinary interventions applicable to prevention of interpersonal violence and homicide in black youth. In *Surgeon General's Workshop on Violence and Public Health* (DHHS Publication No.

HRS-D-MC 86-1, pp. 35–43). Washington, DC: U.S. Government Printing Office.

Prothrow-Stith, D. (1987). *Violence prevention curriculum for adolescents*. Newton, MA: Education Development Center.

Prothrow-Stith, D., Spivak, H., & Hausman, A. J. (1987). The violence prevention project: A public health approach. *Science, Technology, and Human Values, 12*(3 & 4), 67–69.

Prothrow-Stith, D., & Weissman, M. (1991). *Deadly consequences*. New York: HarperCollins.

Spivak, H., Prothrow-Stith, D., & Hausman, A. (1988). Dying is no accident: Adolescent violence and intentional injury. *Pediatric Clinics of North America, 35*(6), 1339–1348.

Stringham, P., & Weitzman, M. (1988). Violence counseling in the routine health care of adolescents. *Journal of Adolescent Health Care, 9*, 389–393.

Wolfgang, M. E. (1958). *Patterns in criminal homicide*. New York: Wiley.

Wolfgang, M. E. (1986). Homicide in other industrialized countries. *Bulletin of the New York Academy of Medicine, 62*(5), 400–412.

PART III

Infants, Youth, and Late Adulthood

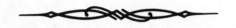

12

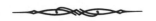

Homeless Women
with Children

Aisha Gilliam

The major purposes of this chapter are threefold: to provide an assessment of current knowledge on the health of homeless black women, to provide a model for treatment services for homeless women based on preliminary research findings, and to propose a research agenda as well as implications for policy. The needs of the homeless in general have generated serious concern; however, the needs of the most disadvantaged sectors of this population—women with children (of whom a vast majority are minorities)—have not received the attention warranted.

Research has suggested that poor women and women of color face many social and economic barriers in their attempts to integrate into the dominant culture, problems that are exacerbated by poor health status. Traditional rigid demarcations between investigations of health, mental status, and work and family roles have generated a limited model of women's health. Women's health is best examined by studying the complex interrelationships between the health of women and their social, political, and cultural situations (Paltiel, 1988).

Socioeconomic dimensions, including the multiple role responsibilities within the family and psychosocial factors (such as chronic life stresses and lack of social support) are critical to an understanding of the health status of poor and minority women, including homeless women representative of both categories. The emerging picture suggests that the lowest income groups are more likely to suffer negative effects of risky behavior (alcohol, drug, or tobacco use) generally undertaken as a source of comfort or relief from stressful lives. While access to money is no guarantee of mental health, and its absence does not necessarily lead to mental illness, it is generally conceded that poverty can be a determinant and a consequence of poor mental health (Langer & Michael, 1963). More effective coping behavior might require an investment in time, energy, knowledge, and money that is beyond the capacity of poverty-stricken individuals.

African-American women are disproportionately represented among the poor and the homeless. In 1983, 47 percent of all African-American families were headed by women, and over half had incomes below the poverty level, compared to 30 percent for all female-headed households and 7 percent for the nation's two-parent households. Recent studies indicate that an overwhelming majority of homeless families in major cities are headed by single females of color having as their major source of income Aid to Families with Dependent Children — substantially under the poverty level (Roth & Fox, 1990; Hu, Covell, Morgan, & Arcia, 1989).

Review of Literature on the Homeless

Researchers have estimated that homeless women make up between 18 and 25 percent of the homeless population and that the numbers will continue to increase (Bachrach, 1987; Bassuk, Rubin, & Lauriat, 1986; Ropers & Boyer, 1987). This growing population of women has been described as being unable to form and maintain stable relationships, as having poor or nonexistent work histories, and as having experienced difficulties in parenting (Bassuk, 1986). This group is comprised of young and middle-aged (seventeen- to forty-nine-year-old) single women and their children. Single-parent families have been estimated to comprise more than 20 percent of the total homeless population (Bassuk et al., 1986). These single-parent families are increasingly susceptible to situations that exacerbate poverty, such as lack of education, inadequate job skills, lack of job opportunities, poor health, and racism (Lauriat, 1986; Bassuk et al., 1986). Investigators have also found that a large percentage of homeless families were minorities who received some type of federal aid, experienced relationship problems, and tended to reside within their own communities for two or more years (Ropers & Boyer, 1987).

Alcohol and Other Drugs

The results of recent research on the prevalence of alcohol and other drugs among the homeless population indicate that 30 percent of homeless people have alcohol problems and an additional 10 percent or more have histories of other drug use (Wright, Knight, Weber-Burdin, & Lam, 1987; Milburn, 1989). The use of alcohol and other drugs by homeless persons often leads to acute and chronic physical disorders. Homeless individuals experience inordinately high rates of respiratory ailments, trauma, cardiovascular disease, and diseases directly linked to alcohol and other drugs (Filardo, 1985; Wright et al., 1987). Persons of low economic status who have a problem with alcohol and other drugs are at especially high risk for homelessness. Individuals with alcohol and other drug problems face physical and psychiatric disorders that further contribute to the problem of homelessness (Gilliam, Scott, & Thomas, 1989).

Stress, Social Support, and Health

Studies have revealed that unmarried women are more vulnerable to life stresses, economic stress, and social isolation than men are (Aneshensel, 1986). Thus, they are more likely to develop depression. In addition, Aneshensel notes that parental responsibilities can compound other sources of stress, such as unemployment, lack of housing, and health concerns. Lazarus (1984) provides some clues to the coping styles of the poor and women by recognizing denial as a palliative form of coping. Denial, as a form of selective inattention or escapism, may be healthy in one context but risky and even life threatening in another, when it interferes with actions necessary to survival or constructive change.

In reference to stress and coping behavior, Antonovsky (1979) has coined the term *salutogenesis*, which means a sense of coherence among individuals and groups involving a perception of one's environment as predictable and comprehensible. The stronger people's sense of coherence, he argues, the more adequately they will cope with the eminent stressors in life and the more likely they are to maintain their position on the health continuum. For poor homeless African-American women, the lack of housing and the movement from one shelter or relative to another entail adjusting to new individuals with varying rules and regulations, possibly creating an environment with a lack of coherence and unpredictability of daily life situations. The death of a relative or close friend, employment loss or changes in living or housing conditions, changes in marital status, and changes in numbers of family members in households (Holmes & Rahe, 1967) are other stressful life events that are daily occurrences in the homeless population (Muhlenkamp & Sayles, 1986). Prolonged stress can cause a breakdown in coping mechanisms (Holmes & Rahe, 1967), which is a common occurrence among the homeless.

Empirical evidence increasingly suggests a positive relationship between social networks and social support, and physical and mental health as a means to understand the relationship of homeless persons to contextual factors (Israel & Rounds, 1987). For example, Linn (1986) maintains that lack of social support is associated with a decline in self-reported health status as well as lower self-esteem and that promoting social support to improve the health and well-being of a large number of women may be more feasible than trying to reduce stressors. In addition, peer support may provide individuals with empathy and understanding that professionals cannot offer. Other researchers have shown social support to be an important factor in the maintenance of well-being, in decisions to engage in help-seeking behaviors (Dohrenwend & Dohrenwend, 1984), and in decreasing the adverse effects of life stressors. Wilcox (1981) also observed that group membership was a significant indicator of positive health practices and that social support that existed in groups was reflected in high levels of self-esteem. Although social support has a demonstrated relationship to mental health, further investigation is needed to examine the relationship between mental health, social support, and social network characteristics. For example, there may be different forms of social support and networks, such as social programs and social services (Bassuk et al., 1986) or informal networks of kin and friends (Lovell, 1988) that can be perceived, valued, or utilized differently by individuals or groups.

Interventions

There is little research on interventions for homeless women, particularly homeless African-American women. From a practical perspective, the needs of this group can be addressed through methods that have worked with women living under stressful conditions in various settings. These include alleviation of anxiety, reduction of and desensitization to stressful conditions, goal clarification and development of awareness of alternatives through building self-esteem and self-efficacy, and exposure to problem-solving techniques in making decisions about parenting and seeking employment and housing (Berman-Rossi & Cohen, 1988; Breton, 1988; Gilliam et al., 1989).

In one study of homeless women in hotels in New York City, Chavkin, Kristal, Seabron, & Guigli (1987) offered intervention for improving the mental and physical health status of homeless women. They noted that these women delivered infants of lower birth weight than women in the general population. Recommendations from this study included on-site health education accompanied by on-site health care, and social services such as income maintenance and nutrition supplementation. In his work with depressed patients, Crockett (1986) outlined four phases of a process that resulted in more positive affect and increased self-efficacy for patients over the course of a few months: venting anger and frustration, agreeing to behavioral contracts, becoming motivated to change by using imagery exercises, and developing social and negotiation skills in order to gain more control over the environment.

Additionally, research on the prevention of AIDS among drug abusing women indicates that increasing self-reliance, communication skills, assertiveness, and problem-solving skills and utilizing peer groups are effective approaches for supporting behavioral change among women (Williams, 1986; Mondanaro, 1987). These strategies are similar to those offered by Breton (1988) and Berman-Rossi & Cohen (1988), where a high degree of shared needs and the potential for mutual aid have been found to be particularly strong and helpful to this client population.

Depression in Women

Maternal and child well-being have been found to be influenced by such factors as depression (Brown & Harris, 1978), chronic stress (Holmes & Rahe,

1967), and lack of social support (Kessler, Price, & Wortman, 1985). Seligman (1974) links helplessness to the sociological reality of powerlessness, and depression in women to women's perception of powerlessness in society—a feeling that action is futile. Contrary to many other theorists, Seligman maintains that it is not the loss of reinforcement, but the loss of control over reinforcement that causes depression. The prevention of learned helplessness depends on the person's previous experiences in mastering reinforcements in his or her own behavior. People who have been victimized with few opportunities to change their uncomfortable situation are particularly susceptible to depression. According to the sociopsychological explanation for depression, we could expect to find the highest rates of depression among the group of people who experience the greatest number of stressful life demands and at the same time the fewest actual possibilities for mastery of them. Homeless African Americans represent such a group who have few experiences in gaining mastery over their environment. It is no wonder that rates of depression are high among this group (Gilliam et al., 1989).

Several studies have measured the significance of specific aspects of social support in the development of depressive symptoms in both general and at-risk populations (Israel & Rounds, 1987; Kessler et al., 1985). This research indicates that individuals with low social support are at much greater risk for the development of depressive symptoms. Flaherty, Gaviria, Black, Altman, & Mitchell (1983) have provided data showing that social support factors have considerably greater predictive power for depressive symptoms than does measurement of life events. Thus, one can conclude that homeless African-American women—especially those who have endured the most difficult conditions for long periods—are at great risk for depressive symptoms, anxiety, and poor self-esteem.

Empowerment and Self-Esteem

Empowerment has surfaced as a recurrent theme in the literature on planning and implementation of successful programs for the homeless. Gross and Rosenberg (1987) define empowerment as increasing influence over one's life circumstances and decisions. Approaches using this definition are directed at influencing individuals to take a more responsible and assertive role in determining their own actions in various situations. Some programs stress a "step-by-step" self-management process for empowerment, in which the participants learn techniques of self-observation, goal setting, imaging, modeling, considering alternatives, rehearsal, feedback, and behavior shaping (Gilliam, Scott, & Troup, 1988; Gilliam, Hollander, & Overby, 1990).

Groups for building social supports and assisting in the decision-making process have been used in work with the homeless (Martin & Neyowith, 1988). This process involves women meeting together in a supportive atmosphere where they examine their own experiences as women. The outcomes of consciousness-raising groups include increases in self-esteem and decreases in guilt, self-hatred, and feelings of inadequacy; improved intellectual and personal autonomy; increased sense of community with other women; and a reduction in feelings of loneliness, isolation, and alienation.

Health and Functioning of African-American Women

The traditional value system of black America has promoted the black woman as caring, nurturing, loving, and fighting for black men and their children. This has included a strong work ethic in order to provide for themselves and family members. Historically, African-American women have had to respond to distorted and debilitating images of themselves projected by the popular media and rooted in a society steeped in racism. Today, more than one-third of single mothers with children under the age of six have incomes below the poverty line (Ladner, 1971; Pearce & McAdoo, 1981). Given this state of affairs, it is no coincidence that African-American single-parent families are disproportionately represented among the homeless.

The psychological implications and consequences of this phe-nomenon of poverty and homelessness are great, since most homeless African-American women with children are poor single heads of households. In her social essay, Bennett (1987) writes that each of these circumstances can engender stress. The stresses of being single are aggravated by the demands of motherhood, a role that is complex and demanding even under the best economic and social conditions. The situation is more difficult for poor women with limited financial and social resources. For the woman who finds herself homeless with children, the demands, responsibilities, and strains and stresses of motherhood can become overwhelming. If they are not dealt with, the consequences can often result in child abuse and neglect that can range from verbal to physical assault (Gilliam et al., 1989). If the circum-stances are resolved positively or if there is adequate coping, the woman can enjoy mental health. If they are not resolved or resolved negatively, she may experience emotional distress or even mental illness.

One of the strongest black cultural patterns is that of extensive help systems. This social network provides emotional support, mutual aid, eco-nomic supplements, social interaction, and protection of the family's integ-rity from assault by the external environment (Billingsley, 1968; Hill, 1972). This supportive network is especially essential to the mother rearing children alone where needs are extensive and go beyond individual resources (McAdoo, 1980). Homeless women with children often find themselves out-side this network for a host of reasons, some having contributed to their homelessness. Many of these homeless mothers may be suffering from lim-ited positive life experiences, few experiences with success, and a legacy of poverty with limited visions of future possibilities for their children. For homeless black women with children, the situation is made more difficult because of the inability to provide positive male role models and because of their own loss of status as a role model due to the inability to provide housing for their family.

African-American women share a disproportionately large responsibility for the care, nurturing, and support of themselves and their children. These are the same women who are in the poorest health themselves, are likely to experience the greatest psychologically induced symptoms or illnesses, and are likely to face the highest medical risks, particularly during pregnancy and childbirth (U.S. Department of Health and Human Services, 1985). At each step of the way, the homeless African-American woman is faced with complex responsibilities. She often encounters multiple barriers while being responsible for maintaining wellness and preventing illness for her family under socioeconomic conditions that promote mental and physical illness. Zambrana (1988) points out that poor women and women of color must sort out those health concerns that are more appropriately alleviated through traditional support, such as information and assistance from family and community, and those that are best served by modern medicine and institutional providers. She must learn how the health care system is organized, where to seek appropriate care, and how to linguistically and culturally translate her concerns into information that will be meaningful to health professionals.

A Study of Homeless African-American Women

The study described in the following paragraphs was undertaken as part of an evaluation to determine the needs of the changing population of homeless women in a shelter in the Washington, D.C., metropolitan area. The major objective was to make recommendations for implementing program changes, deletions, or additions to the services offered by the shelter.

Methodology

The focus of this study was to describe the characteristics of 337 homeless women with children residing in a shelter located in metropolitan Washington, D.C. Particular emphasis was placed on characteristics related to physical and mental health status, health care utilization, relationships between physical abuse and substance abuse, and health status of homeless women. In addition, this study explored other needs, such as restoration and maintenance of social functioning among homeless women with children.

Data were collected by shelter staff from records maintained on each resident. Records included results of the Beck Depression Scale and the State and Trait Anxiety Scales collected on each woman when she entered the shelter. Records also reflected residents' cooperation and adherence to shelter rules (as measured by a ten-item Likert-type social function scale), participation in training and location of permanent housing programs, medical concerns, health care and emergency room utilization, and social problems such as histories of physical and substance abuse.

Subjects included a sample of predominately African-American women (99 percent), with a mean age of 25.6 (range 18–55). Educational background ranged from less than a high school education ($N = 135$) to some college education ($N = 41$ or 14 percent); 3 percent were college graduates. Fifty-four percent were dependent upon public assistance, while only 19 percent were employed while they lived in the shelter. The number of children residing in the shelter with their mothers ranged from zero to six. Slightly more than 50 percent of the women had one child in the shelter, whereas close to 40 percent had two children.

Findings

Findings from this study are consistent with much of the previous literature. Reported here are findings related to health care utilization. Results from analysis of depression, anxiety, and social functioning follow.

Health Care Utilization. The women who participated in this study remained in the shelter for an average of 74.3 days. The mean average number of days was 40.5 in 1984 and 90 in 1989, representing a steady increase throughout the five years covered by this study. The number of hospital and emergency room visits made by residents and their children was used as a measure of health status. A total of seventy-five women, 22 percent of the study population, had made at least one hospital/emergency room visit. Twenty-six percent ($N = 87$) of these women had a history of physical abuse. Twenty-three, or 30 percent, of these women had a history of drug abuse. It is also important to note that 30 percent ($N = 101$) of the study population had children who were hospitalized or visited the emergency room.

Depression, Anxiety, and Social Functioning. Results from analysis of a social function scale (alpha = .88) demonstrated that women who had histories of drug abuse ($N = 75$) had lower mean scores (mean = 31.64, SD = 6.9) when compared to the 182 women with no history of substance abuse (mean = 34.18, SD = 7.02). No significant differences were found on the Beck Depression Scale and the State/Trait Anxiety Inventory. However, it should be noted that the overall mean Beck Depression Scale score was 15.2 (mild to moderate depression), the State Anxiety Inventory score was 80.2, and the Trait Anxiety score was 78.2. These results suggest that the study population experienced mild to moderate depression and elevated levels of anxiety on entering the shelter. These findings have implications for the need to provide coping skills and parenting skills as an integral part of health education services in the shelter.

Child abuse and child neglect have been documented among mothers who are experiencing a great deal of stress and who have low self-esteem.

Therefore, an attempt was made to measure the incidence of child abuse in this homeless population. While child abuse and neglect are common in this population, further research is needed to determine the relationship among these variables and the health and social functioning of homeless women.

Recommendations

The findings of this study corroborate those in the literature that emphasize the higher incidence of depression among homeless women, a condition that strongly impacts on social functioning. Over a fourth of the women in the sample have a history of physical abuse (26 percent), which erodes self-esteem and contributes further to feelings of helplessness that women experience. In addition, the results indicate that those with a history of physical abuse scored lower on the social functioning scale, which may in fact be related to the high degree of depression among this group. The incidence of substance abuse can be evaluated in the context of maladaptive coping when there is an inability to effectively deal with the stresses and strains of poverty, motherhood, and homelessness, compounded by the problem of abusive relationships. Women who have been abused are at risk for abusing their children; thus, one sees the occurrence of child abuse and neglect in this population as a situation exacerbated by homelessness.

The Model

Based on the findings of the study just described (Gilliam et al., 1988, 1990), a model was developed to do the following:

- Help homeless women overcome the dysfunctional consequences of substance abuse, especially abuse of alcohol.
- Provide training in negotiation and conflict resolution skills to help homeless women gain more control over their environment and to overcome the dysfunctional consequences of physical abuse.
- Provide a forum for developing problem solving and alternative means of discipline as necessary parts of the parenting skills needed in this population.
- Provide opportunities that are self-reinforced in order to increase self-esteem and self-efficacy.
- Increase the likelihood of self-health action for improving the health of women and their children.

Description of Model

The proposed model is interactive and seeks to provide a framework for designing programs and activities to address key issues identified in the literature and clinical factors pertinent to working with homeless women and children. The model consists of five dimensions that are dynamically interrelated and interdependent; thus, it is known as the *S-5 model*. These dimensions are social support, self-esteem, self-efficacy, stress reduction, and self-health action (see Figure 12.1). The model has been successfully used to develop a comprehensive program for serving the needs of homeless women with children. Such a program will typically include a relocation component; a counseling component; weekly women's support groups; weekly health education groups; a day-care component with parent counseling and parent training; and resource networking where women are empowered to advocate on their behalf.

The first dimension of the S-5 model is *social support*. It is based on the premise that social ties are important to social adjustment. Old ties should be explored and new ties developed to facilitate positive relationships with significant others, thereby reinforcing social acceptance. Nurturing that may be received from significant others (for example, kinship members, peers, or health personnel) may serve as a reinforcing factor in the maintenance of healthful attitudes and behaviors.

The second dimension is *self-esteem* and is buttressed by the internalization of social acceptance. Moreover, social acceptance is needed to pursue self-adjustment, because lack of acceptance and identity turmoil can hinder personal motivation to change. Attachment has a supportive role for both adults and children (Bowlby, 1969); it increases the likelihood of developing social skills as well as promoting a degree of satisfaction that motivates people to change their condition.

The third dimension of the S-5 model is *self-efficacy*. Self-efficacy, or the evaluation of one's actions as positive and worthwhile, builds on the development of (1) social strengths—which are necessary to establish and maintain close relationships; (2) intellectual strengths—which include the ability to learn, understand, and make sound decisions and which are necessary to be successful in tasks and occupations; (3) emotional strengths—which include inner strength to deal constructively with one's own feelings and those of others and the ability to achieve one's goals; (4) spiritual strengths—which are important in understanding values, improving self, and contributing to the human condition with concern and empathy; and (5) physical strengths—which include the ability to maintain health, stamina, and physical attractiveness. The three components already mentioned (S-1–S-3) represent program activities designed to impact the stressors in one's life.

The fourth dimension of the S-5 model is *stress reduction*. This component of the model deals with the ability of the individual to handle stress on different levels, so that it does not become overwhelming and lead to feelings of powerlessness and meaninglessness. Stress can occur as a result of social disadvantages and lack of social support. It can also be compounded by previous experiences that influence the individual's interpretation of life events and by social isolation, social rejection, and status inconsistency

Figure 12.1. Conceptual Model for Health and Social Functioning of Minority Homeless Women with Children.

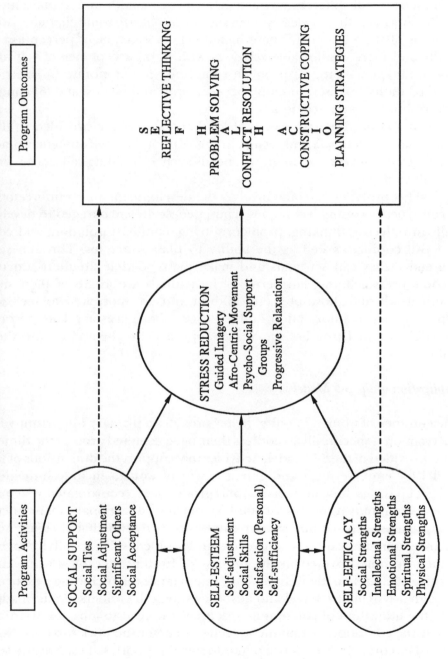

(Selye, 1974; Lazarus, 1984). The stress reduction component also includes specific intervention parameters, as detailed in the oval (see Figure 12.1).

The fifth dimension of the model is *self-health action*. Maslow (1982) identified several different characteristics of self-health and actualization. Those working with homeless women should emphasize some characteristics in terms of the S-5 model. These include (1) more efficient perception of reality and more comfortable relations with it, (2) acceptance of self and others, (3) spontaneity, (4) problem centering, (5) autonomy, (6) interpersonal relations, (7) discrimination between ends and means, and (8) continued freshness of appreciation.

In a home, the basic needs of food and shelter are provided so that individuals can feel safe and secure. In this supportive environment, women can begin to concentrate on growth needs such as building self-esteem and self-sufficiency.

This program outcome involves the development and reinforcement of constructive coping techniques. Thus, people are encouraged to develop skills in reflective thinking, problem solving, conflict resolution, and constructive coping, as well as the ability to plan strategies. Through self-awareness, they can set goals and make plans so that situations do not become overwhelming. Furthermore, individuals are aware of their own health needs and those of their children and are motivated to seek the appropriate help, information, and resources when necessary. They become positively attuned to a holistic health approach for themselves and their children.

Application of the S-5 Model

The entrance of women into the shelter provides a primary opportunity for intervention — specifically to address their need centered around the dimensions provided in the S-5 model. Activities that support the dimensions of the model for empowerment and enhancement of women include individual and group counseling, women's support groups, and a coordinated system to utilize community resources for employment and educational enhancement. Comprehensive programs should emphasize activities that increase self-reliance, communication, assertiveness, and problem-solving skills by having women become involved in the process of finding housing and making positive changes in their lives. The importance of including resources through a system of referral and advocacy should be underscored. In addition, the utilization of community resources can lead to jobs, job training, and/or the educational attainment needed to enter the work force.

The converging evidence points to social support, self-esteem and self-efficacy as variables that mediate between stressful life events and the ability to cope. The model identifies these as important components to be included when planning any comprehensive program for homeless women with children. For instance, developing parenting skills through training classes that include involvement of mothers as day-care aides in settings where their children are placed is one way to increase mothers' self-efficacy in parenting (Gilliam et al., 1988). This interactive model to increase self-health action requires that social, behavioral, and environmental variables be clearly defined and examined both in designing activities and in evaluating their effectiveness. Input from the women is important and feedback is necessary at each step of the way to ensure appropriateness as well as cultural and regional sensitivity. Participation by the women and responsibility for setting individual goals (as in a counseling component) and a group agenda (for example, in a support group) allows for growth, self-esteem building, and group cohesiveness. By utilizing the extensive time spent in the shelter system to enhance their skills, women who do find housing are more able to effectively maintain that outcome and reduce the revolving door to the shelter system.

Implications

African-American homeless women with children represent a portion of the homeless population with a broad array of problems and needs. Studies have consistently cited the lack of affordable housing as a major precipitating factor. The present study illustrates that many of the problems of homeless women with children are brought on as a result of a cycle of poverty, with homelessness as the end result. Contributing to the homeless problem for single women and their dependent children is a lack of adequate housing, unemployment, and decreasing federal income combined with inflation (Kozol, 1988). Therefore, policies that provide financial support for housing emergencies may help prevent families from becoming homeless.

Because of the differing needs of the homeless population, policies that emphasize prevention, comprehensiveness in service delivery, and collaboration are needed. These policies should address prevention through income support programs, the provision of low-income housing, basic skills training programs, and health service delivery. Programming developed to serve the homeless population must address the effects of homelessness on children. Homelessness helps to perpetuate the underclass and poverty. For the cycle to be broken, government, private foundations, and business must work together to develop and implement innovative programs aimed at reducing risks to these children, as well as educational programs that emphasize skill development and esteem building such as that put forth in the S-5 model.

Further research is needed to understand access issues to health care among poor and minority women; socioeconomic, cultural, and systemic factors must also be considered. For example, homeless minority women with children may be handicapped by a lack of education, information, and health insurance. While an increasing number of studies point to a relationship between health status and social roles, class and cultural variables as causal factors remain poorly understood aspects of the health behavior of low-income and minority women. Therefore, these need to be further investigated. Researchers also need to become aware of the situational factors that affect poor women's health status.

Analytical frameworks such as the Health Belief Model (Hochbaum, 1958; Rosenstock, 1960, 1966, 1974a, 1974b; Becker, 1974) and Aday and colleagues' Access to Care Model (1980) — developed to examine preventive health behavior — have emerged from the study of the dominant-culture middle-class populations. Therefore, models that interpret data in meaningful ways must expand their parameters to take into account clearly defined socioeconomic, cultural, racial, and regional variables that address the relationship between health status, social functioning, chronic life stress, social support, work status, and occupational history. Social and environmental variables must be clearly defined and examined, both in designing studies and in interpreting the data on poor and minority populations. Models such as the S-5 model need to be further tested so that there is more information about their applicability as interventions for sustained behavioral change. Moreover, this author emphasizes the need to design comprehensive programming to enhance women's sense of self-worth, particularly as a strategy for helping them retain housing. Overall, applied models that give guidance to the design and implementation of programs are as essential as those that provide theoretical frameworks for understanding, broadening, and reforming the conceptualization of women's situations and the frameworks from which they operate.

Conclusion

The recognition that homeless women have special needs beyond the need for housing is not new. The proposed schema for positive health action is based on a distillation of salient studies presented in the literature as well as experiences in working with homeless women in the metropolitan area of the District of Columbia. Research should seek to look at the relationships of the variables outlined by the S-5 model, with particular emphasis on comprehensive programs that work and that empower women to maintain housing by developing the necessary skills to function in society. In addition, political, social, and economic actions will be required to alleviate poverty and thereby have an impact on the abundance of health problems that afflict homeless African-American women and their children.

References

Aday, L. A., Andersen, R., & Fleming, G. V. (1980). *Health care in the U.S.: Equitable for whom?* Newbury Park, CA: Sage.

Aneshensel, C. S. (1986). Marital and employment role-strain, social support, and depression among adult women. In S. E. Hobfoll (Ed.), *Stress, social support, and women* (pp. 99–114). Washington, DC: Hemisphere.

Antonovsky, A. (1979). *Health, stress, and coping: New perspectives on mental and physical well-being*. San Francisco: Jossey-Bass.

Bachrach, L. L. (1987). Homeless women: A context for health planning. *Millbank Quarterly, 65,* 391–396.

Bassuk, E. L. (1986). Homeless families: Single mothers and their children in Boston shelters. In E. L. Bassuk (Ed.), *The mental health needs of homeless persons* (pp. 45–53). San Francisco: Jossey-Bass.

Bassuk, E. L., Rubin, L., & Lauriat, A. S. (1986). Characteristics of sheltered homeless families. *American Journal of Public Health, 76,* 1097–1101.

Becker, M. H. (1974). (Ed.). The Health Belief Model and personal health behavior. *Health Education Monographs, 2,* 326–327.

Bennett, M.B.H., (1987). Afro-American women, poverty and mental health: A social essay. *Women and Health, 12*(3/4), 213–229.

Berman-Rossi, T., & Cohen, M. B. (1988). Group development and shared decision making: Working with homeless mentally ill women. *Social Work with Groups, 11*(4), 47–61.

Billingsley, A. (1968). *Black families in white America*. Englewood Cliffs, NJ: Prentice-Hall.

Boone, M. S. (1982). A socio-medical study of infant mortality among disadvantaged blacks. *Human Organization, 41*(3), 227–236.

Bowlby, J. (1969). *Attachment and loss*. New York: Basic Books.

Breton, M. (1988). The need for mutual aid groups in a drop-in center for homeless women: The sistering case. *Social Work with Groups, 11*(4), 63–78.

Brown, G. W., & Harris, T. (1978). *Social origins of depression*. New York: Free Press.

Chavkin, W., Kristal, A., Seabron, C., & Guigli, P. E. (1987). The reproductive experience of women living in hotels for the homeless in New York City. *New York State Journal of Medicine, 87*(1), 10–12.

Crockett, M. S. (1986). Depression: A case of anger and alienation. *American Journal of Nursing, 86*(3), 294–298.

Dohrenwend, B. S., & Dohrenwend, B. P. (1984). Life stress and illness: Formulation of the issues. In B. S. Dohrenwend & B. P. Dohrenwend (Eds.), *Stressful life events and their contexts*. New Brunswick, NJ: Rutgers University Press.

Filardo, T. (1985). Chronic disease management in the homeless. In P. Brickner (Ed.), *Health care of homeless people*. New York: Springer.

Flaherty, J., Gaviria, M., Black, E., Altman, E., & Mitchell, T. (1983). The role of social support in the functioning of patients with unipolar depression. *American Journal of Psychiatry, 140*(4), 473–476.

Gilliam, A., Hollander, R., & Overby, L. (1990). The use of relaxation techniques, guided imagery, and Afro-centric movement to reduce stress and increase body image in homeless women. Unpublished report, Howard University, School of Graduate Studies, Washington, DC.

Gilliam, A., Scott, M., & Thomas, S. B. (1989, October). *Health and social functioning of minority homeless women with children: Implications for program development*. A research presentation on the effects of poverty, substance abuse, and homelessness on the health and health care of women and their children. American Public Health Association, Chicago.

Gilliam, A., Scott, M., & Troup, J. (1988). *Health education needs and social functioning of homeless women and their children* (technical report). Hyattsville, MD: Institute of Minority Health and Human Development.

Gross, T. P., & Rosenberg, M. L. (1987). Shelters for battered women and their children: An under-recognized source of communicable disease transmission. *American Journal of Public Health, 77*, 1198–1201.

Hill, R. (1972). *The strength of black families*. Washington, DC: National Urban League.

Hochbaum, G. M. (1958). Public participation in medical screening programs: A sociopsychological study (PHS Publication No. 572). Washington, DC: U.S. Government Printing Office.

Holmes, T. H., & Rahe, R. H. (1967). The social readjustment rating scale. *Journal of Psychosomatic Research, 11*(2), 213–218.

Hu, O. J., Covell, R. M., Morgan, J., & Arcia, J. (1989). Health care needs of children of the recently homeless. *Journal of Community Health, 14*(1), 2–10.

Israel, B. A., & Rounds, K. A. (1987). Social networks and social support: A synthesis for health educators. *Advances in Health Education and Promotion, 2*, 311–351.

Kessler, R., Price, R., & Wortman, C. (1985). Social factors in psychopathology: Stress, social support, and mental health in community samples. In L. Syme (Ed.), *Social support and health* (pp. 83–103). San Diego, CA: Academic Press.

Kozol, J. (1988). *Rachel and her children: Homeless families in America*. New York: Crown.

Ladner, J. A. (1971). *Tomorrow's tomorrow: The black woman*. New York: Doubleday.

Langer, T. S., & Michael, S. T. (1963). *Life stress and mental health*. London: Collier-Macmillan.

Lauriat, A. L. (1986). Sheltering homeless families: Beyond an emergency response. In E. L. Bassuk (Ed.), *The mental health needs of homeless persons* (pp. 87–94). San Francisco: Jossey-Bass.

Lazarus, R. S. (1984). The costs and benefits of denial. In B. S. Dohrenwend & B. P. Dohrenwend (Eds.), *Stressful life events and their contexts*. New Brunswick, NJ: Rutgers University Press.

Linn, M. W. (1986). Elderly women's health and psychological adjustment: Life stressors and social support. In S. E. Hobfoll (Ed.), *Stress, social support, and women* (pp. 223–233). Washington, DC: Hemisphere.

Lovell, A. M. (1988, November). *Networks, mental health status, and the context of homelessness in New York City*. Paper presented at the 116th annual meeting of the American Public Health Association, Boston.

McAdoo, H. P. (1980). Black mothers and the extended family support network. In La Frances Rodger-Rose (Ed.), *The black woman*. Newbury Park, CA: Sage.

Martin, M. A., & Neyowith, S. A. (1988). Creating community: Group work to develop social support networks with homeless mentally ill. *Social Work with Groups, 11*(4), 79–93.

Maslow, A. H. (1982). *Towards a psychology of being* (2nd ed.). New York: Van Nostrand Reinhold.

Maza, P. L., & Hall, J. A. (1988). *Homeless children and their families: A preliminary study*. Washington, DC: Child Welfare League of America.

Milburn, N. (1989). Drug abuse among the homeless. In J. Momeni (Ed.), *Homeless in the United States* (Vol. 11). Westport, CT: Greenwood Press.

Mondanaro, J. (1987). Strategies for AIDS prevention: Motivating health behavior in drug dependent women. *Journal of Psychoactive Drugs, 19*(2), 143–149.

Muhlenkamp, A. F., and Sayles, J. A. (1986). Self-esteem, social support and positive health practices. *Nursing Research, 35*(6), 334–338.

Paltiel, F. L. (1988). Is being poor a mental health hazard? *Women and Health, 12*(3,4) 189–211.

Pearce, D., & McAdoo, H. P. (1981). *Women and children: Alone in poverty.* (Monograph). Washington, DC: National Advisory Council on Economic Opportunity.

Ropers, R. H., & Boyer, R. (1987). Perceived health status among the new urban homeless. *Social Science and Medicine, 24*, 669–678.

Rosenstock, I. M. (1960). What research in motivation suggests for public health. *American Journal of Public Health, 50*, 295–301.

Rosenstock, I. M. (1966). Why people use health services. *Milbank Memorial Fund Quarterly, 44*(3), 94-124.

Rosenstock, I. M. (1974a). The Health Belief Model and preventive health behavior. *Health Education Monographs, 2*(4), 354–386.

Rosenstock, I. M. (1974b). Historical origins of the Health Belief Model. *Health Education Monographs, 2*, 354–386.

Roth, L., & Fox, E. R. (1990). Children of homeless families: Health status and access to health care. *Journal of Community Health, 15*(4), 275–284.

Seligman, M. (1974). Depression and learned helplessness. In R. J. Freedman & M. Katz (Eds.), *The psychology of depression: Contemporary theory and research.* Washington, DC: Winston & Sons.

Selye, H. (1974). *Stress without distress*. Philadelphia: Lippincott.

U.S. Department of Health and Human Services. (1985). *Report of the Secretary's Task Force on Women's Health Issues* (Vol. 2). Washington, DC: U.S. Government Printing Office.

Wilcox, B. L. (1981). Social support, life stress, and psychological adjustment: A test of the buffering hypothesis. *American Journal of Community Psychology, 9*, 371–386.

Williams, L. S. (1986). AIDS risk reduction: A community health education intervention for minority high risk group members. *Health Education Quarterly, 13*, 407–421.

Wright, J. D., Knight, J. W., Weber-Burdin, E., & Lam, J. (1987). Ailments and alcohol: Health status among the drinking homeless. *Alcohol Health and Research World, 11*(3), 22–27.

Zambrana, R. E. (1988). A research agenda on issues affecting poor and minority women: A model for understanding their health needs. *Women and Health, 12*(3/4), 137–161.

13

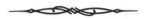

"Too Soon, Too Small, Too Sick": Black Infant Mortality

Virginia Davis Floyd

According to the U.S. Department of Health and Human Services (1991a), "The birth of a healthy infant to a healthy woman is the most important goal for our nation." Thus, infant mortality— the number of children out of every 1,000 born who do not live to reach their first birthday— is a very critical issue for the nation. In this country, the first year of life is, in fact, the most dangerous until one reaches the age of sixty-five. In 1988, 38,408 U.S. babies died before they reached the age of one, providing the nation with an infant mortality rate of 10.0 deaths per 1,000 live births. As many as half of these deaths could have been prevented with current knowledge and available services. In 1981, the United States ranked sixth in infant mortality rates among developed countries. Currently, our nation ranks twenty-second in the developed world for infant mortality outcome. The United States ranks behind Japan, Germany, Sweden, Canada, Spain, Australia, England, and fourteen other developed countries. For a nation that expends a greater percentage of its gross national product on health care than any other country and that maintains an elaborate technological health care system, this low standing is nothing less than an international disgrace.

An analysis of the nation's infant mortality problem utilizing race-specific information reveals the long-standing reality that in this nation black infants die at twice the rate of white infants within the first year of life. This black-white infant mortality gap has always existed and, alarmingly, it has continued to increase since the 1920s. Thus, the infant mortality problem is a serious concern to the African-American community and must be addressed if the health status and total well-being of this community are to improve.

Contrary to conventional thought and ongoing practices, infant mortality should not be dealt with by means of the medical model alone but requires cultural and health perspectives as well. Such an approach recognizes the social, economic, and cultural components that result in poor health outcomes. The infant mortality crisis in the African-American community reflects the complex quality-of-life issues that converge and subsequently cause children to die.

This chapter will discuss the multiple reasons for the alarming fact that black babies are dying at twice the rate of white babies, and often needlessly. It presents race-specific national infant mortality data, surveys risk factors for infant mortality, and makes recommendations for program and policy changes based on a comprehensive culture and health model perspective.

Data Overview

Black infant mortality rates in the United States have consistently been nearly double the white rates. The 1988 black U.S. infant rate is 17.6 deaths per 1,000 live births, as compared to the white rate of 8.5 deaths per 1,000 live births. The 1988 black infant mortality rate is equal to the infant mortality rate of the white population in 1970. On the average, 11,000 black infants die annually before the age of one. The *Report of the Secretary's Task Force on Black and Minority Health* (U.S. Department of Health and Human Services, 1985) estimates that over 50 percent of that number, or 6,178 black infant deaths, were "excess deaths" (or deaths that would not have occurred if black and white infant mortality rates were the same). If similarity in rates occurred, the United States would rise from twenty-second in the developed world to thirteenth. If one were to consider the black infant mortality rate only, the United States ranking would fall to thirty-second.

The secretary of the Department of Health and Human Services set objectives for the nation for the year 1990. The gap in race-specific infant mortality rates was so great that two separate and unequal objectives were established: (1) an overall infant mortality rate of 9 deaths per 1,000 live births by the year 1990, and (2) a black infant mortality rate not to exceed 12 deaths per 1,000 live births by the year 1990. The white population achieved the goal of 9 deaths per 1,000 live births in 1986, with an infant mortality rate of 8.6 deaths per 1,000 live births. The black population fell far short of both goals, with an infant mortality rate of 17.6 deaths per 1,000 live births in 1988 — the lowest black infant mortality rate in the history of the country. There is no evidence to suggest that the nation would have succeeded in reaching the goal of 12 for the black population by 1990 (U.S. Department of Health and Human Services, 1991b). The national health objectives for the year 2000 outline an infant mortality goal of 7.0 deaths per 1,000 live births.

In analyzing total infant mortality rates, a geographic pattern termed the nation's "infant mortality belt" can be discerned. Of the ten states where infant mortality rates are the highest, eight were in the South in 1987, as noted below.

Washington, D.C.	19.3
Mississippi	13.7
Georgia	12.7
South Carolina	12.7
Alabama	12.2

North Carolina	11.9
Louisiana	11.8
Tennessee	11.7
Delaware	11.7
Illinois	11.6
Maryland	11.5

This infant mortality belt is also the poverty belt, the undereducation belt, the rural belt, the minority belt, and the unemployment belt of the nation. All of the top-ranking states in infant mortality rates have black populations significantly higher than the national average of 12.1 percent. Table 13.1 shows similar but more inclusive data for the following year, 1988. Figure 13.1 depicts national infant mortality rates by race for the period 1980–1988.

If one examines the geographic pattern of black infant mortality, a different picture emerges. Regionally, for the period 1985–1987, black infant mortality was highest in the East North Central Region (Michigan — 22.2 deaths/1,000 births and Illinois — 21.4 deaths/1,000 births). States having the lowest rates were found in the Mountain Region (Arizona — 14.3 deaths/1,000 births) and Pacific Region (Washington — 13.8 deaths/1,000 births).

The major cause of infant mortality is low-birthweight babies born too soon (prematurity), too small (low birthweight and intrauterine growth retardation), and too sick. Collectively, low birthweight (defined as weighing less than 2,500 grams) and very low birthweight (defined as weighing less than 1,500 grams) are utilized as the major risk factor of infant mortality. Although the evidence reveals a slow but continual decline in the nation's infant mortality rates, we have not seen a similar pattern in percentage of low-birthweight births. In 1988, 6.9 percent of all births were low birthweight — weighing less than 2,500 grams or 5½ pounds. This percentage was 7.1 in 1978 and declined to 6.7 in 1984. The recent alarming trend reveals movement in an upward direction. The decline in infant mortality rates over the past two decades has been due to health providers' ability to provide intensive care to premature infants and establishment of regional neonatal intensive care units (NICUs) and not the health care industry's ability to prevent low-birthweight births (McCormick, 1985). Low-birthweight infants comprise 6.9 percent of the births yet account for two-thirds of neonatal deaths, and very-low-birthweight infants account for half of neonatal deaths (Klein & Goldenberg, 1990).

The black-versus-white infant mortality gap parallels the gap in low-birthweight and very-low-birthweight births between the two populations. Blacks contribute 17.2 percent of all live births in the nation (672,435), but 30.8 percent of all low-birthweight and 38.4 percent of very-low-birthweight infants (see Figure 13.2). In 1988, 13.0 percent of all black births were low birthweight compared to only 5.7 percent of white births. For very-low-birthweight births, blacks have a three-times-greater risk, with 2.8 percent compared to only 0.9 percent for white infants. The Healthy People 2000 objectives set a total low-birthweight rate goal of not more than 5 percent and

Table 13.1. Infant Mortality Rates by Race, 1988.

State	Rates			Black/White Rate Ratio
	Total	White	Black	
Alabama	12.1	9.3	17.2	1.84
Alaska	11.6	9.8	a	a
Arizona	9.7	9.4	17.9	1.90
Arkansas	10.7	8.7	17.4	1.99
California	8.6	8.2	15.9	1.95
Colorado	9.6	9.6	12.0	1.25
Connecticut	8.9	8.0	15.5	1.95
Delaware	11.8	9.1	21.1	2.33
District of Columbia	23.2	19.9	26.0	1.31
Florida	10.6	8.5	17.4	2.03
Georgia	12.6	9.2	18.9	2.06
Hawaii	7.2	7.2	a	a
Idaho	8.8	8.5	a	a
Illinois	11.3	8.7	20.7	2.39
Indiana	11.0	9.9	19.9	2.00
Iowa	8.7	8.3	19.9	2.40
Kansas	8.0	7.0	16.5	2.37
Kentucky	10.7	10.0	17.4	1.75
Louisiana	11.0	9.0	14.3	1.59
Maine	7.9	8.0	a	a
Maryland	11.3	8.5	17.8	2.10
Massachusetts	7.9	7.3	15.4	2.12
Michigan	11.1	8.6	21.9	2.55
Minnesota	7.8	7.2	19.5	2.71
Mississippi	12.3	8.7	16.1	1.85
Missouri	10.1	9.0	16.2	1.80
Montana	8.7	8.8	a	a
Nebraska	9.0	8.1	22.4	2.75
Nevada	8.4	7.5	18.7	2.51
New Hampshire	8.3	8.4	a	a
New Jersey	9.9	7.9	18.5	2.35
New Mexico	10.0	9.7	a	a
New York	10.8	8.9	18.1	2.04
North Carolina	12.5	9.6	19.5	2.04
North Dakota	10.5	10.0	a	a
Ohio	9.7	8.6	15.9	1.84
Oklahoma	9.0	9.3	12.6	1.37
Oregon	8.6	8.5	14.7	1.72
Pennsylvania	9.9	8.1	19.8	2.43
Rhode Island	8.2	7.5	13.8	1.83
South Carolina	12.3	9.6	16.6	1.73
South Dakota	10.1	9.7	a	a
Tennessee	10.8	8.2	18.6	2.25
Texas	9.0	8.3	14.2	1.72
Utah	8.0	7.9	a	a
Vermont	6.8	6.7	a	a
Virginia	10.4	8.1	17.9	2.21
Washington	9.0	8.7	16.1	1.85
West Virginia	9.0	8.5	a	a
Wisconsin	8.4	7.5	16.4	2.20
Wyoming	8.9	8.8	a	a
U.S. Total	10.0	8.5	17.6	2.10

a States with less than 1,000 births to black women.
Source: Adapted from U.S. Vital Health Records, National Center for Health Statistics, 1989.

Figure 13.1. Infant Mortality Rates by Race, United States, 1980–1988.

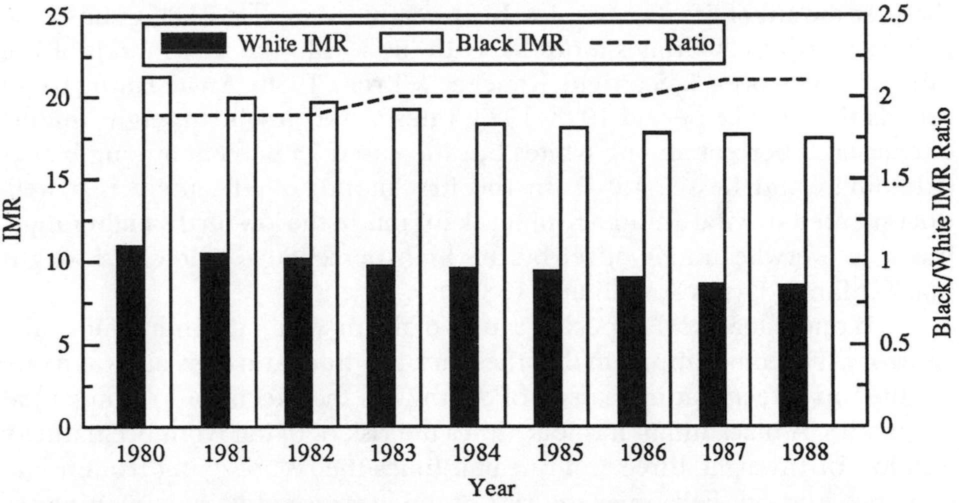

Source: Adapted from U.S. Vital Health Records, National Center for Health Statistics, 1989.

a very-low-birthweight rate of no more than 1 percent of all live births. The separate and unequal goal for black mothers is set at 9 percent low birthweight and 2 percent very low birthweight of black births.

The data clearly outline the strong association between low birthweight and increased infant mortality. Infants with low birthweight (< 2,500

Figure 13.2. Live Births by Weight, Women Age Fifteen to Forty-Four Years, United States, 1988.

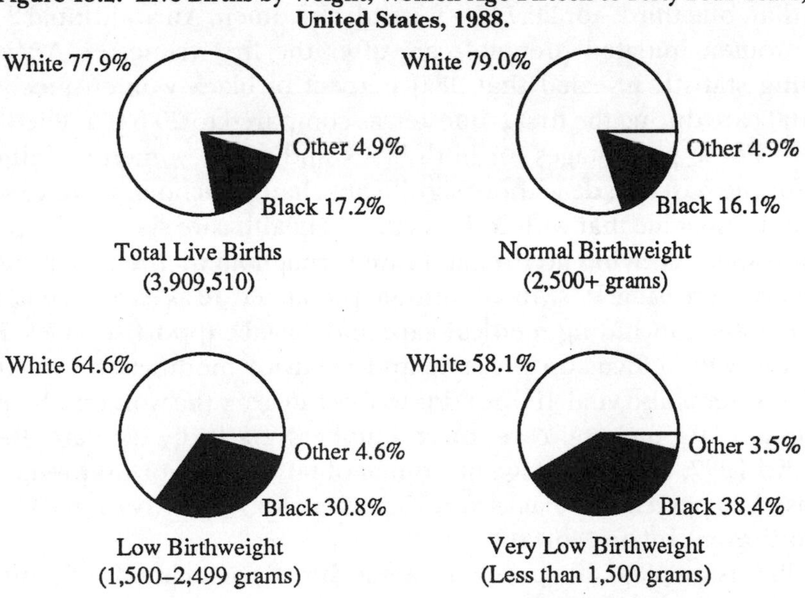

White 77.9%
Other 4.9%
Black 17.2%
Total Live Births
(3,909,510)

White 79.0%
Other 4.9%
Black 16.1%
Normal Birthweight
(2,500+ grams)

White 64.6%
Other 4.6%
Black 30.8%
Low Birthweight
(1,500–2,499 grams)

White 58.1%
Other 3.5%
Black 38.4%
Very Low Birthweight
(Less than 1,500 grams)

Source: Adapted from U.S. Vital Health Records, National Center for Health Statistics, 1989.

grams) are forty times more likely than normal-weight infants to die within the first month of life. For very-low-birthweight infants (< 1,500 grams), the risk increases to 200 times more likely to die within the first month of life (Shapiro, McCormick, Starfield, Krischer, & Bross, 1980). An alarming trend reveals that for the period 1973–1983, rates of very-low-birthweight infants decreased 3 percent among whites but increased 13 percent among blacks (Kleinman and Kessel, 1987). In the first month of life, there is a well-documented survival advantage of black infants in the low-birthweight range, but it is overwhelmingly offset by the high percentage of low-birthweight black infants (Jaynes & Williams, 1989).

If one examines the specific causes of death within the infant mortality category, it becomes apparent that the black-to-white ratio is greater than one for the top fifteen leading causes of death with the exception of congenital anomalies. A black infant has four times the risk of dying from prematurity and low birthweight, three and one-half times the risk of dying from homicide, two and one-half times the risk of dying from infections (meningitis, pneumonia, influenza, septicemia), and twice the risk of dying from newborn infections, maternal complications, and accidents. What makes these statistics unacceptable is the fact that the majority of these causes of deaths where inequality exists are either preventable or treatable (Children's Defense Fund, 1991).

The Role of Prenatal Care

What factors contribute to a baby being born too soon, too small, and/or too sick? In 1987, 74,087 women received no prenatal care in this country, and more than one-third — or 26,743 — were black women. An additional 215,003 black women initiated prenatal care after the first trimester. An equally alarming statistic revealed that 38.9 percent of black women received no prenatal care during the first trimester, as compared to 20.6 percent of white women. These percentages for both black and white women remained the same for the past decade without significant change (Schoenborn, 1988). It is difficult to imagine that with today's current health care system, the percentage of women receiving no prenatal care throughout their entire pregnancy is actually increasing! It is vital to initiate prenatal care as early as possible in the pregnancy, including medical care and social support services. Health education with a focus on life-style and behavior modification during the first trimester is also vital. If one adds to this category the women who receive inadequate late prenatal care, these numbers markedly escalate. Between 1980 and 1987, the percentage of women obtaining late or no prenatal care increased 26 percent for blacks and 17 percent for whites (National Commission to Prevent Infant Mortality, 1990).

Provision of quality prenatal care is directly associated with improved birth outcomes. Many risk factors of low birthweight and prematurity can be identified through the prenatal care process, and steps designed to alter them can be implemented. A pregnant woman who receives no prenatal care is three times as likely as others to have a low-birthweight baby.

Two major national reports produced by the Institute of Medicine (IOM) and the National Commission to Prevent Infant Mortality (NCPIM) presented similar recommendations on how to alleviate the infant mortality problem in the United States. They urged that provision be made for universal access to prenatal care and delivery services for all pregnant women regardless of class, race, or ability to pay. In short, the only eligibility criterion for receiving quality perinatal care services in this nation should be the fact that one is pregnant (Institution of Medicine, 1988; National Commission to Prevent Infant Mortality, 1988). The goal of universal access to prenatal care and delivery of services must be met if significant change is to occur in the infant mortality problem within the African-American community.

If the goal is universal access to prenatal care and delivery of services for all pregnant women and comprehensive well-child care for all children, then services must truly be accessible. Services must be where people are, at a time that is convenient and delivered in a specific manner that is culturally sensitive. This will require that the present system (both private and public) make radical changes in its health care delivery mechanisms. Until this happens, "true access" will continue to be an elusive outcome.

No current scientific data support a genetic basis for the infant mortality gap between the races. Thus, a solution based solely on the medical model will not correct the infant mortality problem. A truly comprehensive approach is required. To fail to address the effects of poverty, unemployment, lack of educational opportunities, and racism on the overall infant mortality rate is to doom proposed solutions to failure.

Maternal Risk Factors

Recognizing the importance of individual responsibility in determining one's health outcome, we must become concerned with the new morbidities associated with adverse maternal practices. The first step in producing a healthy infant is to begin with a healthy mother. Maternal health status, both in general and during pregnancy, is of paramount importance.

Nutrition

Maternal nutrition plays a major role in prevention of low birthweight, mental retardation, and failure to thrive on the part of babies. Recent findings (Buescher, Larson, Nelson, & Lenihan, 1991) show that pregnant women's participation in the Women's, Infants', and Children's Supplemental Nutrition Program (WIC) leads to improved birth outcomes. In Georgia, a study of 111,000 WIC births revealed that, in general, WIC mothers were disproportionately African American and had a lower infant mortality rate than the average Georgia mother. Infant mortality rates were halved by WIC participation when compared to African-American non-WIC mothers. Additionally, it was found that mean birthweight rose steadily with longer WIC participation: to 150 grams at seven or more months participation (Rafferty, 1990). Similar findings have been obtained in studies conducted in North Carolina and Pennsylvania (Beuscher et al, 1991; Pennsylvania Department of Health, 1991). These findings support the premise that one of the critical determinations in reducing infant mortality is access to services. They also speak to the issue of expanding a program with proven value to serve all who qualify. Currently, WIC services are available to only half of all eligible women in the nation.

Maternal substance abuse is an increasingly important risk factor for infant birth outcome. Much attention has recently been focused on the increased use of illegal drugs by women of reproductive age. In addressing the issue of black infant mortality, investigators must carefully examine all substances, both legal and illegal, that are in fact killing black children.

Tobacco

Tobacco use is a major killer of Americans in all age groups, and it is a significant contributor to infant mortality and morbidity in the United States. It is currently reported that between 21 and 30 percent of all pregnant women smoke throughout their pregnancy. According to Schoenborn (1988), the association between maternal smoking during pregnancy and low birthweight (both prematurity and intrauterine growth retardation) is well established. The most consistent finding is a reduction in birthweight of 150 to 300 grams (Floyd, Zahniser, Gunter, & Kendrick, 1991). Smoking during pregnancy is also associated with increased risk of spontaneous abortion, abruptio placenta, placenta previa, bleeding during pregnancy, and sudden infant death syndrome. Smoking by mothers and fathers increases the risk of early childhood bronchitis, pneumonia, and respiratory-related hospitalizations.

A breakdown of smoking statistics reveals that black women smoke less frequently than white women. In general, the prevalence of smoking among married women is higher among white women than black women and is higher for women under twenty years of age irrespective of race (Mullen, 1990). Smoking cessation programs have been shown to be effective with groups of women of reproductive age. It is estimated that low birthweight rates would be decreased by 10 to 30 percent and infant mortality rates by 10 percent if pregnant women would not smoke during pregnancy. Recognizing these statistics and other negative health effects of tobacco use, African-Americans must speak out against the tobacco industry's assault on the black community.

Alcoholism and Fetal Alcohol Syndrome

Alcoholism is the other legal drug that is severely influencing infant mortality and morbidity. Maternal alcohol consumption is associated with miscarriage, mental retardation of the infant, low birthweight, and fetal alcohol syndrome. In 1989, the Surgeon General reported that there were at least 5,000 infants born each year with fetal alcohol syndrome and 50,000 with fetal alcohol effects (National Commission to Prevent Infant Mortality, 1990). Alcohol abuse is the primary preventable cause of mental retardation. Given its effect on birth outcome as well as its association with child abuse and neglect, alcohol education and cessation programs must become a priority agenda item for the African-American community.

Drug Abuse

A great deal of attention has been directed toward illegal substance abuse among pregnant women. The nation is witnessing an explosion of drug-exposed infant births and associated morbidities. One study surveyed thirty-six hospitals across the country and found that one out of every eleven infants was born to a woman who abused illegal drugs (cocaine, heroin, methadone, amphetamines, PCP, and/or marijuana) during pregnancy. Based on this survey, it is estimated that as many as 375,000 infants may be affected annually by maternal consumption of illegal substances (National Association for Perinatal Addiction Research and Education, 1988). Illegal drug use during pregnancy is associated with poor pregnancy outcomes, including spontaneous abortion, placental abruption, low birthweight, neuro-behavioral problems, sudden infant death syndrome, and genito-urinary tract malformations. The minor problems of learning disabilities, attention deficit disorders, and behavioral problems will become increasingly evident as this cohort of drug-exposed infants becomes older. Due to the lack of required reporting, voluntary testing, and location of published studies, valid statistics by race are not available. It is believed that the incidence of drug abuse during pregnancy among middle- and upper-income women is widely underestimated. One study found no significant difference between the rate of drug use among women receiving care at public clinics and those utilizing the private sector. The National Commission to Prevent Infant Mortality (1990) reported that white women were slightly more likely to abuse drugs during pregnancy than black women. Regardless of the baseline prevalence data, the rising trend in maternal consumption of illegal substances is alarming for the African-American community.

Sexually Transmitted Diseases

Directly associated with the substance abuse increase in the black community is the parallel rise in sexually transmitted diseases and perinatal AIDS. An epidemic of syphilis is occurring in the black community with a resurgence of congenital syphilis. Infants born infected with syphilis are at an increased risk of premature death, low birthweight, mental retardation, and chronic health problems. Congenital syphilis is completely preventable when detected and treated in the mother.

The AIDS epidemic is truly devastating to the African-American community and has a special impact in the maternal and child population. Approximately 70 percent of all children and women with AIDS are children and women of color (Centers for Disease Control, 1991). To address this devastating problem, the African-American community must confront the substance abuse issue head on.

More than half of the six million annual pregnancies in the United States are unintended. One of the best predictors of a healthy birth outcome is whether the birth is a wanted one. Family planning services allow children to be born at the appropriate time—when they are wanted and loved. It must be noted that the risk of unintended pregnancies is not uniformly distributed. The rate of unintended pregnancy is 2.5 times greater for black women than for white women, and twice as high for teenagers as for older women (World Health Organization, 1988). Comprehensive family planning services that are culturally based, religiously sensitive, and truly accessible are mandatory for the African-American male and female population. Comprehensive family planning services are a mandatory part of the overall infant mortality solution.

What needs to be apparent is the role that individual actions and choices play in whether a pregnant woman decides to practice risky health behaviors such as use of illegal substances, smoking, and engaging in unprotected intercourse. The need for personal responsibility must be addressed within the African-American community. At least one Afrocentric social scientist interprets the epidemic of drug abuse, violence, teen pregnancies, divorces, and some current economic problems as symptoms of African-American "lives out of control" (Akbar, 1985). The control of one's life begins with the knowledge of one's self, one's history, and one's culture. Culture displacement and nonrecognition contribute to the disproportionate share of infant deaths experienced by the black community. For a pregnant woman to be motivated to seek services for herself and her unborn child, she must understand who she is and what she wants. The mental health/spiritual well-being of women is often overlooked in the provision of health care services to minority populations. Unless health care providers seek to understand the cultural norms of the African-American community and all of its individual subsets, true access will continue to be unobtainable for the black population.

There are many maternal and family risk factors that are outside the control of the individual that must be considered to achieve reductions in the excess infant mortality rates of the black community. The large social issues of poverty, educational access, employment opportunities, housing, and institutional racism have a significant impact on whether babies live or die within the African-American community. Programs must address these larger structural issues in addition to merely providing traditional health care to mothers and children. This awesome task of attacking the "big issues" must not be avoided because of the enormity of the issues; instead, it must be a constant focal point of all health programs irrespective of their magnitude. The health status of African Americans will not improve unless these problems are addressed forthrightly (Boone, 1989).

Conclusion

An infant death is a tragic event that occurs within a spectrum of maternal, social, and environmental events. To ensure a positive birth outcome, we must address all the components along the continuum, beginning prior to conception and continuing throughout the woman's reproductive life. Family planning services must be accessible to all who wish to plan for children. An unintended pregnancy is the first step in an unwanted pregnancy, which significantly contributes to poorer birth outcome. Preparation for pregnancy requires maintenance of good health habits, such as establishing proper nutrition, avoiding harmful substances, and obtaining adequate exercise. Likewise, along with physical readiness, there must be an accompanying mental readiness to become a parent. For African-American women, this healthy mental readiness requires both a knowledge of self and a comfort with their Afrocentric culture and self-image.

Comprehensive prenatal care services are the foundation of any programmed effort to address the high rate of black infant mortality. Prenatal care must be more than merely the provision of standard health care services. Social service case management is a vital part of the continuum of services. This component—which includes transportation, child care, parenting education, and literacy skill building—is especially required for hard-to-reach and low-income populations. Intensive educational and outreach campaigns must become a standard ongoing activity within the continuum. These campaign efforts must be culturally specific and sensitive to address the special needs of the African-American population. A successful effort must have both "the right message and the right messenger." The nation must continue to address the severe shortage of minority health personnel, given its impact on the health status of minority and underserved communities. Health and social services delivered by African-American providers should be a high priority in establishing service programs.

Universal access to prenatal care and improved delivery of services are mandatory components of a successful campaign to reduce infant mortality. Removal of financial barriers to access, especially for low-income women, is critical to this success. Expansion of the federal Medicaid program, employer-sponsored insurance programs, and state universal health insurance programs are a few of the mechanisms to be utilized. African-American women are disproportionately represented in the low-income, underinsured, and noninsured categories. Also, access must not be hindered because of geography, service hours, language difficulty, provider attitude, or bureaucratic red tape.

To reduce infant mortality, moreover, special attention must be focused on the infant at birth and on the provision of postpartum services to both mother and child. Additionally, the development of parenting skills, accident prevention, early development education, and mother/father/child bonding require attention. Provision of well-child care and necessary high-risk care is mandatory. Finally, reestablishment of postpartum family planning services is critically important for both mothers and fathers.

More generally, community empowerment efforts are essential (Braithwaite and Lythcott, 1989). Business as usual has not and will not solve the infant mortality problem for the black community. The comprehensive health care team needs new members drawn from community-based organizations, churches, self-help groups, local governments, and black civic organizations. The political will to mobilize the forces and address this and other crises must be found within the African-American community. Change agents and health providers must continue to address the issues of class and race that impact negatively on black health outcomes. Children are the most precious resource of the African-American community. All children, born and yet to be born, deserve nothing less than a full promise of tomorrow.

References

Akbar, N. (1985). *The community of self* (rev. ed.). Tallahassee, FL: Mind Productions.

Boone, M. S. (1989). *Capital crime: Black infant mortality in America*. Newbury Park, CA: Sage.

Braithwaite, R., & Lythcott, N. (1989). Community empowerment as a strategy for health promotion for black and other minority populations. *Journal of the American Medical Association, 261*(2), 282–283.

Buescher, P. A., Larson, L. C., Nelson, M. D., & Lenihan, A. J. (1991). *An evaluation of the impact of prenatal WIC participation in birth outcomes and Medicaid costs in North Carolina* (Studies Report Series No. 55). Raleigh: North Carolina Department of Environment, Health, and Natural Resources.

Centers for Disease Control. (1991). *HIV/AIDS Surveillance Report*. Atlanta, GA: Author.

Children's Defense Fund. (1991). *The state of America's children, 1991*. Washington, DC: Author.

Floyd, R. L., Zahniser, C., Gunter, E. P., & Kendrick, J. S. (1991). Smoking during pregnancy: Prevalence, effects, and intervention strategies. *Birth, 18*(1), 48–53.

Institution of Medicine. (1988). *Prenatal care: Reaching mothers, reaching infants*. Washington, DC: National Academy Press.

Jaynes, G. D., & Williams, R. M. (Eds.). (1989). *A common destiny—blacks and American society*. Washington, DC: National Academy Press.

Klein, L., & Goldenberg, R. L. (1990). Prenatal care and its effect on preterm birth and low birth weight. In I. R. Merkotz & J. E. Thompson (Eds.), *New perspectives on prenatal care* (pp. 501–530). New York: Elsevier.

Kleinman, J. C., & Kessel, S. S. (1987). Racial differences in low birth weight. *New England Journal of Medicine, 317*, 749–753.

McCormick, M. C. (1985). The contribution of low birth weight to infant mortality and childhood morbidity. *New England Journal of Medicine, 312*, 82–90.

Mullen, P. P. (1990). Smoking cessation counseling in prenatal care. In I. R. Merkotz & J. E. Thompson (Eds.), *New perspectives on prenatal care* (pp. 161–176). New York: Elsevier.

National Association for Perinatal Addiction Research and Education. (1988). Innocent addicts: High rates of prenatal drug abuse found. *ADAMHA News, 14*, 7.

National Commission to Prevent Infant Mortality. (1988). *Death before life: The tragedy of infant mortality* (Commission Report and Appendix). Washington, DC: Author.

National Commission to Prevent Infant Mortality. (1990). *Troubling trends: The health of America's next generation* (Commission Report). Washington, DC: Author.

National Commission to Prevent Infant Mortality. (1991). *One stop shopping: The road to healthy mothers and children.* (Commission Report). Washington, DC: Authors.

Pennsylvania Department of Health, State Health Data Center. (1991). *Statistical News: WIC & Birth Files Linked for Analysis, 14*(2), 1–3.

Rafferty, M. (1990). *There is wisdom in WIC.* Unpublished manuscript, Georgia Division of Public Health, Atlanta.

Schoenborn, C. A. (1988). *Health promotion and disease prevention: United States, 1985* (DHHS Publications No. PHS 88-1591). Washington, DC: U.S. Government Printing Office.

Shapiro, S., McCormick, M. C., Starfield, B. H., Krischer, J. P., & Bross, D. (1980). Relevance of correlates of infant deaths for significant morbidity at 1 year of age. *American Journal of Obstetrics and Gynecology, 136*, 363–373.

U.S. Department of Health and Human Services. (1985). *Report of the Secretary's Task Force on Black and Minority Health.* Washington, DC: U.S. Government Printing Office.

U.S. Department of Health and Human Services. (1991a). *Caring for our future.* Hyattsville, MD: Public Health Service.

U.S. Department of Health and Human Services. (1991b). *Health United States, 1990* (DHHS Publication No. PHS 91-1232). Washington, DC: U.S. Government Printing Office.

World Health Organization, Collaborating Center on Perinatal Care and Health Service Research in Maternal and Child Care. (1988). *Unintended pregnancy and infant mortality/morbidity: Closing the gap.* Geneva, Switzerland: Author.

14

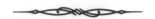

Lead Poisoning:
A Modern Plague Among
African-American Children

Wornie L. Reed

Lead poisoning is of special significance for African-American children, who are much more likely than white children to have elevated levels of lead in their blood. It is more dangerous than some forms of cancer — yet it is virtually ignored by the American public. Lead poisoning has seriously afflicted a much higher segment of the population than some diseases that were called "epidemics" — but it has received little public attention. There has been a public failure to recognize that this disease is a serious threat to improved health status. Lead poisoning has permanently damaged tens of thousands of babies, children, and adults in this nation, and the list of victims is still growing (Jordan, 1985).

Lead present in paint, dust, and soil is possibly our most significant toxic waste problem in terms of the seriousness and the extent of human health effects. Millions of dollars have been spent to clean up hazardous waste sites involving toxic substances whose health effects are still controversial. Yet lead — a toxic substance with confirmed damaging and permanent health effects on extremely large numbers of children in urban areas — has not been targeted for aggressive cleanup action.

Lead poisoning in humans has been identified as a cause of high blood pressure, heart disease, birth defects, complications in pregnancies, and developmental problems in infants. It is a health problem of epidemic proportions in the black community. This serious health problem is yet another example of the production of "illth" — injurious consumer commodities — in modern society. As the means of production create wealth for some sectors of society, they also create illth for other sectors: "At the present time refuse produced in this country is estimated to be increasing about four percent per year; . . . about the same as the yearly increase in the Gross National Product" (Cole, 1971, p. 33).

It is apparent that lead in the environment can be considered undesirable refuse. Just as the health and wealth of society accrue to some groups more than others, so does the illth. The black community — as usual — gets a

178

disproportionate share of the latter. Society is showing a disinterest in those who are the most likely victims of lead poisoning: small black children from poor and minority families living in old housing in dilapidated inner-city areas. In affluent and middle-class suburbs, only 3 percent of white children have dangerous levels of lead in their blood, compared to 30 percent of inner-city black children.

Background

As a result of industrialization, lead is ubiquitous in the human environment. Having no known physiological value, lead can only produce harm. Children are particularly susceptible to its toxic effects. Excessive absorption of lead is one of the most prevalent and preventable childhood health problems in the United States today (Centers for Disease Control, 1975).

Since 1970, the means of detecting and managing lead exposure by children has changed substantially. Before the mid 1960s, a level below 60 micrograms of lead per deciliter (μg/dl) of whole blood was not considered dangerous enough to require intervention (Chisholm, 1967). By 1975, as a result of more experience with this phenomenon, the level at which intervention is suggested had declined 50 percent—to 30 μg/dl. In that year, the Center (now Centers) for Disease Control (CDC) published the study *Increased Lead Absorption in Young Children: A Statement by the Center for Disease Control.* Since then, many studies have indicated that lead is toxic at levels previously thought to be nontoxic (Smith, Grant, & Sors, 1989). In 1990, the blood level at which intervention was recommended was 25 μg/dl or greater, and the CDC recommended that it be reduced to 15 by 1991. Furthermore, it is now generally recognized that lead toxicity is a widespread problem—one that is neither unique to inner-city children nor limited to one area of the country. However, its most prevalent occurrence is in old inner-city areas.

Average blood levels for the U.S. population have been established by the Second National Health and Nutrition Examination Survey (National Center for Health Statistics, 1981), and lead-contaminated soil and dust have emerged as important contributors to blood lead levels, as has leaded gasoline through its contribution to soil and dust lead levels. An increasing body of data supports the view that lead, even at levels previously thought to be "safe," is toxic to the developing central nervous system (Smith et al., 1989).

Obviously, a major public health objective would be the prevention of lead poisoning. One major advance in primary prevention has been the reduction of lead in gasoline. This action is probably responsible for the findings of reduced average blood lead levels in children nationwide (Annest et al., 1983) and in two major cities (Rabinowitz & Needleman, 1982; Billick, Shier, & Current, 1980; Kaul, Davidow, Eng, & Gewirtz, 1983). In addition, lead is no longer allowed in paint for residential dwellings, furniture, and toys.

The primary sources of lead are air, water, and food. Despite a 1977 ruling by the Consumer Products Safety Commission that limits the lead content of newly applied residential paints, millions of housing units still contain leaded paints that were applied before the ban. Older houses that are dilapidated or that are being renovated are a particular danger to children. In many urban areas, lead is found in soil (Mielke et al., 1983) and house dust (Charney, Kessler, Farfel, & Jackson, 1983). Consequently, screening programs — a form of secondary prevention — are still needed to minimize the chances of lead poisoning development among susceptible young children.

A nationwide survey conducted from 1976 to 1980 showed that children from all geographic areas and socioeconomic groups are at risk for lead poisoning (Mahaffey, Annest, Roberts, & Murphy, 1982). Data from that survey indicate that nearly 4 percent of all U.S. children under the age of five years had blood lead levels of 30 μg/dl or more. Extrapolating this figure indicates that an estimated 675,000 children six months to five years of age had blood lead levels of 30 μg/dl or more.

There are, however, race and class differences in lead poisoning. Two percent of white children had these high blood lead levels, but 12.2 percent of black children had such levels. The levels for some black children are even higher: among black children living in the cores of large cities and in families with annual incomes of less than $6,000, the prevalence of levels of 30 μg/dl or more was 18.6 percent. Among white children, those in lower-income families had eight times the prevalence of elevated blood lead levels that those in families with higher income had. This difference is a function of residential areas.

In the past decade, knowledge of lead toxicity and its effects has increased substantially. Previously, medical attention focused on the effects of severe exposure to lead and clinically recognizable signs and symptoms of toxicity. It is now apparent, however, that lower levels of exposure may cause serious behavioral and biochemical changes. Results of a growing number of studies indicate that chronic exposure to low levels of lead is associated with altered neurophysiological performance and that young children are particularly vulnerable to this effect (Needleman, Gunnoe, & Leviton, 1979; Winneke, 1982; Yule, Lansdown, Mitlar, & Urbanowicz, 1982).

Many factors can affect the absorption, distribution, and toxicity of lead and put children at greater risk than adults. Children, for instance, are more exposed to lead than older persons because their normal hand-to-mouth activities introduce many nonfood items into their bodies (Lin-Fu, 1973). Once absorbed, lead is distributed throughout soft tissue and bone. Young children absorb and retain more lead on a unit-mass basis than adults. Their bodies also handle lead differently; higher mineral turnover in bone means that more lead is available to sensitive systems in children. Since lead accumulates in the body and is only slowly removed, repeated exposures to small amounts over many months produce elevated blood lead levels. In fact, this is the most probable means of acquiring lead poisoning from soil and dust.

Lead toxicity is mainly evident in the red blood cells, the central and peripheral nervous systems, and the kidneys. Lead also has adverse effects on reproduction in both males and females (Lane, 1949), and recent data (Needleman, Rabinowitz, Leviton, Linn, & Schoenbaum, 1984) suggest that prenatal exposure to low levels of lead may be related to minor congenital abnormalities. In fact, the margin of safety for lead is very small compared with other chemical agents (Royal Commission on Environmental Pollution, 1983).

The effects of lead toxicity are nonspecific and not readily identifiable. Any number of behavioral and biochemical changes may result. Parents, teachers, and clinicians may identify altered behaviors in children that result from lead toxicity as attention disorders, learning disabilities, or emotional disturbances. Because of the large number of children susceptible to lead poisoning, these adverse effects are a major cause for concern.

Some of the symptoms of lead poisoning include fatigue, pallor, malaise, loss of appetite, irritability, sleep disturbance, sudden behavioral change, and developmental regression. More serious symptoms include clumsiness, muscular irregularities (ataxia), weakness, abdominal pain, persistent vomiting, constipation, and changes in consciousness due to early encephalopathy (disease of the brain). Children who display these symptoms need urgent and thorough diagnostic evaluations and prompt treatment should the disease be confirmed.

Lead Poisoning as a Child Health Problem

Lead poisoning among children has changed over the past decade. Previously, it was a disease often presented as encephalopathy associated with children ingesting peeling lead paint. This often led to severe overt effects, effects that are readily detectable in both humans and animals. Prior to the development of chelation therapy for lead poisoning, the mortality rate of encephalopathy was approximately 65 percent. The most severe effects of lead poisoning (acute encephalopathy, seizures, coma, and death) occur at very high blood lead levels — 80 to 100 μg/dl and over (Office of Environmental Affairs, 1985).

Now lead poisoning has become a largely "asymptomatic" condition characterized by an elevated blood lead level linked with many sources of exposure and affecting a broader range of children. Even moderately elevated blood lead levels (13–25 μg/dl) have effects on central nervous system functioning. These less obvious effects occur in such central nervous system functions as intelligence, behavior control, fine motor coordination, neurological dysfunction, and motor impairment. Further, metabolic effects occur in children with blood lead concentrations as low as 7 to 12 μg/dl. Recent studies strongly suggest that even at subclinical levels of lead intoxication, children sustain permanent cognitive and behavioral damage that manifests itself in poor school performance and a variety of learning disabilities (Smith et al., 1989).

To many, the phrase *lead poisoning* evokes an image of a child eating paint chips peeled off the walls of a deteriorated inner-city dwelling. To be sure, children living in such circumstances are at greatest risk of lead poisoning, and the ingestion of leaded paint is the route that yields the most concentrated exposure to this metal. Like most stereotypes, however, this one has proven to be far too simplistic a characterization of the problem. In the past decade, advances in our understanding of the epidemiology of childhood lead exposure have led to an increasing acceptance of the existence of a syndrome of "subclinical" or "silent" lead toxicity. In other words, children with lead levels that are not high enough to produce clinical symptoms may nevertheless suffer serious health effects.

Young children are the group at greatest risk of lead poisoning. Because of their behavior and physiology, they generally experience greater exposure than do adults living in the same environment. For instance, their blood lead levels rise more than adults' in response to an increase in dietary or air lead levels because, on a body weight basis, they eat more and breathe a greater volume of air. Most children also engage in some hand-to-mouth activity, an age-appropriate form of exploratory behavior. This may cause a child to ingest lead-bearing materials, such as household dust or yard soil, that pose little danger to adults. A smaller number of children engage in pica, the pathological ingestion of nonfood items. These children are at especially high risk because they may consume a leaded paint chip. A thumbnail-size chip that is 50 percent lead and weighs one gram will deliver a dose of 50,000 micrograms; this is far above the safe daily intake of 5 micrograms per kilogram of body weight.

The metabolism of lead differs in children and adults. Children's absorption of lead through the stomach and intestines is more efficient, especially if there are certain nutritional deficiencies (for example, iron, calcium, zinc) present as well, which is often the case. A greater fraction of a child's total body lead burden is metabolically active rather than sequestered in bone. In general, while lead's toxicity in adults is expressed as peripheral nervous system dysfunction (for instance, motor weaknesses), effects in children usually involve the central nervous system. The developing nervous system is especially vulnerable because lead has greater access to the brain prior to the complete development of the cellular barrier that protects this critical organ from toxic substances in the blood. The greater cellular metabolism of the immature brain makes it vulnerable to the adverse effects of lead on cell respiration and oxygen transport. Excessive exposure may alter the number or organization of connections between neurons, or the communication between them, perhaps resulting in irreversible changes in structure and function.

Subclinical lead intoxication is especially troublesome because it is asymptomatic. Parents, for instance, find it difficult to understand lead hazards when their children do not appear to be "sick." In addition, since long-term exposure is cumulative over time, toxicity occurs without the parents' recognition. Probably the most significant implications of lead's distribution in the body are its high degree of accumulation with repeated exposure and its slow rate of removal when exposure occurs.

Sources of Lead Exposure

Children may be exposed to lead from a wide variety of sources, including tap water, canned food, air, and paint. All children in the United States are exposed to lead in the air, in soil and dust, and even in the normal diet. While lead may come from such sources as water from piping and water distribution systems and from lead leaching from the seams of soldered cans, probably the most critical sources are lead-based paint, airborne lead, and soil and dust.

Lead-Based Paint

Direct ingestion of lead paint — the most concentrated source of lead — is most often the cause of high- or urgent-risk symptomatic or asymptomatic lead poisoning. Lead-based paint is the major source of high-dose lead exposure and symptomatic lead poisoning for children in the United States. The interior of about twenty-seven million households in this country are contaminated by lead paint that was produced before the amount of lead in residential paint was controlled. Since the 1977 ruling by the Consumer Products Safety Commission, household paint must contain no more than 0.06 percent lead. However, before 1977 some interior paints contained in excess of 50 percent lead. A further complicating factor is that lead-based paint is still available for industrial, military, and marine usage. Occasionally, this paint is used in homes.

Quite often, lead poisoning occurs in children under six years of age who live in deteriorated housing built before World War II. Children in this age group often mouth and/or swallow peeling paint chips. This practice of pica — the ingestion of nonfood substances — is normal behavior for young children. It is not race or class based. However, since poor families and black families are the principal occupants of such housing, children in these families have more adverse health effects from this form of normal childhood behavior. In recent years, this kind of lead poisoning has been reported among "urban homesteaders," who are moving from the suburbs into the cities and rehabilitating old houses.

Airborne Lead

Inhalation of airborne lead is also a means of poisoning children. Although inhalation is a minor means, airborne lead that gets deposited in soil and dust is a major source of lead poisoning. This airborne lead is produced by automotive and industrial sources. Studies have shown that children living within 100 feet of major roadways have higher blood lead levels than those living farther away (Caprio, Margulis, & Joselow, 1974). Low-income families and black families often tend more than others to live near such major roadways.

Soil and Dust

Soil and dust that contain lead are also extremely important sources of lead exposure for children. Lead in soil and dust comes from particles of airborne lead produced by automotive, industrial, and similar sources. Flaking lead paint also plays a part in contaminating the soil around homes. The potential health effects of lead in dust and dirt are increased by small particle size, which enhances absorption, and by its continuing presence in children's environments. In particular, hand-to-mouth transfer of lead-contaminated dust and dirt occurs through normal play (Barltrop, 1966; Sayre, Charney, Vostal, & Pless, 1974). This activity often produces subclinical chronic lead intoxication, which constitutes over 90 percent of all childhood lead poisoning cases.

Effects of Lead

Studies in the 1940s demonstrated that there are lasting neurotoxic effects of lead poisoning and that children with previous lead poisoning made unsatisfactory progress in school. More recent studies of nonovert lead intoxication of children have revealed a number of adverse effects. For example, one study found that seven times as many lead-exposed children were repeating grades in school or being referred to the school psychologist. High-risk lead-exposure groups have been found to score less on IQ or other types of psychometric tests than referent control groups with lower lead exposures (Grant & Davis, 1989).

In studies of nonovertly lead intoxicated children, lower lead body burdens (7–12, low; and 13–24, elevated) are examined by psychometric measures, particularly IQ tests. In a pioneering study by Needleman et al. (1979), the deciduous teeth of children were studied, and significant differences were found between the low- and elevated-lead groups on decrements in IQ scores. Other studies of children in general pediatric populations have found significant differences between those with low levels and those with elevated blood lead levels in IQ scores, developmental skills, and behavior (usually as measured by the classroom teacher). Although some of these studies had methodological weaknesses, especially the early ones conducted in the 1970s, more recent studies have improved on the methodologies and reached similar results. These effects are reduced when potential confounding variables are controlled (Smith, 1989).

That lead can affect the survival and development of the fetus and infant has been known for more than 100 years (Smith et al., 1989). This knowledge, however, was based on relatively high levels of exposure to lead. More recently, researchers have uncovered adverse health effects to fetuses and infants from relatively low levels of exposure. Some studies show effects such as decreased birthweight, shortened gestation, and stillbirths. Gestational age, birthweight, and postnatal neurobehavioral development have been found by several prospective studies to be affected by low and elevated blood lead levels (Grant & Davis, 1989).

Studies in Boston, Cincinnati, Cleveland, and Port Pirie (South Australia) found similar results using the Mental Development Index (MDI) of the Bayley Scales of Infant Development in a two-year follow-up study of infants (Grant & Davis, 1989). They each measured the maternal blood lead at delivery or at a prenatal clinic visit and tested the infants at six-month intervals. The deficit in the Bayley MDI scores was fairly consistent across studies: there were 2 to 8 points deficit per 10 μg/dl increase in blood lead level. Each of these studies of infants with low and elevated blood lead levels controlled for long lists of potential confounders such as maternal IQ, maternal alcohol usage, maternal age, ethnicity, SES, father's education, mother's and father's workplaces, child birth rank, parental relationship, and so on. These studies are consistent in their conclusions: intrauterine lead exposure results in impaired postnatal neurobehavioral development. They show that lead concentrations of 10 to 15 μg/dl, and possibly lower, are related to developmental deficits from early exposure.

The duration of gestation is reduced as a function of lead exposure in two of these studies. At blood lead levels above 14 μg/dl, the risk of preterm delivery was 4.4 times that at 8 μg/dl or below. Another study, which reexamined the Cincinnati data, concluded that birthweight is affected starting at blood lead levels of 12 or 13 μg/dl (Grant & Davis, 1989). The implications of these findings are straightforward. About 27 percent of the women of childbearing age had blood lead level concentrations of 10 μg/dl or more in 1980 (National Center for Health Statistics, 1981). Thus, nearly one million infants may have been born in the United States in 1980 to mothers with maternal lead levels high enough to put the infants at risk for developmental impairments.

MDI scores have been moderately but significantly correlated with later IQ test scores. A four-point change in the MDI score for an individual child would not generally be considered clinically important. On the other hand, a four-point downward shift in a normal distribution of MDI scores results in 50 percent more children scoring below 80 on the IQ test.

Prevention

Current childhood lead poisoning prevention programs have a case finding and treatment focus. These programs were established in the late 1960s and early 1970s when the accepted threshold levels for toxic effects of lead were much higher than today. It was believed that if the lead levels in children did not reach these thresholds, they would not suffer any serious or permanent health effects. At that time, the emphasis was on screening children for lead poisoning, providing medical treatment, and removing the sources of lead (that is, lead paint). This approach was based on the assumption that with early detection and intervention, lead encephalopathy and the resultant brain damage would be prevented. The early detection and intervention would keep children's lead levels from becoming very high. This approach was successful in that many of the more severe consequences of lead poisoning—including death and mental retardation—were reduced. On the other hand, the lower levels of lead continued to cause serious, but asymptomatic, health effects. It is now known that screening and medical and environmental treatment—important secondary prevention methods—do not provide primary prevention.

All children diagnosed as having lead poisoning require continual medical treatment, environmental assessment, and educational monitoring. Obviously, lead-poisoned children must be treated. It should be noted that medical treatment, which is essential, is painful for the child and distressing for the family. The failure to treat a child, however, subjects him or her to permanent damage. The environmental evaluation and deleading are necessary prior to returning an already-poisoned child to the home environment. The child should also be carefully monitored and evaluated by the educational system, since the effects of lead poisoning on the central nervous system may cause such problems as attention disorders, learning disabilities, and emotional disturbances.

Substantial preventable costs result from continuous neglect of primary prevention. Treating only already-poisoned children is a costly way of dealing with the problem. Primary prevention of lead poisoning would protect children before they are poisoned; however, the problem is continually dealt with only after children are lead poisoned. The probable permanent effects of this practice on the central nervous system are quite serious.

Until more focus is placed on lead poisoning as a serious public health problem and until all babies are screened and home environments tested, some cautionary measures can be taken. Parents can have their young children screened by available inexpensive tests so that any lead found can be immediately removed from the child and the home. While the blood tests for lead are simple, the removal of lead from the blood of a child is not. The process, called *chelation*, in which chemicals are combined with lead in the bloodstream to facilitate the excretion of lead, is often painful and much of the aforementioned neurological damage may have already been inflicted.

The Race Effect

The city of Boston provides an example of how blacks are affected disproportionately by lead poisoning. Lead poisoning, while occurring throughout this city, is to a surprising degree concentrated within very limited geographic areas. Four neighborhoods—Dorchester, Roxbury, Jamaica Plain, and Mattapan—are the highest in the number and percentage of children poisoned. These neighborhoods account for 87 percent of the city's lead-poisoned children and only 56 percent of the at-risk population (nine months to six years of age). Further, sixteen of the census tracts in these neighborhoods—containing less than 18 percent of the city's at-risk children—account for 41 percent of Boston's lead-poisoned children. These neighborhoods contain a major portion of the black population of Boston. Although blacks make up only 20 percent of the population of the city of Boston, they are 78 percent of Roxbury, 81 percent of Mattapan, and over 20 percent of Dorchester residents.

It is not surprising, then, that as the primary inner-city dwellers, blacks have excess amounts of lead poisoning. Data from the late 1970s show that black children are more than six times as likely as white children (12.2 percent to 2 percent) to have elevated levels of lead in their blood. In Boston, children nine months to six years old living in twenty-eight discrete areas in predominantly black neighborhoods have nearly 30 percent of Boston's childhood lead poisoning, yet they constitute only 4.4 percent of the children in this age group. About one out of every four children in each of these areas has been poisoned (Office of Environmental Affairs, 1985).

Generally speaking, greater amounts of lead occur in urban areas—areas where blacks have been "forced" to live. Housing discrimination, along with the national urbanization of blacks, has led to what some call the development of black "ghettos." The National Advisory Commission on Civil Disorders, which was established after the widespread rioting in black communities in the mid 1960s, reported in 1968 that "what white Americans never understood, but what the Negro can never forget, is that white society is deeply implicated in the ghetto. White institutions created it, white institutions maintain it, and white society condones it" (*Report of the National Advisory Commission on Civil Disorders*, 1968, p. 2).

Consequently, blacks and now Hispanic children have higher levels of lead exposure than white children. In fact, the mean blood lead level of black children age six months to five years who live in large urban areas is 23 μg/dl, nearly matching the level now regarded as elevated (Bellinger, 1989).

This is not strictly a class issue. For example, it has been demonstrated that some of the excess black infant mortality is independent of class: there is a race effect over and above the class effect (Reed, 1986). In very recent years, we have learned that lead affects the fetuses of pregnant women and that these effects may lead to adverse birth outcomes, including infant mortality. It is highly possible that the excess infant mortality of middle-class blacks who live in poor urban neighborhoods is a result of forces that lead to residential segregation.

Conclusion

The Boston Childhood Lead Poisoning Prevention Program oversees the abatement of lead paint hazards and monitors the blood lead levels of young children throughout the city. The deleading of poisoned children's homes appears to contribute significantly to the reduction of their blood lead levels. However, even six to twelve months after deleading, about 50 percent of the children tested still had lead levels over 30 μg/dl (59 percent of those originally with levels over 50 μg/dl and 46 percent of those initially under 50 μg/dl). Clearly, then, for many children lead-based paint is not the only significant source of lead. Because lead-contaminated soil has been found to be a major contributor to elevated lead levels in children, it is quite likely that for many of the children whose lead levels do not steadily decline to safe levels after the removal of lead paint, soil is a significant source of lead exposure. The pattern of sustained toxicity almost certainly undermines cognitive and central nervous system development in these children. Consequently, there is a pressing need to remove lead-contaminated soil and to do so in a preventive manner.

The Special Commission on Lead Poisoning Prevention for the Commonwealth of Massachusetts has made a number of recommendations for improving the prevention of lead poisoning. Of these, perhaps the two most important are the following:

1. The addition of inspections and, where appropriate, removal of leaded soil
2. The initiation of a program of primary prevention in geographic areas with extremely high rates of lead poisoning

Since lead is clearly an important toxic waste, the Health Department of the city of Boston appealed to the Environmental Protection Agency (EPA) for funds to remove lead-contaminated soil in the highest-risk areas of Boston. Legislation was offered in the U.S. Senate to provide an additional $45 million (in the reauthorization of the EPA Superfund Program) to initiate lead-contaminated soil removal in up to three major cities. Three cities — Boston, Baltimore, and Cincinnati — requested funds for lead cleanup efforts; however, the EPA persuaded Congress to limit the appropriation to a total of $15 million for pilot programs in these three cities.

Since the EPA Superfund only addresses exterior pollution problems, the pilot programs are directed at soil removal from sites with high concentrations of lead. The federal government is requiring that the pilot programs prove that the removal of soil makes a difference. This requirement appears to be a reasonable goal for the pilot projects until the programs are examined in the context of the EPA's other Superfund work. In other EPA Superfund projects, there is no such requirement to demonstrate a positive effect following the removal of toxins. The rule is to remove hazardous material if it exists. Furthermore, if there is an imminent threat to humanity, the hazardous material must be removed within a year. All of this is done whether or not there is any evidence of exposure or whether there is any consistently strong evidence of human health effects. For example, there was recently a $45 million Superfund project in Holbrook, Massachusetts, to remove contaminants that have no comparable immediate impact on human health. Yet the Boston City Health Department could not obtain adequate funds to remove lead—a proven contaminant—from the most contaminated residential areas in Boston. In fact, $45 million would clean up the highest-risk areas of Boston.

All children under six years of age are at risk for lead poisoning. Consequently, children should be screened for blood lead each year until they are past this age. It is important to do this screening to detect low, but dangerous, levels of lead in children who do not exhibit any symptoms. On the other hand, the most effective primary prevention strategy would be to remove lead from a child's environment before, not after, a child is poisoned. This would involve the inspection, by the local health department, of each dwelling unit containing a child less than six years of age. Owners of units with exposed lead would be required to delead—inside and outside the house. The EPA Superfund should be used to remove lead-contaminated soil outside the house. Deleading home interiors is more complicated, since homeowners are required to pay for that expensive process—a situation that leads to very few homes being deleaded. Consequently, some mechanism is needed to provide public assistance to homeowners who delead.

While we wait for public health programs to be developed to handle the serious issue of lead removal, parents of preschool children who live in older, deteriorating neighborhoods should be informed—by local health departments—about the need to have their children screened periodically and about how to protect them from lead-infested environments. For example, parents could frequently wet mop and vacuum accessible paint flakes and dust to reduce potential lead hazards in the child's environment.

Such actions, although seemingly simple, can make an important difference in children's exposure to lead poison. The reduction of disease and death from lead poisoning will certainly require a concerted effort by environmental regulatory authorities. Until such policy implementation is realized, African-American children will remain disproportionately at risk for this preventable public health problem.

References

Annest, J. L., Pinkle, J. L., Makuz, D., Neese, J. W., Bayse, D. D., & Koyar, M. G. (1983). Chronological trend in blood count levels between 1976 and 1980. *New England Journal of Medicine, 308*, 1373–1377.

Barltrop, D. (1966). The prevalence of pica. *American Journal of Disease in Children, 112*, 116–123.

Bellinger, D. (1989). Prenatal/early postnatal exposure to lead and risk of developmental impairment. In N. Paul (Ed.), *Research in infant assessment* (March of Dimes Birth Defects Foundation, Original Articles Series, Vol. 25, No. 6, pp. 73–97). White Plains, NY: March of Dimes Defects Foundation.

Billick, I. H., Shier, D. R., & Current, A. S. (1980). Relation of pediatric blood lead levels to lead in gasoline. *Environmental Health Perspectives, 34,* 213–217.

Caprio, R. J., Margulis, H. L., & Joselow, M. M. (1974). Lead absorption in children and its relation to urban traffic densities. *Archives of Environmental Health, 28,* 195–197.

Centers for Disease Control (CDC). (1975). *Increased lead absorption in young children: A statement by the Center for Disease Control.* Atlanta, GA: Author.

Charney, E., Kessler, B., Farfel, M., & Jackson, D. (1983). Childhood lead poisoning: A controlled trial of the effect of dust-control measures on blood lead levels. *New England Journal of Medicine, 309*(18), 1089–1093.

Chisholm, J. J. (1967). Treatment of lead poisoning. *Modern Treatment, 4*(4), 710–720.

Clark, K. (1965). *Dark ghetto.* New York: HarperCollins.

Cole, L. C. (1971). Playing Russian roulette with biogeochemical cycles. In H. P. Dreitzel (Ed.), *The social organization of health.* New York: Macmillan.

Grant, L. D., & Davis, J. M. (1989). Effects of low-level lead exposure on pediatric neurobehavioral development: Current findings and future direction. In M. A. Smith, L. D. Grant, & A. I. Sors (Eds.), *Lead exposure and child development: An international assessment* (pp. 49–118). Boston: Kluwer.

Jordan, R. (1985, July 27). Ignored and deadly. *Boston Globe,* p. 17.

Kaul, B., Davidow, B., Eng, Y., & Gewirtz, M. (1983). Lead, erythrocyte, protoporphyrin, and ferritin levels in cord blood. *Archives of Environmental Health, 38*(5), 296–300.

Lane, R. E. (1949). The care of the lead worker. *British Journal of Industrial Medicine, 6,* 125–143.

Lin-Fu, J. S. (1973). *Preventing lead poisoning in children today* (DHEW Publication No. HSM 73-115). Rockville, MD: Maternal and Child Health Services.

Mahaffey, K. R., Annest, J., Roberts, J., & Murphy, R. S. (1982). National estimated blood lead levels: United States 1976–80: Association with selected demographic and socioeconomic factors. *New England Journal of Medicine, 307,* 573–579.

Mielke, H., Anderson, J., Berry, K., Mielke, P., Chaney, R., & Leech, M. (1983). Lead concentration in inner-city soils as a factor in the child lead program. *American Journal of Public Health, 73*(112), 1366–1369.

National Center for Health Statistics. (1981, July). Plan and operation of the Second National Health and Nutrition Examination Survey, 1976–80. *Vital and Health Statistics* (Series 1, No. 15) (DHHS Publication No. PHS 81-1317). Washington, DC: U.S. Government Printing Office.

Needleman, H. L., Gunnoe, C., & Leviton, A. (1979). Deficits in psychologic and classroom performance of children with elevated dentine lead levels. *New England Journal of Medicine, 300,* 689–695.

Needleman, H. L., Rabinowitz, M., Leviton, A., Linn, S., & Schoenbaum, S. (1984). The relationship between parental exposure to lead and congenital abnormalities. *Journal of the American Medical Association, 251,* 2956–2959(22).

Office of Environmental Affairs. (1985). *Boston child lead poisoning: Request for immediate clean-up of lead-contaminated soil in emergency areas.* Boston: Department of Health and Hospitals.

Rabinowitz, M. B., & Needleman, H. L. (1982). Temporal trends in the lead concentrations of umbilical cord blood. *Science, 216*(4553), 1429–1431.

Reed, W. (1986). Suffer the children: Some of the effects of racism on the health of black infants. In P. Connor and R. Kerr (Eds.), *Critical perspectives in the sociology of health and illness* (2nd ed., pp. 34–44). New York: St. Martin's Press.

Report of the National Advisory Commission on Civil Disorders. (1968). New York: Bantam Books.

Royal Commission on Environmental Pollution. (1983, April). *Ninth report: Lead in the environment* (report presented to Parliament by Her Majesty). London: Her Majesty's Stationery Office.

Sayre, J. W., Charney, E., Vostal, J., & Pless, I. B. (1974). House and hand dust as a potential source of childhood lead exposure. *American Journal of Disease of Children, 127,* 167–170.

Smith, M. A. (1989). The effects of low-level lead exposure on children. In M. A. Smith, L. D. Grant, & A. I. Sors (Eds.), *Lead exposure and child development: An international assessment* (pp. 3–48). Boston: Kluwer.

Smith, M. A., Grant, L. D., & Sors, A. J. (Eds.). (1989). *Lead exposure and child development: An international assessment.* Boston: Kluwer.

Winneke, G. (1982, September 4). Neurobehavioral and neuropsychological [effects of lead] [Letter to the editor]. *Lancet, 2*(8297), 550.

Yule, W., Lansdown, R., Mitlar, I. B., & Urbanowicz, M. A. (1982). The relationship between blood lead concentrations, intelligence, and attainment in a school population: A pilot study. *Developmental Medicine and Child Neurology, 23,* 567–761.

15

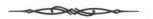

Sickle Cell Anemia and
African Americans

Charles F. Whitten

Sickle cell disease is a serious health problem that disproportionately affects African Americans. As with any health problem, the ultimate goal is to prevent its occurrence or to cure it after onset. Another goal is to improve treatment protocols to enable people to live lives that are least compromised. The primary purpose of this chapter is to assess the current situation with respect to achieving those goals. First, however, it is necessary to describe the various sickle cell conditions and how they are acquired.

In 1904, a black student from Grenada who was attending the Chicago College of Dental Surgery became ill. His physician, on examining his blood under a microscope, discovered that some of his red blood cells were sickle shaped rather than round, as is normal (Herrick, 1910). This was the beginning of the medical profession's recognition of sickle cell anemia (SCA), but there is evidence that the disease had been present for centuries. In several West African ethnic groups, there are indigenous names for the disease that reflect some of its characteristics. For example, for the Ga of Ghana, the name Chwechweechwe reflects the relentless, repetitious, and gnawing nature of the pain that individuals with SCA experience (Konotey-Ahulu, 1968). A Ghanaian specialist in sickle cell disease has established, through oral history, that SCA has probably been present in nine generations of one family dating back to 1670 (Konotey-Ahulu, 1974).

The Sickle Cell Conditions

The basis for the occurrence of sickle-shaped red blood cells is the presence of a special type of hemoglobin designated as sickle hemoglobin. Red blood cells contain hemoglobin, a substance that carries oxygen from the lungs to the various organs and tissues that require oxygen to live and carry out their functions. Red blood cells that contain normal hemoglobin remain round when they release oxygen, whereas cells that contain sickle hemoglobin can assume a sickle shape. This occurs because on the release of oxygen, the millions of minute hemoglobin particles (molecules) in the cells tend to join together, forming "rods" that distort the cells into the shape of a sickle.

Sickle cells have two undesirable characteristics: they are rigid and fragile. Normal red blood cells are soft and pliable and are able to squeeze through small blood vessels easily; because of their rigidity, sickle cells tend to plug blood vessels, thereby obstructing the flow of blood from time to time. This can result in tissue and organ damage. Normal red blood cells have a life span of about 120 days. Sickle cells last only from six to thirty days, and the bone marrow cannot produce cells fast enough to completely replace those that are destroyed. The result is a constant anemia (that is, a smaller-than-normal quantity of red blood cells and hemoglobin).

SCA is a genetic disease. That is, it is determined by genes that govern the type of hemoglobin produced. For the purpose of understanding the sickle cell conditions, the type of hemoglobin a person has is determined by two hemoglobin genes, one from each parent. Those who have inherited a gene for sickle hemoglobin from both parents have SCA. Virtually all of their hemoglobin is sickle hemoglobin, and rod formation and sickling readily occurs when oxygen is released to the organs and tissues. Inheritance of the gene from only one parent results in sickle cell trait (SCT), in which only about one-half of the hemoglobin is sickle hemoglobin. This amount is too small for rod formation and sickling to occur when oxygen is released to organs and tissues. Thus, SCT is a carrier state and not a disease.

If both parents have SCT, they each have a gene for normal hemoglobin and for sickle hemoglobin. Therefore, in each pregnancy there is a 25 percent chance for the child to inherit the sickle hemoglobin gene from both parents and to have SCA, a 50 percent chance of inheriting the normal hemoglobin gene from one parent and the sickle hemoglobin gene from the other and to have SCT, and a 25 percent chance of inheriting the gene for normal hemoglobin from both parents and to be normal with respect to sickle cell conditions. These odds or risks are present in *each* pregnancy. Obviously, if only one parent has SCT, the couple cannot have a child with SCA. There are two other major types of sickle cell disease: sickle cell–hemoglobin C disease, a condition in which the individual has inherited the gene for sickle hemoglobin from one parent and for hemoglobin C from the other, and sickle cell–thalassemia disease, in which the individual has inherited the gene for sickle hemoglobin from one parent and the gene for thalassemia from the other. The thalassemia gene decreases the production of normal hemoglobin. These two diseases tend to be milder in severity than SCA.

In the United States, sickle cell conditions occur primarily in blacks; approximately one of twelve black Americans is born with SCT and about one of 600 with SCA. Far less frequently, sickle cell conditions occur in other U.S. populations, primarily those of Puerto Rican, Cuban, and southern Italian ancestry. It is clear that a disease of this severity and prevalence creates a major challenge for health care professionals and scientific investigators.

So what has been the response? Three distinct periods in the biomedical response to the challenge are identifiable.

Sickle Cell Research

From 1910, when the disease was first reported in the medical literature (Herrick, 1910) to 1940, sickle cell research can be largely characterized by efforts of patient care specialists to gain a better understanding of what constituted SCA and how it could be differentiated from other diseases. From 1941 to 1970, biochemists and geneticists became involved and three major discoveries were made. First was the recognition of the genetic difference between SCT and SCA; that is, one sickle hemoglobin gene is inherited in SCT and two in SCA (Beet, 1949; Neel, 1949). The second was the discovery by Nobel Laureate Linus Pauling that there is a chemical difference in the hemoglobin molecule of those who have a sickle cell condition (Pauling, Itano, Singer, & Wells, 1949). Indeed, SCA has a prominent place in medical history as the first identified molecular disease (the hemoglobin molecule is the causative agent). The third was the recognition that there has been an advantage to having sickle cell trait in West African countries (Allison, 1954). In these countries, a form of malaria has been responsible for many thousands of deaths in young children. Young children who have SCT are less likely to contract malaria and die from it, and hence more likely to live and ultimately pass the gene on to their children. This survival of the fittest has been the major factor in the development of a high frequency of SCT in black West Africans and their descendants wherever they live. Obviously, though, having SCA has not been advantageous.

Despite those three landmark advances, this period has been characterized as one of benign neglect, for few dollars were available for research and little effort was made to have the black population gain the benefit of what was known about the inheritance of the disease. During those thirty years, no effort was made to detect and educate carriers so that they could decide whether they wished to take the chance of having a child with SCA. As late as the early 1970s, virtually every parent who had a child with SCA became aware of their potential for having a child with the disease after the birth of the first child having the disease.

During the period from 1971 to 1990, there was significant progress in research, in the provision of services, and in the level of funding by the National Institutes of Health. The direction of research has included attempts to gain a better understanding of the formation of sickle cells, the behavior of sickle cells when they flow through blood vessels, and the characteristics of sickle cells after they sickle. These areas of investigation are required in order to determine the types of drugs that can prevent, inhibit, or reverse the sickling process. A large number of drugs have been tested in the laboratory, a smaller number in animals, and a few in individuals who have SCA. Unfortunately, at this time we do not have a drug on the horizon that is likely to be effective in treating all individuals who have SCA. However, very promising research is being conducted with the ultimate goal of having individuals with SCA produce normal hemoglobin rather than sickle hemoglobin. Two approaches are being explored—bone marrow transplantation and gene therapy.

Red blood cells are manufactured in the bone marrow. So one approach to a cure is to destroy all of the patient's bone marrow and replace it with bone marrow from a donor who does not have SCA (Kirkpatrick, Barrios, & Humbert, 1991). Several children in the United States (Mentzer, Packman, Wara, & Cowan, 1990) and twelve in Belgium (Vermylen, Robles, Juane, & Cornu, 1988) have had successful transplants. Currently, though, the risk for the host to destroy the donor's transplanted marrow (graft rejection) or for the donor's marrow to attack the host (graft-versus-host disease) is too high to recommend this approach for general use. Substantive research is underway to determine how to reduce the incidence of these two complications. In the interim, criteria are being established to decide which children might be better served by taking the risk of transplantation rather than allowing the disease to run its course. The first group of children who are likely to be recommended for transplants are those who have had a stroke and have a genetically compatible sibling to serve as the donor. Currently, children who have had a stroke are placed on a transfusion program, receiving transfusions every three to four weeks to prevent a recurrence. Recurrence is prevented because a high percentage of red blood cells are transfused normal red blood cells that cannot sickle. But transfusion therapy is not free of disadvantages. Hemoglobin contains iron, and when the transfused red blood cells break down, iron is released. Unfortunately, the human body does not have an effective mechanism for excreting iron, and eventually the retained iron damages the heart, liver, and pancreas. There are drugs called *chelators* that when administered by pump can effectively aid in the excretion of iron by the kidneys. Both the transfusions and chelation are difficult to maintain and seriously impair the quality of life. On the other hand, strokes can recur after years of transfusion therapy because of the persistence of a narrowed vessel in the brain (a major factor in the occurrence of strokes). We can anticipate that in the near future, less severely affected patients will be offered transplantation as methods to reduce the risk of graft rejection and graft-versus-host disease complications.

In gene therapy, the gene for sickle hemoglobin is replaced with a gene for normal hemoglobin. Significant advances have been made in gene therapy research, but it is not at a point where patient application is possible (Banks, Markowitz, & Lerner, 1989). Although most of the research that has been conducted has basically provided a better understanding of the complex sickle cell phenomenon, there have been a few discoveries that have been beneficial to parents and patients. For example, it has been shown that the daily administration of penicillin can prevent sudden death from bacterial infections in infancy and early childhood (Gaston et al., 1986) and that the diagnosis of SCA can be made early enough in pregnancy to give a woman the option of whether to continue or terminate the pregnancy (Rowley, 1989).

The following sections discuss service needs and programs. Individuals with sickle cell conditions have service needs that if unmet can result in unfavorable physical, psychological, social, and economic consequences. Considered here are SCT and SCA.

Sickle Cell Trait Service Needs

SCT is not a disease, and knowledge of having it is basically of no value to one's health status or care, but, as indicated, couples who both have SCT have a 25 percent chance of having a child with SCA in *each* pregnancy. If they are not aware prior to childbearing that they both carry the sickle cell gene, the first child of one out of approximately 600 black couples will have SCA. Thus, these parents will be faced with the psychological, social, and economic burden of caring for a child with an illness that is currently incurable and that reduces life expectancy without having had an opportunity to exercise options with respect to mate selection or taking the risk.

Since the risk of an SCT couple having a child with SCA is well established and there are reliable and relatively inexpensive tests to identify carriers, individuals with SCT have a right to have their sickle cell status determined and to know its implications for the health of their children. Thus, one of the objectives of SCT services is to identify and counsel individuals with SCT during the childbearing years so that they can make informed decisions in their best interest regarding family planning.

In the early 1970s, the recognition of the need for blacks to be informed, tested, and counseled accelerated the development of community organizations (the first was founded in 1955). These organizations were funded by the private sector and/or the federal government. Federal government support consisted of grants to twenty-six community organizations. Though limited in scope, this pilot program was very effective. With the move by the federal government to incorporate genetic disease funding in Block grant awards to the states rather than funding organizations directly, these programs were discontinued or their capacity to function effectively was seriously diminished. Few states continued to support these efforts with state funds. Community organizations—including the seventy members of the National Association for Sickle Cell Disease, Inc. (NASCD)—are attempting to carry out programs primarily with private sector funding, augmented in some instances by state, municipal, or United Way support. Also, there is a public education, testing, and counseling component in the ten National Institutes of Health–supported Comprehensive Sickle Cell Centers. Some testing is done, too, by private physicians and those working in health maintenance organizations (HMOs), but typically such testing is not accompanied by substantive counseling. Overall, it is evident that the available services are grossly inadequate to meet the need.

There is another dimension to the need for trait carriers to receive appropriate service. Effective SCT counseling (which is better labeled sickle cell education, because giving advice is prohibited) requires transmission of the information that will enable clients to make informed decisions. That body of information is easily defined (Whitten, Thomas, & Nishiura, 1981). Thus, there should be a basic curriculum that is not significantly altered by the whims and views of individual counselors, and individuals should be trained to implement the curriculum. Furthermore, training is required to ensure that the counseling is nondirective—that is, that neither opinions of the counselors nor perceived societal preferences are communicated in any way, either verbally or nonverbally. The objective is for the information received in counseling sessions to play an unbiased role in some of the most critical decisions individuals make, namely, selection and family planning. Thus, it is disturbing to note that (1) we do not have a basic universally used curriculum, (2) some counselors have not had formal training, (3) many counselors are not periodically and systematically monitored and evaluated, and (4) a certification process is not in place. The expertise is available to develop these efforts. What is lacking are the funds to support them.

There is another set of circumstances in which there is a need for SCT services. As indicated earlier, a diagnosis of SCA can be made early in pregnancy. This gives a woman an opportunity to decide whether to continue or terminate the pregnancy in time for a safe and legal abortion. This is an extremely valuable advance, because prior to this development, SCT couples who wished to be certain that they would not have a child with SCA had to forgo having their own biological children.

Technically, prenatal diagnosis requires a specimen of the developing placenta to be obtained by inserting a biopsy instrument through the vagina into the uterus (chorionic villus sampling). This can be done at about nine weeks after conception. Or a sample of the amniotic fluid can be obtained by insertion of a needle through the abdominal wall into the amniotic sac that surrounds the developing fetus (amniocentesis). This can be done at about fifteen weeks after conception. In either case, the DNA of the cells obtained can then be analyzed to determine whether or not the fetus has SCA. Unfortunately, offering this technology has not become a part of the standard of care for pregnant women who are at risk for SCT.

In the absence of guidelines, some physicians fail to inform their patients of available services (in part because of their attitudes about the appropriateness of abortion). In the absence of informed choices, there are two adverse consequences. Some women will be faced with the care of a child with SCA, a child that they would not have had if they had been provided with counseling (received the appropriate information). Conversely, some women will have an abortion that would have been unnecessary if they had received appropriate counseling. These are unacceptable consequences, because each stems from abridgment of two fundamental rights—the right to know and the right to decide.

The Scientific Advisory Committee of NASCD has developed a position paper on prenatal diagnosis that includes goals, guidelines, and implementation steps and procedures. The recommendations have been endorsed by three national black professional organizations (the Obstetrics and Gynecology section of the National Medical Association, the Association of Black Psychologists, and the National Association of Black Social Workers). It was not accepted for inclusion in a technical bulletin published by the American College of Obstetrics and Gynecology.

The committee proposes that the goal of sickle cell prenatal diagnosis should be to have all women who are pregnant with a child that has SCA make informed decisions that they believe are in their best interests with respect to continuing or terminating the pregnancy. This goal is based on the principle of self-determination. It is not intended to be articulated or perceived as preventive. However, there is an inherent preventive by-product in that it prevents the birth of children with SCA to parents who elect to avoid that outcome. It follows from the goal that success of prenatal diagnosis and counseling should not be determined by the number of pregnancies that are terminated (that is, the decline in the birth of children with SCA), but rather the extent to which informed self-interest decisions are made.

The achievement of informed self-interest decision making also applies to the associated decisions that women will have to make with respect to the service elements. Decisions include whether to have the initial sickle cell test, whether to have the mate tested, and whether to have a prenatal diagnostic test including those instances in which the father refuses to be tested. Implicit in the goal is that women exercise their options in an environment that does not evoke guilt or recrimination with respect to their decisions. Women who decide to have an abortion ought to be able to do so without being exposed to verbal comments or nonverbal behavior that indicates that hospital personnel disapprove of their decision. Similarly, women who decide to continue their pregnancies and later have a child who experiences a great deal of difficulty with the disease should not be humiliated by insensitive health care providers who believe that a chance was missed by not aborting.

To achieve the proposed goals of prenatal diagnosis, the following must occur. Pregnant women who have SCT must be given a sickle cell test. If it is positive, they must be counseled — that is, informed about the nature of the carrier state, the manifestations of SCA, the potential burden on affected persons and parents, the management of the disease, how the disease is transmitted, the reproductive odds, and available options. It must then be determined whether to have the father tested. If the father also has SCT, he must also be counseled. Subsequently, both parents can decide whether they wish to ascertain whether the fetus has SCA. If so and the results are positive, they must have a counseling session that is designed to arrive at a decision.

NASCD recognizes that there are a number of noncognitive or affective factors that will probably influence or determine the decision. The primary care physician has the obligation to offer prenatal sickle cell testing to women, to provide basic information about the disease, and to offer sickle cell testing to the father. Whether the primary care physician provides the necessary cognitive/affective counseling or refers the patient to appropriately trained personnel should be the physician's option, depending on his or her training.

The cognitive/affective counseling requires individuals who have been specifically trained for this function. Currently, medical geneticists, genetics counselors, and some obstetricians and family practitioners are qualified. Training programs are needed to enable primary care physicians, social workers, public health nurses, and others (with appropriate backgrounds) to become qualified. The individual who conducts the cognitive/affective counseling should be trained and available to conduct postabortion counseling.

Sickle Cell Anemia Service Needs

With respect to SCA, there are significant health problems that occur primarily from the obstruction of blood flow, rapid destruction of sickle cells, and anemia. Recurrent, unpredictable pain attacks that are a result of SCA may be severe enough to require narcotics and hospitalization. It is the only disease with a lifetime propensity for pain attacks, and the pain most frequently involves the abdomen and chest but may be generalized. Other conditions include anemia, lowered exercise tolerance, painful swelling of hands and feet in infancy, sudden pooling of blood in the spleen in infancy (which can be a cause of sudden death), susceptibility to overwhelming pneumococcal infections, leg ulcers, breakdown of the head of the femur (the major bone in the hip joint), growth retardation, delayed onset of puberty, prolonged painful erection of the penis, gallstones, and strokes.

Individuals with SCA also may have to cope with a number of psychosocial stresses, including a lifetime of unpredictable occurrence of pain, growth retardation, delayed onset of puberty, repeated hospitalization, unpredictable interruption of important activities, lack of a cure, decreased life expectancy, limited job opportunities, and uncertainty about the desirability of marriage and having children (Whitten & Fischhoff, 1973).

It needs to be emphasized that no one has all of these physical and psychosocial problems. There is a wide and varied spectrum in the clinical expression of SCA with respect to the frequency, duration, and severity of pain attacks; the incidence of complications; and the impact on psychosocial and functional status and the life span. Furthermore, there is no basis for predicting the severity of the disease. Even a person's past history is unreliable for predicting the future course of the disease.

With respect to the management of SCA, physicians can do very little to prevent or reverse the processes that create the physical problems. They cannot prevent cells from sickling, reverse their shape after they have sickled, restore the life span of sickle cells to normalcy, prevent sickle cells from plugging blood vessels, or unplug blood vessels that are blocked with sickle cells. The thrust of medical care with respect to the physical manifestations of the disease is to minimize physical disability. This is accomplished by prompt treatment of pain (with whatever pain killer is necessary, up to and including morphine), by giving transfusions when anemia is severe or when there is sudden pooling of blood in the spleen, by treating infections with antibiotics, by removing gallstones, by preventing recurrent strokes with regularly administered transfusions, and by preventing infections with vaccines and antibiotics.

There is recognition in the health care field that the lives of individuals with chronic illnesses are frequently more negatively impacted by psychosocial factors than by the physical manifestations. That is true of SCA. Thus, appropriate health care extends beyond relief of symptoms to efforts to prevent or ameliorate the debilitating psychosocial effects of the disease. Supportive services can help individuals to live productive fulfilling self-supportive lives compromised only by the sickle cell health problems that cannot be prevented.

The quality of life of far too many adults with SCA is considerably lessened because of lack of economic self-sufficiency. At least 50 percent of adults with SCA are not employed on a full-time basis (Farber, Koshy, & Kinney, 1985) and are dependent on public assistance and/or their families for subsistence. This state of affairs exists despite their ability, if appropriately educated or trained, to handle any job or vocation that does not entail heavy manual labor.

There is an external factor that contributes to this high rate of unemployment. Employers are reluctant to hire individuals who have the potential for having a rate of absenteeism that might make it impossible for them to carry out their duties on a daily basis. Although all individuals with SCA are at risk for pain attacks that are unpredictable in their frequency, severity, and duration, the majority do not have pain attacks frequently enough to disqualify them for employment. Employers are encouraged not to take a class action position on the question of employment. Rather they should treat each person with sickle cell disease as an individual. Thus, they should employ individuals with SCA and ascertain whether the pattern of the individual's disease is or is not compatible with employment.

However, if all adults with SCA who are job trained were suddenly employed, it would have limited impact on the problem, because the vast majority of those who are unemployed lack marketable skills. Thus, an internal factor exists that is a greater determinant of the unfavorable employment status of this group than the external factor is. Children with SCA tend to be overprotected and therefore raised as though they are invalids. In an effort to be compassionate, parents tend to inadvertently raise children with a chronic disease such as SCA in a manner that leads to the development of an "ill" rather than "well" mentality. They become "programmed" to live a life of dependency rather than one of self-sufficiency. This results in many having neither the education nor the vocational skills that would render them employable.

We know that parents in general need but receive little education and guidance with respect to the task of raising children. Since the task of successfully raising children with a chronic illness is extremely difficult, the need for specific instructions is critical. Unquestionably, some parents intuitively raise their children effectively or need little help; many, however, require ongoing advice, counseling, and support.

During the course of children's lives from infancy on, programs are needed to provide disease education, anticipatory guidance, and counseling on adjustment and coping for both children and their parents. Other needs include the following: tutoring if the frequency and duration of pain attacks result in excessive absences, assistance in resolving school-related problems, social case work to help in the resolution of general problems of living that are compounded by having a chronic illness, academic and career guidance, and assistance in obtaining scholarships or vocational training grants. For those who have not been fortunate enough to have received these services, there is a great need for comprehensive vocational rehabilitation.

One other observation needs to be made with respect to medical management. There is a need to develop a universally practiced approach to patients who seek relief of pain in hospital emergency rooms. Some patients do have pain attacks that for periods of time occur very frequently and require narcotics for relief. When they seek care at emergency rooms, too often they are suspected of being drug abusers; this affects attitudes toward them and how their treatment is managed. This is a complaint voiced by patients all over the country. The problem is compounded by the fact that we have no objective way of determining whether the pain felt is sickle cell related. Unquestionably, there are some substance abusers in the adult sickle cell population, but they are the exception. Nationwide, to sum up, there are very few programs that address all of the needs of the sickle cell disease population.

Newborn Screening

There is another aspect of the service needs of the SCA population. Infants and young children have a markedly reduced ability to prevent exposure to bacteria (pneumococcus) that cause pneumonia from proceeding to an overwhelming infection and death. A landmark study funded by the National Institutes of Health convincingly demonstrated that twice-daily administration of penicillin could virtually eliminate this tragic outcome (Gaston et al., 1986). Because infection and death can occur before symptoms that could lead to the recognition of SCA become evident, participants in a national conference sponsored by the National Institutes of Health arrived at a consensus that sickle cell testing should be covered by state laws that require testing of newborns for other conditions (metabolic diseases) that have the potential for avoidable tragic outcomes (Consensus Conference, 1987).

For this approach to be effective, all black newborns have to be tested. Parents have to be located and notified. The infants have to be retested, and once the diagnosis is confirmed, parents have to be brought under the care of health providers so that they understand the nature of the disease and the value of penicillin administration. Since it has been fully documented that at all educational and socioeconomic levels of our society, health knowledge is not always translated into appropriate health behavior, there is a need for personnel to advocate continuously for compliance and to resolve barriers.

With regard to the conference recommendations, forty states have passed laws that require sickle cell testing in newborns. However, not all of them have actually provided the funding to implement the activities that are required to make testing programs successful.

Although the conference participants recognized the value of community sickle cell organizations, few states are using this resource for follow-up programs. When one considers that for some families, aggressive but sensitive and skillful efforts are required to maintain penicillin compliance, the experience, credibility, and acceptability of staffs of community organizations enhance the probability of achieving a high level of compliance.

The identification of SCA in newborns provides a golden opportunity to save their lives. In addition, it provides an opportunity to impact their development and adjustment early enough, and over a long enough period, to allow this generation of individuals with SCA to become self-sufficient and productive. Unfortunately, only a few cities have programs in place to achieve that objective.

The National Association for Sickle Cell Disease (NASCD)

A successful and effective approach to the resolution of a multifaceted health problem such as sickle cell conditions requires more than research initiatives and the direct provision of services. Some entity has to be responsible for direction, coordination, policy setting, presenting credible and respected positions on controversial issues, continuous assessment and refinement of needs, and overall advocacy.

The need for those functions has been particularly great for the sickle cell movement because this is the first disease for which there has been a national effort to identify carriers of a genetic disease prior to the birth of an affected child and to provide counseling thereafter. As can be expected, a number of sensitive social and ethical issues have had to be resolved for this program to be acceptable and effective.

Intense interest in the development of programs to serve the needs of the sickle cell population was one of the foci of the civil rights movement of the 1960s. A number of black voluntary groups began to provide public education and testing. Their interest and commitment were laudable, but some of their efforts were misguided (use of inaccurate and misleading literature, misinterpretation of test results, and use of an inadequate sickle cell test) because of the lack of adequate information. Thus, there was a need to harness, coordinate, and direct those efforts into an appropriate unified program so that they would be maximally beneficial and effective. In 1971, NASCD was organized to assume that responsibility.

NASCD's contributions to the sickle cell movement can be classified under eight headings (resolution of untoward "thrusts," educational materials, visibility, standards and guidelines, training, conferences, technical assistance, and youth scientific career motivation). The organization's value to the black community extends beyond its contributions to the resolution of the sickle cell problem. The health, social, and economic problems confronting the black community are so extensive and complex that programmatic efforts must extend beyond resolution of individual problems. A mission of those who undertake program development must be to deal with problems in a way that enhances the overall development and well-being of the black community. NASCD has accomplished many of these goals. It has established effective models for dealing with problems that disproportionately affect the black community. It is the only national black health organization developed to address SCA issues. It also expanded job opportunities for blacks through encouraging its member organizations to employ individuals as program directors, social workers, career development and tutorial coordinators, trait counselors, secretaries, and data entry clerks.

NASCD has also made a contribution to our society at large. The capacity exists to identify carriers of genetic diseases that occur predominantly among whites. NASCD has already resolved some of the issues that could potentially threaten the acceptability and viability of screening and counseling programs, thus benefiting a broader segment of the population.

Conclusion

The prospects for a cure through bone marrow transplantation and gene therapy are excellent. Fortunately, funding for the perfection of these approaches for SCA patients is not dependent on monies for specific sickle cell research, since each of these modalities is of value for other diseases (for example, bone marrow transplantation is an answer for some forms of leukemia, and gene therapy is an answer for the several hundred genetic diseases).

With respect to developing effective treatment approaches, there has been a decline in the response of researchers to the challenges of sickle cell conditions, as reflected by the number of applications for research grants from the primary source of research support (the National Institutes of Health). There were seventy-one applicants in 1982 but only thirty-two in 1990. A section of the U.S. Congressional Orphan Drug Act that was passed in 1982 states that "the Secretary of Health and Human Services shall provide for the development and support of not less than ten comprehensive centers for sickle cell disease." The centers are funded primarily to conduct basic and clinical research. The level of funding is capped at one million dollars per year. This level of funding has not kept pace with other initiatives of the division that fund and administer the sickle cell programs (the Division of Blood Diseases and Resources of the National Heart, Lung, and Blood Institute). Sickle cell patients are primarily dependent on these two groups of researchers — that is, those funded through investigator-initiated awards and those funded in the comprehensive sickle cell centers for significant improvement in treatment modalities.

Finally, with respect to meeting the nonmedical needs of the sickle cell population, successful models have been developed. Full or widespread implementation is primarily limited by a lack of adequate funding. This also applies to the activities and programs of NASCD. The organization is capable of markedly increasing the number of effective sickle cell community organizations, but the dollars to do so are not available. Thus, future progress toward the mission of an enhanced quality of life for those with sickle cell conditions is highly dependent on a substantial increase in governmental and private sector funding. The role of government in addressing the unmet needs of health problems such as sickle cell conditions is paramount (Whitten & Nishiura, 1985).

References

Allison, A. C. (1954). Protection afforded by sickle cell trait against subtertian malarial infection. *British Medical Journal, 1*, 290–294.

Banks, A., Markowitz, D., & Lerner, N. (1989). Gene transfer — A potential approach to gene therapy for sickle cell disease. *Annals of the New York Academy of Science, 565*, 37–43.

Beet, E. A. (1949). The genetics of the sickle cell trait in a Bantu tribe. *Annals of Eugenics, 14*, 279–284.

Consensus Conference: Newborn screening for sickle cell disease and other hemoglobinopathies. (1987). *Journal of the American Medical Association, 258*(9), 1205–1209.

Farber, M., Koshy, M., & Kinney, T. (1985). Cooperative study of sickle cell disease: Demographic and socioeconomic characteristics of patients and families with sickle cell disease. *Journal of Chronic Diseases, 38*, 495–505.

Gaston, M. H., Verter, J. I., Woods, G., Pegelow, C., Kelleher, J., Presbury, G., Zarkowsky, H., Vichinsky, E., Iyer, R., Lobel, J. S., Diamond, S., Holbrook, C. T., Gill, F. M., Ritchey, K., & Falletta, J. M. (1986). Prophylaxis with oral penicillin in children with sickle cell anemia. *New England Journal of Medicine, 314*(25), 1593–1599.

Herrick, J. B. (1910). Peculiar elongated and sickle shaped red blood corpuscles in a case of severe anemia. *Archives of Internal Medicine, 6*, 517–521.

Kirkpatrick, D., Barrios, N., & Humbert, J. (1991). Bone marrow transplantation for sickle cell anemia. *Seminars in Hematology, 28*(3), 240–243.

Konotey-Ahulu, F.I.D. (1968). Hereditary qualitative and quantitative erythrocyte defects in Ghana: A historical and geographical survey. *Ghana Medical Journal, 7,* 118–119.

Konotey-Ahulu, F.I.D. (1974). The sickle cell diseases: Clinical manifestations including the "sickle cell crisis." *Archives of Internal Medicine, 133,* 611–619.

Mentzer, W., Packman, S., Wara, W., & Cowan, M. (1990). Successful bone marrow transplant in a child with sickle cell anemia and Morgueo's disease. *Blood, 76,* 69A.

National Association for Sickle Cell Disease. (1988). *Position paper on prenatal diagnosis.* Los Angeles: Author.

Neel, J. V. (1949). The inheritance of sickle cell anemia. *Science, 110,* 64–66.

Pauling, L., Itano, H. A., Singer, S. J., & Wells, I. C. (1949). Sickle cell anemia: A molecular disease. *Science, 110,* 543–548.

Rowley, P. T. (1989). Prenatal diagnosis for sickle cell disease. *Annals of the New York Academy of Sciences, 565,* 48–52.

Vermylen, C., Robles, E. F., Juane, J., & Cornu, G. (1988). Bone marrow transplantation in five children with sickle cell anemia. *Lancet, 1,* 1427–1428.

Whitten, C. F., & Fischhoff, J. (1973). Psychosocial effects of sickle cell disease. *Archives of Internal Medicine, 133,* 681–689.

Whitten, C. F., & Nishiura, E. N. (1985). Sickle cell anemia. In N. Hobbs & J. M. Perrin (Eds.), *Issues in the care of children with chronic illness: A sourcebook on problems, services, and policies* (pp. 236–260). San Francisco: Jossey-Bass.

Whitten, C. F., Thomas, J., & Nishiura, E. N. (1981). Sickle cell trait counseling: Evaluation of counselors and counselees. *American Journal of Human Genetics, 33*(5), 802–816.

16

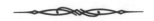

Adolescent Pregnancy
in the African-American
Community

Joyce A. Ladner
Ruby Morton Gourdine

Adolescent pregnancy is considered to be an epidemic in the United States. For African-Americans, the problem of teenage pregnancy is particularly devastating because of the sociomedical consequences experienced by this group. National data, as well as data from the nation's capital, are used to highlight the problem of teenage pregnancy. An exploration of the consequences is necessary because they are so varied and because the teen parent's adjustment is dependent on supportive family services and policies.

A key element in the situation of teenage pregnancy is poverty. Poverty impacts the African-American community in ways that often cause a ripple effect in terms of social consequences. In many cases, these consequences are manifested in black youth who are poorly educated or who drop out of school. Additionally, increased medical problems, poor socialization, and parenting skills that produce children who find it difficult to become a part of mainstream society exacerbate the problem. New social problems (for example, AIDS and crack addiction) that were not apparent ten years ago are tremendous problems now. African-American teenagers represent a group at risk for developing AIDS and/or addiction to crack. These health concerns coupled with teen parenting hold grave consequences for the children of teen parents.

A child born to a teenage parent often faces a bleak future. The future becomes even bleaker with the risk of AIDS infection and drug addiction. The tremendous technological resources of the United States must be tapped to more effectively facilitate the African-American community's efforts to combat these societal ills. This chapter presents a review of selected programs that can assist the African-American community in dealing with the problem of teenage pregnancy and the attendant social and medical ills.

It is important to examine teenage pregnancy from a national perspective, since such a focus defines the feasibility of solutions to combat the problem. Data from the District of Columbia will be presented, since this area has a large community of African-American citizens. A discussion of causal factors is necessary because these factors and the public response to them affect policies and programs. Specific needs of teens and their off-spring will also be addressed. A review of existing programs will provide the reader with a basis for interpreting the thesis presented, as well as an opportunity to view an array of current efforts related to the problem. It is also the intention of this review to invite the reader to develop new research and programmatic strategies toward solving the problem.

Teenage pregnancy and childbearing rates are higher in the United States than in other Western nations (Jones et al., 1985). This has been attributed to the fact that some of these areas, such as Western Europe, have focused on teenage pregnancy rather than teenage sexuality (Furstenberg, Brooks-Gunn, & Morgan, 1987).

The problem of teenage pregnancy within the African-American community is particularly poignant. Urban areas such as the District of Columbia, Chicago, Los Angeles, and New York experience especially high rates of teenage pregnancy. For example, in the District of Columbia, two in ten teenagers become pregnant each year. In 1986, 4,180 District of Columbia teenagers had pregnancies that terminated in birth, abortions, or miscarriages (Office of Policy and Planning, 1988). In the District of Columbia, the rate of teenage pregnancies for girls twelve to fifteen years of age increased between 1984 and 1986, while the rate for teens fifteen to nineteen years of age remained stable. An even more dramatic statistic from 1986 is the observation that 309 adolescents in the District of Columbia gave birth to a second child, while 49 gave birth to a third child (Office of Policy and Planning, 1988).

Data from the District of Columbia's Office of Policy and Planning (1988) indicate that the rate of teenage pregnancy remained relatively stable over a three-year period. These rates were 17.8 percent, 17.0 percent, and 16.3 percent for 1985, 1986, and 1987, respectively. For the period 1984–1986, the rate of pregnancies for teens under fifteen increased from 17.3 to 27.1 percent. For the same time period, the rate for teens over fifteen years of age shifted slightly, from 42.3 percent in 1984 to 41.9 percent in 1986. These pregnancy rates remained fairly stable, albeit higher than what would be an expected rate of teenage pregnancy.

The high teenage pregnancy rates in the District of Columbia are attributed to a set of circumstances that result from at-risk behaviors. These risky behaviors include (1) early sexual activity with multiple partners, often without effective use of birth control; (2) drug abuse; and (3) lack of appropriate information on birth control advice and devices. The high rate of teen pregnancy and the continued exhibition of risky behaviors are of particular concern, because—in spite of a proliferation of programs, information, and research—there appears to be little impact on teenage pregnancy rates and related problems in the nation's capital and across the country. Researchers argue that the reason the rate remains constant is that there is no sole criterion for determining causes and/or devising solutions to the problem of teenage pregnancy. One must also realize that the targeted group (teen parents) may view the problem differently than mainstream society. Therefore, one must be mindful that the wider societal view and expectations of an appropriate time to procreate is not in sync with the realities of life for those teens who become pregnant.

Social Consequences of Teenage Pregnancy and Parenthood

According to McAdoo (1986), the legacy of slavery has prevailed in certain sectors of the African-American community. These members of society are caught up in, and have no hope of removing themselves from, their dejected status (McAdoo, 1986). The pathos of the African-American community and family life is a much-debated topic (Moynihan, 1968; Gutman, 1976; McAdoo, 1986; Ladner, 1971; Glasgow, 1981). In light of these varied views, culturally sensitive researchers have demonstrated that the African-American family cannot be viewed in a monolithic context. African-American communities must be viewed in a holistic manner in which both strengths and weaknesses are discussed. This is a preferable approach because it allows the social scientist to more closely examine problem areas with regard to African-American lives as well as to pose workable solutions.

Generally, social scientists view changes in our society's mores and norms as a major contributor to the pervasiveness of the problem of teenage pregnancy (McAdoo, 1986; Ladner & Gourdine, 1984; Furstenberg et al., 1987). Consider that not much more than a generation ago, pregnancy without the sanction of marriage was taboo. Sexual relationships were generally reserved for persons who were "courting" with the intention of marriage. This relationship between partners was considered preparatory to marriage. Today, it is generally accepted that sexual relationships do not necessarily lead to marriage. The sexual revolution of the 1960s is credited with an expression of freedom that has had an impact on family life that in some instances has been devastating. Gone are the days when a girl became pregnant and delivered a child and it was considered a mistake, and that mistake was forgiven and families and communities assisted the young woman in reconstructing her life so that she could reenter school, find employment, and later marry (Ladner & Gourdine, 1984).

The sexual revolution has affected family life in general, but of grave concern for many social scientists is the devastating impact the sexual revolution has had on the lives of African Americans. The African-American family is in crisis. Approximately 50 percent of African-American households are headed by a woman (Matney & Johnson, 1983). Single parenting and poverty are viewed as a causal factor in destabilizing the African-American family. Single female–headed households tend to be poorer than their counterparts. African-American families may have been the trend-setters in terms of single-parent status (Furstenberg et al., 1987). The increase in female-headed households has created a so-called "feminization of poverty." "Being born into poverty is regarded by many researchers as tantamount to a life sentence of adult disadvantage" (Furstenberg et al., 1987).

Causes of Adolescent Pregnancy

Adolescent pregnancy has complex causes. Researchers have examined various factors in studying this problem.

Socioeconomic status

For African-American teen parents, most of whom are poor, economics offers a plausible explanation for being parents too soon (Ladner, 1987). Economic factors are further impacted when teenagers fail to complete school or fail to gain skills while in school that are salable in a technologically oriented job market. Available jobs for the poorly prepared are often low-paying service jobs that offer little opportunity for career advancement. The fact that many teens remain unmarried contributes to their lower economic status. An unmarried, underaged, or uneducated teen parent's economic future is unstable and exacerbates the problems associated with raising children and obtaining economic parity with others who do not become parents and who complete school.

Teen parents often rely on their parents or public assistance to sustain them and their children. While public assistance is a notable program that offers support to the unemployed and assists the needy, it does little in terms of providing economic stability and increasing economic status for families. In fact, it is seen by some as a causal factor in family and economic destabilization. A common perception of those who receive public assistance is that it is a crutch they learn to rely on. This often results in a false sense of security that is characterized by dependency and complacency. Unfortunately, teens—let alone their parents, who may be poor themselves, whether they receive public assistance or belong to the working poor—rarely understand the "system" and how it works. African Americans are subjected to a "double standard" that is imposed on them in terms of having unequal access to opportunities (that is, jobs, housing, education). This double standard may be evidenced when teen parents reject the "world of work" and accept public assistance for a life that appears to some to be one of immediate gratification without many responsibilities. If they do not choose this option, they may be forced to take jobs with low pay and little advancement because of their limited educational background. These jobs may be disappointing, in that the teens soon realize that the positions are leading them nowhere. They come to understand that the standards for parenthood and self-sufficiency imposed by American society are ones they cannot meet. The reality is that parenting is difficult under the best of circumstances.

The public views teenage pregnancy as a certain path to poverty and welfare dependency (Furstenberg et al., 1987). Findings show that the earlier a teen becomes a parent with little or no family support, the more likely the teen parent and child are to face a bleak economic future. Further, according to Furstenberg et al. (1987), the family size is also a predictor of receiving public assistance. Other factors, such as living in unsafe neighborhoods, attending poor-quality schools, associating with peers who do not value education, and delaying sexual activity, are equally compelling (Furstenberg, 1976; Furstenberg, Brooks-Gunn, & Morgan, 1987).

Education

Education is viewed as an escape from poverty, yet to the poor, it may seem elusive. The dropout rate among African-Americans has been recorded as being as high as 61 percent in some urban areas (Hammack, 1986). Education is usually truncated among teens who become parents. This situation impacts directly on their socioeconomic status and how they impart the importance of education to their offspring.

     School performance may be the most significant of the outcomes of early parenthood, since failure in school is a potent predictor of economic dependency (Furstenburg et al., 1987). The offspring of teen parents generally fare as well as their counterparts when they initially enter school. However, when school performance is viewed over a period of time, there tends to be massive school failure (Furstenburg et al., 1987). In the Furstenburg study, at least one-half of the subjects had repeated a minimum of one grade. Grade failure and discipline showed a high correlation. This study also showed the pervasive effects the mothers had on the child's academic performance in school. Similar data consistently demonstrate that the worse the student does in school, the more likely he or she will be to drop out. If students do poorly in school, the more likely they are to become teen parents and drop out of school. If they drop out of school, the more likely they are to be poor. Being poor starts the vicious cycle over again.

Consequences of Adolescent Pregnancy

Teenage pregnancy can have a wide range of social and medical consequences. A host of complications is related to this problem.

Social Circumstances

Not all families that experience out-of-wedlock pregnancy view the consequences the same way. Burton (1990) conducted a study in a small African-American community that offers a perspective different from what we might expect. Her investigation, carried out in a culturally sensitive context, found that the subgroup she was studying reflected an alternative life-course strategy, unlike the common perception that teenage childbearing is considered a violation of expected social behavior that produces negative outcomes. Burton asserts that alternative life-course strategies met the needs of the community because young mothers were valued parts of the community's functioning and survival. This community of intergenerational teen parents relied on each other for child rearing and monetary and familial support. They also provided assistance for the elderly. The elderly in this population (in their mid fifties) did not constitute aged populations in the conventional or gerontological sense (that is, those sixty-five or over), but rather were defined in terms of their poor health status and low life expectancy (mid fifties).

Because this community was self-contained, it remained viable. However, this system did not allow family members to be upwardly mobile and to seek "mainstream" lives. Findings on intergenerational teenage motherhood indicate that grandmothers who ranged in age from late twenties to early forties acted much older than they were (Ladner & Gourdine, 1984). Their family roles were hampered by a myriad of health problems, including hypertension, obesity, diabetes, and other ailments. These health problems, along with social isolation, led them to live more sedentary lives than would be expected (Ladner & Gourdine, 1984). However, these life-styles were not necessarily preferred, but were ones that the families accepted in a resigned manner.

Burton (1990) asserts that expectations of the African-American families in her study appeared to be defined by the limited experiences of their community. Members of the community were not allowed movement out unless the female left to work to support the family. Males in this community, however, were allowed to move out since they were not viewed as viable to the family structure.

Probably a more practical explanation for the alternative life-course strategy Burton presents is that it creates a family style that becomes functional in view of the diminished availability of marriageable mates due to incarceration and high mortality rates. Another strategy addressed by Burton is the age-condensed generational family structure. This emerges when teenage pregnancy/parenthood is consistent across generations and families (Ladner & Gourdine, 1984; Burton, 1990). Burton states that the fourth strategy is the child-rearing system of grandmothers who expected and desired to raise their grandchildren. This role was one that was ascribed to grandmothers in this community. Mothers were not expected to raise their own offspring. This delayed parenting for the grandparents in this community appeared to be desired and emotionally fulfilling.

However, our findings were different from Burton's (Ladner & Gourdine, 1984). The mothers were more reluctant to raise their grandchildren because many of them were still bearing children and found it difficult to care for several infants at the same time. They looked forward to a time when they could stop parenting. While they expressed supportive feelings and concerns for their teen daughters and grandchildren, they really saw themselves more in a role of "coparenting" than as grandmothers in a traditional sense.

Findings from these two studies suggest ways in which the African-American family defines itself. The self-contained community may be apparent throughout parts of the United States. However, a more likely pattern is families who experience intergenerational teen pregnancy and reside in urban areas where poverty is pervasive and opportunities limited. The migration from the South to the North, integration, and immigration have affected the African-American family in vastly different ways. These poor families continue to exist with little opportunity to escape the socioeconomic problems that have held their families hostage for several generations. The extended family as a resource has not been guaranteed for African-American families anymore (Martin & Martin, 1978).

Medical Consequences

The most important factor affecting pregnancy outcome is the mother's age and her gynecological history (Birch & Gussow, 1972). Consultation with the doctor prior to pregnancy is considered ideal. Teenagers tend to underestimate the consequences of their sexual activity, and once they suspect they might be pregnant, they hide their pregnancy from their parents for a variety of reasons. This behavior puts a teenage mother at risk medically.

Medical problems associated with teenage pregnancy are intrinsically linked, thus supporting a need for interdisciplinary approaches to the problem (Morton, 1984). Sociomedical problems surface during teen pregnancy. Stepto (1975) notes that pregnancy early after the onset of menarche causes the greatest risk for teenage girls due to their gynecological immaturity. The onset of menarche for girls is now at age 12.5 (Stepto, 1975). The statistics cited earlier in this chapter document that the pregnancy rate for teenagers under fifteen years of age is increasing.

Psycho-Socio-Medical Problems: The Ante Goes Up

The problem of adolescent pregnancy is more complicated than it may initially appear. All too often the teen parent's problem is viewed as a problem that speaks more to her morality than to the myriad of problems that encompass teen pregnancy/parenthood. Teen pregnancy/parenthood is more than just a medical, educational, or psychosocial problem. It is a problem that affects the "whole" family, community, and society. While it has been documented that African-American girls' rate of teen pregnancy is almost twice as high as that of whites, African-American girls do not find it any easier to resolve the issues of pregnancy (Shouse, 1975).

African Americans are very concerned about the future of their children and grandchildren. They express the same wishes for their children as the wider society does (Ladner & Gourdine, 1984; Shouse, 1975). However, they do view their options for improving their condition as more limited. Teen parents and their mothers may have relationships that are fraught with problems—many of which are developmentally appropriate. What complicates the mother-daughter relationship when a teen pregnancy occurs is the need to resolve the developmental issues as well as the parenting issues. Shouse (1975) is credited with enumerating the reasons that teen mothers become pregnant, namely, for love and acceptance, because of anger and fear, to determine their own adequacy as a female, and to disregard parental and societal standards.

Other explanations are more culturally based. Ladner (1971) raises several issues regarding womanhood in African-American families. She asserts that family socialization is so vastly different among racial and class lines that one cannot assess one without the other. In low socioeconomic African-American families, girls are socialized into womanhood around the age of seven or eight (Ladner, 1971). Their socialization primarily comes from an extended family and peers. Ladner (1971, p. 61) theorizes that in the ghetto, "Childhood is a luxury most parents cannot afford." The result is a "womanchild" who is expected to act and does act in a way that far exceeds her chronological age. This life-style is often viewed as amoral by the wider society. Additionally, it is a life-style that may lead to teenage pregnancy and cause problems for African-American communities (Morton, 1984).

Until recently, the African-American family was viewed by researchers as being without a cultural context. Culture permeates the fiber of all families, and so to discuss any findings without a cultural base should be viewed with suspicion. However, we must also recognize that while cultural similarities are documented for African-American families, greater differences may exist in terms of socioeconomic factors. The common links between African-American families are their culture and their experience with racism. The impact and interpretation of racism may differ among individuals, but racism is systematically reflected in policies and programs that target certain groups. It is probably true that most African-American families desire that their children achieve "The American Dream." The lack of access to the same opportunities whites have and/or the barriers one experiences tend to make African-American families more suspicious of those guaranteed rights of individuals in the United States. Legal intervention has been and continues to be necessary for African Americans to obtain their rights as Americans. In his book *Maggie's American Dream* (1988), James Comer presents an account of his family who worked very hard to see their children get a piece of the "American Dream." The strong, intact African-American family he describes is not a fantasy. African-American families with positive values and a strong sense of achievement do exist. When strengths of African-American families are acknowledged and extolled, the quality of life for all African Americans is improved.

The problems associated with being poor at times appear to be overwhelming. The perplexities of the so-called "underclass" are evidenced by severe income deprivation, unstable employment, low functional skills, and limited access to education and other social services (Cottingham, 1982).

The recent increase in female-headed households has exacerbated the problem. The extended family as we have known it is not as viable in urban areas.
Therefore, the safety net for many African Americans does not exist. Resources for these families become more scarce because of an increase in
single-parent homes by choice or divorce. Family stresses increase as well
(McAdoo, 1986; Morton, 1984).

When we consider the previous discussion of family life-styles, we can
readily understand the tremendous stress the adolescent mother and her
family may experience. With the increase in teen mothers under the age of
fifteen, the likelihood of having more intergenerational teenage mothers
increases. The concept and reality of "children raising children" is a reason
for concern. We must be concerned not only about the pregnancy and birth,
but also with the quality of parenting this generation of children will receive.
A new family life-style may be emerging without established norms either
culturally or generally. Moynihan (1968) described the matrifocal family as
existing in a "tangle of pathology." Many African-American scholars took
exception to this view. Billingsley (1968), Ladner (1971), and Hill (1972)
questioned the methodological and theoretical approaches of research that
focused on the "pathology" of African-American families. However, noting
the debate and variety of viewpoints, we must now look more closely at the
emerging life-styles of African-American families.

Ladner and Gourdine (1984) investigated the area of mother-daughter
relationships. This study examined values, beliefs, attitudes, and life-styles. It
found that social welfare policies (AFDC) discourage the inclusion of the
male in poor families; these families (mothers and children) reject the
presence of the male because of his unstable employment or because they do
not see it as viable for other reasons. This situation causes severe psychological damage for all family members. The grandmothers exhibit a sense of
powerlessness with respect to their children and are somewhat of a "new
breed." They are "young grandmothers" who are still acting out their childhood fantasies; in some instances, they enjoy the same social interaction that
their daughters find pleasurable. At times they appear to have more of a peer
relationship than a mother-daughter relationship. Their role in child rearing
of both their daughters and grandchildren is not necessarily one of adult
to child.

The mothers in our study also showed little confidence in the grandmothers' abilities to affect change for themselves and their children (Ladner
& Gourdine, 1984). Hence, the relationships between the mothers and
daughters were tenuous, since daughters may blame their mothers for their
situation of poverty or powerlessness. The expectation of how men function
in the family needs further exploration. An interesting story arises around
this issue. Most of the teen mothers in this study were happy to describe the
father's involvement as a parent as providing Pampers for the babies. This
minimal demonstration of fatherhood and responsibility appeared to be
acceptable to this group of young women. These situations cause a great deal

of concern among social scientists, who are fearful of what the next generation will be like in terms of family life and structure.

A New Decade—New Trends

In discussing the problem of teenage pregnancy, we must also discuss the
problems that are associated with sexual activity and pregnancy.

AIDS

Sexually transmitted diseases are a consequence of sexual activity. They affect
the health of the mother and child. The emergence of AIDS has been an eye-
opener in the area of sexually transmitted diseases. However, to state that
AIDS is "only" a sexually transmitted disease is perhaps being too casual
about the problem. The ante goes up for teen parents when AIDS is a
consequence of sexual activity.

According to Marsa (1989, p. 18), "As of October 1989, the Centers for
Disease Control (CDC) had recorded 1,908 cases of full blown AIDS among
children under thirteen years old, and this number did not include the 439
cases of teenagers who have full blown AIDS." The number of teenagers with
AIDS has increased by 40 percent in the last two years (Marsa, 1989). This
raises concern, because as of 1986, the Alan Guttmacher Institute (1986)
found that seven out of ten female teens had sexual intercourse before age
twenty, and eight of ten male teens had sexual intercourse by age twenty. One
must also consider the fact that teenagers who are exposed to the virus may
not show symptoms until many years later. It is believed that young adults who
develop AIDS were infected as teenagers. "The CDC refuses to make future
projections or comment on the specter of an epidemic among adolescents"
(Marsa, 1989, p. 18). While it appears that the actual number of AIDS cases
among teenagers is low, the fact that so many adolescents are sexually active is
a grave cause for concern. Sexual activity among teenagers has prompted
school systems and other social service programs to launch AIDS education
programs.

Drugs

AIDS is related not only to sexual activity but also to drug use. In recent years,
the use of crack cocaine has reached epidemic proportions. Not only does
the use of drugs affect the mothers, but it also affects the quality of the life of
her baby in utero as well as after birth.

Adolescent pregnancy is a health hazard for young women who do not
seek prenatal care. The crack and AIDS situations exacerbate the problem.
The probability of a poor pregnancy outcome is significantly increased for
these groups of parents and offspring. The issue of infant mortality and
morbidity is grave. Health problems associated with crack use for babies

include the possibility of a stroke, low birthweight, physical complications, prematurity, and disturbed behavior (Rist, 1990). However, the medical problems present only one side of the picture. The other side is the environmental hazard (Rist, 1990).

Social Environment

Even when adolescents leave the hospital with a healthy baby, environmental circumstances may affect the child's health status. The child's development is often impaired by poor social and environmental circumstances (Morton, 1984). Such practices as cutting the formula to last longer and infrequent changing of diapers affect the child's nutritional and general health status. The nutrition of a newborn is crucial to his or her growth and development.

For any child to make it in society, certain circumstances must exist that provide a protective, nurturing environment. But understanding the problems these children face is often so foreign to the policy makers that it is difficult to plan effective programs. As Norton (1989, p. 2) says,

> If we do not understand the tapestry of the early natural experiences of children, if we do not understand what environmental and societal contextual forces shape their world view, . . . can we really develop meaningful, relevant, and effective services for them and their families?
>
> To be effective, intervention should be based upon what is acceptable and possible within a particular community. It must be based upon understanding the meaning of behavior from the perspective of children and families being served.

The development of programs to effectively meet the needs of families and children may not necessarily reflect the needs of the wider society. Norton (1989) asserts that families of all types and cultures only teach whatever is thought to be needed in their environment. Thus, in a pluralistic society, the family may prepare the child successfully for life in the family's immediate environment but may not provide the child with experiences needed to operate in the wider society (Norton, 1989).

The changing, diverse nature of society in the United States makes it difficult for families to teach the rules and tools of the larger culture, and, in some homes, mothers may be too anxious and needy to provide what is required for survival (Norton, 1989). This is true when we view the modern teenage parent. The important question becomes, How can we devise programs that address divergent cultural needs?

Programs and Policies

This chapter has reviewed a limited number of studies on the causes of adolescent pregnancy and some probable solutions. A plethora of studies exists to support these views and to further document the causes of teenage pregnancy. However, we must pause to ask how this research has been helpful in solving the problem of teenage pregnancy. Are the rates of teen pregnancy decreasing? Are teen parents good parents? Are these programs institutional in approach?

The state of New Jersey has developed programs affiliated with schools in thirty sites across the state. The goals of the School Based Youth Services Program (SBYSP) are to provide at-risk adolescents with opportunities through programming to complete their education, obtain job skills, and lead productive lives (New Jersey School Board, 1989). This program has been in operation since 1987. The services provided at the centers include the following: (1) employment counseling, training, and placement; (2) summer and part-time job development; (3) drug and alcohol abuse counseling; (4) family crisis counseling; (5) academic counseling; (6) primary and preventive health services; (7) recreation; and (8) referrals to health and social services. The purposes of these programs are to augment and coordinate services for teens. There are twenty-nine centers, at least one in each of New Jersey's twenty-one counties. Sixteen are located in schools, and thirteen are located near schools. These sites offer services during and after school, on weekends, and during the summer months. This idea was conceived because of the recognition that school problems are much different than they were years ago. A concerted effort is made by New Jersey to eliminate the artificial boundaries between education and human services and to bring services under one roof (Sullivan, 1987).

Ladner (1987) concurs with the notion that the most effective approaches to teen pregnancy prevention are those programs that emphasize comprehensive services. Those services most often include education and training, jobs, sex education, family life education, life skills training, peer counseling, male responsibility counseling, with equal emphasis on the needs of female and males (Ladner, 1987). Another example of these programs is the Teen Outreach Program in St. Louis. The after-school program is one that focuses on life-management skills. A key component of the program is the requirement that teens participate in community volunteer service. A sense of self-worth and the ability to overcome adversity is the result of the teenagers' volunteer activity (Ladner, 1987).

Most states and/or cities have services for youth. Often these programs are fragmented, and it is difficult to determine who is servicing whom. New Jersey has set an example by using existing programs and adding additional funding to make programs more comprehensive. This is a model other states may need to review. An evaluation of this program should be forthcoming to determine if the New Jersey model has used public and private funds to maximize effectiveness of services to teenagers. In a time of fiscal constraints, legislators must become more innovative and creative in providing services to those in need.

Policy Implications for the African-American Community

The problem of adolescent pregnancy is complex and can only be solved by means of comprehensive approaches. The programs discussed earlier represent ones that are comprehensive. While the authors endorse the programs discussed, other avenues must also be explored. Teenage pregnancy and parenthood strain the fabric of strong African-American families. Therefore, policies implemented to address the problem of teenage pregnancy must meet the needs of the total African-American community.

Policies should provide for health care, child care, and economic and educational parity (McAdoo, 1988). This type of policy will address the continuing needs that all families have, thus strengthening the African-American family and community. These policies should not be punitive. Families who need assistance need not be viewed as having personal deficits.

These policies must also support the stabilization of African-American families. That is, they should not penalize the fathers/males in the family for being unemployed or marginally employed. McAdoo (1988) asserts that the low income of African-American males contributes to the instability of the family. When black males are not a part of the family structure, single mothers rely on the institutional supports provided by the community or the government (McAdoo, 1988).

African-American families must not only deal with any personal problems they face, but also with institutional racism (Burnham, 1985). Therefore, African-American family members — especially single mothers — experience stress (McAdoo, 1988). The stress they experience contributes to the breakdown of the family unit.

Policies must be implemented to address these problems. However, the authors endorse another approach that should also enhance the implementation of policies and programs. This approach is one of community advocacy and support. We must address the problem externally and internally. Historically, African Americans have been able to assist each other (Martin & Martin, 1985). Strength, love, and commitment have helped the African-American community survive. If this community could survive slavery, it can survive the current problems it faces.

Conclusion

"Teenage pregnancy is a national problem that transcends racial and class boundaries and it is a problem that takes a greater toll on African Americans" (Ladner, 1987, p. 242). Female-headed households are on the rise, and a good number of these families live in poverty. Expectations are lower with each succeeding generation when the reality of life is played out by being poor and living in unhealthy circumstances. An escape appears to be more and more elusive. The intense family problems resulting from poor relationships, societal ills (drugs), and life stresses make African Americans more vulnerable now. A generation ago, the typical pregnant teenager did not suffer the multiple exposures experienced by teens today (Ladner, 1987). Today's youth are more likely to have health-related problems, drop out of school, and lack skills or the desire to get and keep employment (Ladner, 1987).

African-American communities have been splintered, and the strong institutions of earlier years are not as stable. Families are more distressed than before, and the incidence and severity of the problems have increased (Ladner, 1987). The higher stakes for adolescent parents are played out in the following scenario: they are more likely to get sexually transmitted diseases, including AIDS, which is a death sentence; they are also more likely to be exposed to drugs, which is a life sentence. The prevalence of AIDS, crack addiction for mother and child, abject poverty, and the hopelessness that results from these situations are not a sentence African Americans desire or deserve. Immediate actions are required to reduce the incidence of disease and the dire social circumstances that propel African Americans to a type of second-class citizenship. The creativity and other strengths of African Americans can make a difference.

References

Alan Guttmacher Institute. (1986). *United States and cross-national trends in teenage sexuality and fertility behavior.* Unpublished data.

Billingsley, A. (1968). *Black families in white America.* Englewood Cliffs, NJ: Prentice-Hall.

Birch, H. C., & Gussow, D. D. (1972). *Disadvantaged children.* Orlando, FL: Harcourt Brace Jovanovich.

Burnham, L. (1985). Has poverty been feminized in black America? *The Black Scholar, 16*(2), 9.

Burton, L. M. (1990). *Teenage child bearing as an alternative life course strategy in multigeneration of black families.* Manuscript submitted for publication.

Comer, J. P. (1988). *Maggie's American dream.* New York: New American Library.

Cottingham, C. (1982). *Race, poverty, and the urban underclass.* Lexington, MA: Lexington Books.

Furstenberg, F. F. (1976). *Unplanned parenthood: The social consequences.* New York: Free Press.

Furstenberg, F. F., Brooks-Gunn, J., & Morgan, S. P. (1987). Adolescent mothers and their children in later life. *Family Planning Perspective, 19*(4), 142–151

Glasgow, D. G. (1981). *The black underclass.* New York: Vintage Books.

Gutman, H. (1976). *The black family in slavery and freedom.* New York: Random House.

Hammack, F. M. (1986). Large school systems dropout reports: An analysis of definition, procedures, and findings. *Teachers College Record, 87*(3), 324–341.

Hill, R. B. (1972). *The strengths of black families*. New York: National Urban League.

Jones, E., Forrest, J. D., Goldman, N., Henshaw, S. K., Lincoln, R., Rosoff. J., Westoff, C., & Wulf, D. (1985). Teenage pregnancy in developed countries: Determinants and policy implications. *Family Planning Perspectives, 17*(2), 53–63.

Ladner, J. A. (1971). *Tomorrow's tomorrow: The black woman*. New York: Doubleday.

Ladner, J. A. (1987). Black teenage pregnancy: A challenge for educators. *Journal of Negro Education, 56*(1), 53–63.

Ladner, J. A., & Gourdine, R. M. (1984). Intergenerational teenage motherhood: Some preliminary findings. *Sage: A Scholarly Journal on Black Women, 1*(2), 22–24.

Marsa, L. (1989, April). Teaching aids. *Omni*, pp. 19–20.

Martin, E., & Martin, J. (1978). *The black extended family*. Chicago: University of Chicago Press.

Martin, E., & Martin, J. (1985). *The helping tradition in the black family and community*. Washington, DC: National Association of Social Workers.

Matney, W. C., & Johnson, D. W. (1983). *America's black population, 1970–1982: A statistical view*. (Special publication PIO/POP-83-1). Washington, DC: Bureau of the Census.

McAdoo, H. P. (1986). Crisis in the family: Teenage pregnancy is not just a black problem. *Youth Policy, 8*(3), 29–30.

McAdoo, H. P. (1988, April). *Changes in the formation and structure of black families: The impact on black women*. Paper presented at Wellesley College, Center for Research on Women, Wellesley, MA.

Morton, R. D. (1984). *Decision-making, locus of control, and pregnancy outcome of black adolescents*. Unpublished doctoral dissertation, Howard University, Washington, DC.

Moynihan, D. P. (1968). *The negro family: A case for national action*. Washington, DC: U.S. Government Printing Office.

New Jersey School Board, Youth Services Program. (1989). *Fact sheet*. (Available from Assistant Commissioner for Intergovernmental Affairs.)

Norton, D. G. (1989, December). *Research theory and design of relevant culturally and ecologically sensitive intervention*. Paper presented at the Biennial Faculty Training Institute of the National Center for Clinical Infant Programs, Washington, DC.

Office of Policy and Planning. (1988). *Interim report to the mayor, Teenage Pregnancy Prevention Panel*. Washington, DC: District of Columbia Government.

Office of Policy and Planning. (1989, October). *Statistics on birth rates, District of Columbia*. Washington, DC: District of Columbia Government.

Rist, M. C. (1990, January). The shadow children. *American School Board Journal*, 19–23.

Shouse, T. W. (1975). Psychological and emotional problems of pregnancy in adolescence. In J. Zackler (Ed.), *The teenage pregnant girl*. Springfield, IL: Thomas.

Stepto, R. G. (1975). Obstetrical and medical problems of teenage pregnancy. In J. Zackler (Ed.), *The teenage pregnant girl*. Springfield, IL: Thomas.

Sullivan, J. F. (1987, December 5). $6 million to go for social services for students in New Jersey. *New York Times*, p. 29.

17

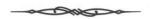

Elderly Issues
in the African-American
Community

Mary S. Harper

In the United States, 6,000 persons celebrated their sixty-fifth birthday in 1989 each day, totaling about 2.2 million persons (American Association of Retired Persons, 1990). The number of Americans sixty-five and older has increased by 21 percent (5.3 million) since 1980, compared to an 8 percent increase for the remainder of the population. The 1990 edition of the American Association of Retired Persons' *A Profile of Older Americans*, which is updated annually, projects that by the year 2030, there will be sixty-six million older persons; they will represent nearly 22 percent of the U.S. population. Persons sixty-five or older numbered 31.0 million in 1989 and represented 12.5 percent of the U.S. population.

In 1989, about 87 percent of persons sixty-five or older were white, and 8 percent (2.1 million) were black. About 2 percent were Native American, Eskimo, Aleut, or Asian and Pacific Islander, and 3 percent were of Hispanic origin. Of the 2.1 million black elderly, 7.5 percent (157,500) were eighty-five or older in 1989. Black elderly form the fastest growing segment of the black population. Between 1970 and 1980, the black elderly population increased 34 percent, but the total black population increased only 16 percent. About one-fifth of black elderly live in rural areas, and over 59 percent are concentrated in the Southeastern states. Ninety-four percent of all elderly are community domiciled, compared to 96 percent of black elderly. More older blacks than whites are widowed, divorced, or separated, and a smaller proportion live with their spouses. However, sharing a home with an adult child, usually a daughter, is a common living arrangement for older blacks. Only 3 percent of all black elderly are institutionalized, whereas 5 percent of white elderly are. Among those eighty-five and older, 12 percent of blacks and 23 percent of whites are in institutions.

Unlike many of the minorities who immigrated to the United States, the black elderly were educated when access to educational resources was severely limited. Yet only 6 percent have no formal education; 17 percent completed high school, as compared to 41 percent among the white elderly.

Thirteen percent of black and white elderly continue to work after age sixty-five. The median income of black elderly men is about $4,113 and of black women about $2,825, as compared to $7,408 for white men and $3,894 for white women. Black elderly are more likely to be sick and disabled and to perceive themselves as being in poor health (American Association of Retired Persons, 1988).

Black adults reach age sixty-five with life histories of a disproportionate prevalence of acute and chronic disease, illness, disability, and "color-coded" access to the health care system. Many of them have had a poorer quality of health care from conception and birth, continuing exposure to greater and more severe environmental risk factors, and the stress of prejudice and discrimination (Cooper, Steinhauer, Schatzkin, & Miller, 1981). Cohort data for cause-specific mortality and morbidity over the past forty years suggest the presence of accumulated deficits across the early life course. These deficits place the black elderly at greater risk for morbidity and mortality than whites of comparable ages.

Old age among blacks, as in the general population, is not a time of inevitable decline (Committee on an Aging Society, 1985; Rowe, 1985). Changes in life-style, reduction of environmental risks in the home and place of employment, and medical intervention can positively affect the quality of life of older black Americans. Survey data (Gibson & Jackson, 1987) reveal that many of the black oldest-old (eighty years and older) are free from functional disability and limitations of activity due to chronic disease or impairments.

Although multiple factors contribute to the persistent disadvantages of blacks, poverty may be the most profound and pervasive. There has been a consistent finding across communities and nations that persons of the lowest socioeconomic status have higher death rates. In a classic study, Kitagawa and Hauser (1973) found that there was a gradient of mortality rates with steady increases from the highest to the lowest social classes. Mortality rates were higher as socioeconomic status declined for both whites and blacks, whether the status was measured by family income, educational level, or occupation. For people of the lowest status, overall mortality was 80 percent greater than for those at the highest socioeconomic level. In addition to increased mortality, almost every form of disease and disability is more prevalent among the poor. Because of the relationship between poverty and health, and because poverty has been a persistent problem for blacks in the United States, it is to be expected that the blacks' greater poverty is responsible for much of the black-white disparity. There has been significant improvement in the social and economic status of older blacks over the past forty years (Jackson, 1981). Although there is disagreement regarding the extent of the improvements in the health status of black elderly, most observers find that the health status of older blacks has improved considerably over the past few decades, particularly with the advent of Medicaid and Medicare in the mid 1960s.

Poverty as an Issue

Poverty, with its deleterious effects on education, self-esteem, quality of life, and life-style, is the major reason why the black elderly have higher cancer rates than their white counterparts (Okie, 1991). So powerful is the impact of poverty that if differences in income, education, and living conditions were eliminated, the pattern would be reversed — blacks would have a lower overall cancer rate than whites. The study also found that people of different races show differences in vulnerability to various tumors. But those differences, whether rooted in heredity or culture, are usually outweighed by the much greater influence of poverty, which raises cancer rates by reducing access to health care and education and by determining where people live.

In the same study, National Cancer Institute researchers correlated cancer incidence rates for blacks and whites in three major metropolitan areas (Atlanta, Detroit, and San Francisco/Oakland) with socioeconomic data from the 1980 census. Poverty accounted completely for the overall excess of cancer seen in blacks. Poverty seems to be a more important risk factor for some kinds of cancer than others. For instance, rates for lung and cervical cancers were very closely tied to income and educational level. Smoking rates are highest among the poorest and least educated Americans. In contrast, cancers of the rectum, stomach, and prostate showed no association with socioeconomic factors (Okie, 1991).

Notably, one of the fastest-growing groups of black elderly is the poor who live in a census-defined poverty area within the central cities. Poverty areas are census tracts with poverty rates over 20 percent in 1980. While not all people who live in poverty areas are poor, Census Bureau data show that the number of poor elderly blacks living in poverty areas grew by 1.5 million or 59 percent between 1980 and 1986 (O'Hare, 1989). With the cost of health care and the high poverty rate for the black elderly, breaking the cycle of 60,000 excess deaths will be extremely difficult. Thirty-nine percent of black elderly lived in poverty in 1981. This represents a decrease from 1959, when 63 percent of black elderly had an income level below the federal poverty line. In 1980, the Census Bureau used different criteria for poverty, designating poor persons as those whose incomes are less than 125 percent of the poverty level. With the change in criteria for poverty, approximately 52 percent of blacks over the age of sixty-five were poor (Chen, 1985). Among the female-headed households, some 69 percent of black elderly were below 125 percent of the poverty level.

Although the black elderly are poorer than their white counterparts, the black elderly pay more out-of-pocket health care expenditures (excluding nursing home care). These expenditures represent only 2 percent of total income in families with income in excess of $30,000, but 21 percent of the total in families with income less than $5,000 (U.S. Congressional Budget Office, 1983). Out-of-pocket health care expenditures for the black elderly range from $500 to $1,500 per year. The black elderly are frequently forced to choose between health care, food, rent, and heat. It is often assumed that the black elderly who are poor have Medicare, Medicaid, and Supplementary Security Income (SSI). However, there are many disparities and barriers to access to health care for the poor black elderly. In 1982, the percentage of Medicare enrollees receiving reimbursement increased for all ages, but a differential between whites (65 percent) and blacks (59 percent) existed (Davis et al., 1989).

The Medicaid law was enacted in 1965 to expand the role of the federal government in financing health care for the poor. Medicaid was designed to help states in improving access to care for the poor and to enable the poor to receive mainstream medical care. Since more than one-third of all blacks are poor, it was assumed that Medicaid would reduce the disparity in access to care by race as well as income.

Medicaid covers 53 percent of the black and 32 percent of the white elderly. Medical benefits are paid unevenly with respect to race and geographic region. Average Medicaid payments per white beneficiary were 50 percent higher than payments per black beneficiary (Davis & Schoen, 1978). The average per-person charge for black Medicaid beneficiaries in 1980 was $598, compared with an average of $878 for white beneficiaries (Howell, Corder, & Dobson, 1985). Black elderly are five times more likely to be on Medicaid.

Medicare coverage is available for 10 percent (2.6 million) of black elderly. Coverage is almost universal. Twenty-eight million elderly persons and three million disabled beneficiaries were enrolled in 1986. Medicare payments exclude glasses, drugs, dental expenses, and hearing aids. Twenty-two percent of the black population over age sixty-five receive support from SSI.

Most income of the black elderly is from governmental sources. Only 5 percent receive any income from savings, in contrast to 36 percent of white elderly. Only 39 percent of black elderly have private insurance, as compared to 58 percent of white elderly. Thirty-seven million Americans are without insurance; 6.3 million blacks (or one out of four) have no insurance (Davis et al., 1989).

Some of the major problems confronting the black elderly include poverty and multimorbidity, with 51 percent having functional limitations (Butler, 1987). Additionally, the black elderly experience longer lengths of stay in institutions, polypharmacy, more physician visits than the white elderly, and access to a "color-coded" health care system.

Life Expectancy

Poverty and unemployment are the two major issues having the most deleterious effect on the black elderly's quality of life. Although both blacks and whites have gained in life expectancy, there has been a persisting lag in gains for blacks. Between 1900 and 1984, the expected remaining years of life at age sixty-five increased from 11.5 to 14.8 for white men, from 10.4 to 13.4 for black men, from 12.2 to 18.8 for white women, and from 11.4 to 17.5 for black women. In 1986, the average life expectancy at birth had increased to 74.8 years. The life expectancy for black Americans has declined for two consecutive years. It was 69.4 years in 1986, having been 69.5 years in 1985 and 69.7 years in 1984 (Sullivan, 1989).

The objectives of Healthy People 2000 (U.S. Department of Health and Human Services, 1990) advocated expansion of life, reduced health disparities among Americans, and access to preventive services for all Americans. In addition to expansion of years of life, a major focus advocated expansion of healthy life. For blacks in 1980, life expectancy was 68 years, whereas years of healthy life was only 56. For whites, life expectancy was 74.4 years and 63 years of healthy life (National Vital Statistics System and National Health Interview Survey, 1990).

Racial Minority Crossover Phenomenon

A mortality crossover exists between blacks and whites in the oldest ages (Manton, Poss, & Wing, 1979; Wing et al., 1985). At about age eighty, black men and women expect to outlive their white counterparts. It has been suggested, but not established, that this crossover in expected years of life is due to the weeding out of all but the hardiest blacks of very old age as a result of their earlier greater susceptibility to illness and violent death (Siegel & Davidson, 1984).

Health Issues Relating to the Black Elderly

Health for the elderly may be conceptualized as the ability to live and function effectively in society and to exercise maximum self-reliance and autonomy; it is not necessarily the total absence of disease (Harper, 1988). According to Rowe (1991), the health of older people has been approached from two different perspectives. The biomedical gerontological and geriatrics model, commonly held by physicians and other medical personnel, defines health in terms of the mechanisms and treatment of age-related diseases and presence or absence of disease. The functional model defines health in terms of older people's level of functioning; it is best summarized by a World Health Organization Advisory Group report: "Health in the elderly is best measured in terms of functioning. . . . Degree of fitness, rather than extent of pathology, may be used as a measure of the amount of services the elderly will need from the community" (World Health Organization, 1959, p. 5). Elderly blacks tend to perceive their health according to their ability to perform activities of daily living and not according to laboratory or x-ray findings. It may be the elderly's assessments and perceptions of their health that give rise to their frequent delay in seeking care or reporting discomfort. Black elderly, regardless of social class and income level, delay in seeking health services. One may ask if this is a form of denial or display of tolerance for the pain and/or discomfort. It has been clearly established that under-reporting and denial of discomfort are unique behaviors of the black elderly—behaviors of which caregivers must be cognizant.

Some of the most common diseases or conditions of the black elderly include hypertension, heart disease, cardiovascular diseases, cancer, diabetes, and chronic diseases (Butler & Hyer, 1990). Woolhandler et al. (1985) estimated that one-third of the excess of 1978 black over white deaths in Alameda County, California, were preventable. They purport that inequalities in the health care services reinforce broader social inequalities and are in part responsible for the disparities in mortality. Cooper et al. (1981) reached a similar conclusion.

There are several unique characteristics of the black elderly, including the (1) tendency to not report or underreport illness and physiological changes, including the fact that they have an enormous pool of tolerated illnesses at any given time, which frequently are ignored, normalized, or left to develop and worsen; (2) tendency to delay reporting of illness; (3) tendency to consider certain physiological changes, such as edema of the legs, morning stiffness, dizziness on rising, constipation, and urinary urgency as part of the process of aging; and (4) tendency to perceive sickness as a sign of weakness.

Health of the black elderly is equally related to public policy and biology. There are several risk factors and life-styles associated with the health of the black elderly. Risk factors such as smoking, use of drugs, unhealthy diets, lack of exercise, and poor stress management increase the risk of consequences of heart disease. Most of these risk factors are socially learned and reinforced aspects of behavior and life-style. Risk of poor health is more likely to be affected negatively by life-style, behavior, and environment than by genetics and biology. Historically, researchers have viewed the aging process as genetically hard-wired and biologically determined. Thus, we have not encouraged thinking in terms of modifying the life-style to improve health or prevent disabling diseases. Many of the illnesses of the black elderly are modifiable; hence, health providers and other caregivers should encourage such behavior. Poverty, ignorance, social isolation, and racism are as deleterious to the aging process and the quality of life for the black elderly as are biological impairments.

The black elderly present disease and/or illness in atypical and altered fashions. A fundamental principle of geriatric care is that many diseases have signs or symptoms in the elderly that differ from those in their younger counterparts. Specific characteristic symptoms of a disease in middle age may be replaced by other symptoms in old age. For instance, acute myocardial infarction studies have suggested that elderly persons are less likely than younger adults to present with chest pain (Pathy, 1967; Rowe, 1989). On the other hand, acute myocardial infarction is not "silent" in older people; there are a variety of other acute symptoms, including syncope and the sudden onset of left ventricular failure (Besdine, 1980). The other difference is that elderly people may present with nonspecific signs and symptoms (Besdine, 1980). Examples include confusion, weight loss or "failure to thrive," disturbance of gait, insomnia, and dehydration (instead of specific symptoms indicating the organ or organ symptom affected). It is not uncommon for the elderly person who has a fecal impaction to present in a state of delirium, or one with hyperthyroidism to present with apathy and cachexia.

Diabetes mellitus and obesity are very common in the black elderly and serve as a "great masquerader." Thirty-eight percent of all people with diabetes mellitus are over sixty-five years of age, including 10 percent of those over sixty-five years old and 20 percent of those over eighty years old. Since this disease can be a great masquerader, it is essential that all health care providers, patients, and family members understand the signs and symptoms of diabetes mellitus and its diagnosis in order to distinguish it from age-related changes in glucose tolerance (Gambert, 1990b).

Diabetes may atypically and nonspecifically present as incontinence, anorexia, delirium, depression, weight loss, and falls, and as an altered sleep-wake cycle. The most common atypical findings of diabetes mellitus in the elderly is an alteration in mentation. This may present as an acute confusional state, delirium, or dementia. It is important that caregivers at all levels observe for atypical presentation of illness, because serious symptoms of treatable diseases often go unreported (Rowe, 1983; Anderson, 1966).

The underreporting or self-destructive behavior often results from the elderly's notion that old age is necessarily accompanied by illness and functional decline, and thus symptoms are expected. Other causes for underreporting are fear of the nature of underlying illness and concern about cost and potential hospitalization. Noninstitutionalized elderly persons have on the average 3.5 important disabilities (Anderson, 1966). Wilson, Lawson, and Brass (1962) found a group of hospitalized elderly persons to have an average of six pathological conditions.

Access and Utilization of Health and Social Services

Access to affordable and quality comprehensive care for all citizens will be the challenge of the twenty-first century. Although significant strides have been made in the delivery of health and social services, great disparities still exist. The health care system in the United States is complex, and until recently, it was very institution-oriented. The institutional orientation deprives the elderly of needed services. Only 5 percent of the elderly aged sixty-five to seventy-nine years of age are in institutions, compared to 20 percent of those eighty and older.

The present health care system needs to recognize the "place" and needs of the community-based elderly as well as the institution-based elderly. It must also recognize that 75 to 80 percent of the noninstitutional care is given by members of the family and significant others, and that 70 percent of the care given in long-term care facilities is given by nursing personnel (primarily nurse aides, licensed practical nurses, and, to a lesser extent, registered nurses). In order to improve the quality of care, we must concentrate on training, monitoring, and supervising the primary care providers. We must promote self-care and mutual care. We must not create iatrogenic dependence. All disciplines and members of the family *must* concentrate on plans of care that foster autonomy and self-direction. Differentials in health and in effective access to health services cannot be considered apart from other dimensions of life, especially where public policy plays a large role. The long-term health care facilities are "driven" by public policies and legislation. These policies are monitored and revised. In contrast to the situation in many other countries, *Notices of Proposed Rule Making* (NPRM) is published in the *Federal Register* for comments. The nursing home industry generally comments, but other health industries and groups (lay and professional) should also comment on the NPRM. NPRM seeks comments on such areas as the use of restraints (physical and chemical), use of psychotropic drugs, training of nurse aides, preadmission screening, and annual reviews and accountability for resident funds. In some areas there has been progress in ending the disparities in health care, while in other areas discontinuities and inequities still prevail. The toppling of barriers of racial segregation has not ensured active inclusion and full participation for many blacks. Among options for public strategy, a combined approach of consensus building, "universality," and efficient "targeting" may make for good policy and good politics.

To redress the remaining differences in equitable access to health care services for the black elderly, the following policy actions are recommended:

- Maintenance or improvement of health status by expanding health insurance coverage under Medicaid and private insurance
- Development of policies that will allow for independence instead of policies requiring institutionalization or bed confinement in the home
- Increased self-care activities
- Modification of the environment to eliminate physical or psychological barriers to desired autonomy
- Maintenance of quality of life
- Achievement of a peaceful death at home
- Active participation of resident and family members in the development and evaluation of the care plan and decision making pertaining to resident care

It has often been claimed that older blacks suffer perceived and actual psychological, social, and structural barriers (Haywood, 1984; Jackson, 1981; Myers, 1984). The usual explanation offered is that low social status is a major impediment to good health care. James et al. (1984) found that regardless of

their socioeconomic background, blacks with hypertension report less frequent use of medical care, more difficulty getting into the health care system,
and greater dissatisfaction with medical care when compared to similarly
afflicted whites.

One of the major barriers to access is the lack of financial resources for
copayment. Other barriers include the lack of quality treatment and medical
staff who will take Medicaid patients. Access to care for Medicaid beneficiaries is impeded because of limited participation in the program by physicians. Ten percent of all primary care physicians provide care to about half of
Medicaid beneficiaries treated in private offices (Mitchell & Cromwell, 1983).
Approximately one out of every four office-based physicians (23 percent)
report that they do not accept Medicaid. About one-third of physicians in the
South (34 percent) and 30 percent in the Northeast and large urban areas
report that they do not accept Medicaid. More than 39 percent of car-
diologists and 40 percent of psychiatrists report that they do not accept
Medicaid. These findings are troublesome, given the concentration of poor
black elderly in the South and urban areas. Only 53 percent of blacks have
Medicaid coverage; 6.3 million are uninsured and have no access to health
services.

Our health care system is driven by policies and practices that raise the
issues of (1) creaming, (2) universality versus targeting, and (3) poverty or
inequality reduction (Miller, 1989). Part of the refusal to admission in long-
term care facilities is due to creaming. Creaming is a policy, intentional or
unintentional, of concentrating on the "easiest cases." The poor black elderly
are frequently considered as outliers (heavy-duty health care services needed)
because of their frequent delay in seeking services. In addition, the black
elderly comorbidity (three to six diseases) gives rise to the use of the "creaming" policy. The assumption is that the methods that led to the improvement
among the "better off" will be equally useful for the worse off who were left
behind. The creaming approach is individualistic; however, it impacts the
black elderly more than it does other elderly groups. Twenty-two percent of
the black elderly are without insurance, 40 percent have medicaid coverage,
and 59 percent are poor. Therefore access to health care is questionable and a
policy of creaming is damaging to the quality of life for the black elderly.

The specific policy questions of how to improve the quality of life for
the black elderly are part of the general policy debate about the competing
principles of universality or comprehensiveness versus "targeting," which
focuses on selectivity or means testing. . . . Targeting is based on income and
needs. These policies raise questions of service utilization in addition to
access for the black elderly. Low-income blacks with health coverage make
twice as many visits to physicians as do the poor without coverage (Davis
et al., 1987).

The utilization issue has three important components related to poverty or inequality reduction. (1) Does medical care make a difference? (2) Will
the black poor take advantage of opportunities for care? For example,

Riessman (1974) found that poor blacks would use health services if they are accessible and appear to be useful. (3) Do finance and delivery systems affect utilization? Davis et al. (1987) concluded that they play a critical role in improvement of access to care for the black elderly.

One of the problems with access is the question of access to what. Is there a positive correlation between the number of physician visits and the health of the client? Little research has been done on quality of care by a provider of the same or different race. Mitchell and Cromwell (1980) found that physicians with large Medicaid practices were less qualified (as measured by board certification, age, and hospital-admitting privileges) than physicians with small percentages of Medicaid patients. Egbert and Rothman (1977) found that between 1952 and 1972, black patients and Medicaid patients in Maryland hospitals were significantly more likely to be operated on by a surgical resident than a staff surgeon. Black elderly use the emergency room and hospital outpatient services more often than they use a regular source of care. Without a regular source for health services, the care is episodic and without continuity and monitoring.

Lang, Kraegel, Rontz, and Krejci (1990) provide guidelines for assessing the quality of care for the black elderly. Accordingly, in order to improve this care, focus must be given to process and outcomes. Quality of care for the elderly is further compromised by misdiagnosis by physicians who are not race and culture sensitive (Lawson, 1986; Rosenfield, 1984; Rosenthal & Carty, 1988).

Assessment

In any assessment of the black elderly, care must be taken in checking the validity and reliability of the measurement instruments. For instance, Adebimpe, Gigandet, and Harris (1981) have questioned the use of the Minnesota Multiphasic Personality Inventory (MMPD) with the black elderly. Similarly, Robinson, Stewart, and Baker (conveyed to the author in a personal communication, May 10, 1990) have questioned the use of the Geriatric Depression Scale (GDS). Interest and concern about the care of the black elderly must extend to boarding and care homes, adult day-care centers, correctional facilities, and highrise apartment buildings. In a study by Roca, Storer, Robbins, Tlasek, & Rabins (1990), in which eighty-five elderly persons residing in four housing buildings were evaluated, 65 percent of the residents were black and low income and 25 percent of the residents evaluated were eighty-five years of age and over. Eighty-nine percent of the residents who were evaluated by the team met criteria for at least one DSM-III-R diagnosis; 63 percent of the disorders had not been previously diagnosed. The most prevalent diagnoses were dementia, depressive syndromes, schizophrenia, and delusional disorders, as well as alcohol abuse or dependence.

Psychiatric disorders are more common among the black elderly

residents of urban public housing. In a recent study, the one-month prevalence of DSM-III-R psychiatric disorders in this population was 31.4 percent
(Rabin, Fischer, & Shapiro, 1986), more than twice the one-month prevalence
(12.3 percent) found among community-dwelling elderly persons in the
United States in general (Regier, Boyd, & Burke, 1988). There is a danger that
untreated, unrecognized disorders of the elderly may give rise to behavior
that may cause eviction, as demonstrated in previous studies (Barker, Mitteness, & Wood, 1988; Bernstein, 1982). Thus, it is imperative that counseling
and supportive services be provided to the large elderly populations who
reside in public housing.

The black elderly constitute a very heterogeneous group. Not only are
they different from other groups, but there are differences within the group.
Gibson and Jackson (1989) found a group of sixty-five to seventy-four-year-old
black elderly who were more disabled than those aged seventy-five to seventy-
nine, and a group of individuals aged eighty to eighty-four who were more
disabled than those aged eighty-five and over. This finding parallels that of
Manton and Saldo (1985). This uniqueness of within-group differences must
be taken into consideration in planning and assessment of care plans.

Rural Black Elderly

Parks (1988) conducted an extensive study of 510 black elderly in three
Southern states (Mississippi, Arkansas, and Tennessee). He found that this
group had a poverty rate of 41.7 percent. In each state, about 80 percent of the
rural blacks aged sixty to sixty-four lived in families, about 2 percent were in
nursing homes, 12 to 15 percent worked, and the median income was $5,656.
Several counties had no physician, and the average physician was about ten
miles away. Transportation was a problem. In several rural areas and inner-
city areas, nurse-managed clinics provided primary care. In several states,
nurses had authority to prescribe medication.

Social Cost of Unemployment

The social cost of unemployment, inflation, and poverty becomes apparent
in the dramatic increase in the levels of disability among the black elderly.
Most black elderly retire because of disability; however, they continue to work
on a second job after retirement. Presently, they are experiencing an increase
in unemployment. Brenner (1977) has calculated that each 1 percent increase in the unemployment rate is accompanied by a 2 percent increase in
mortality rate, about a 2 percent increase in cardiovascular deaths, 5 to 6
percent increase in suicides, 5 percent increase in imprisonment, and 3 to 4
percent increase in admissions to state mental hospitals. Brenner further
calculated that there is an unemployment rate of 20.2 percent for blacks forty
years of age and older. Thus, one must consider unemployment as a physical
and mental health issue for the black elderly. Unemployment impacts the

black elderly's sense of worth and self-esteem. In one study, 50 percent of the black elderly could not perceive themselves as retired (Gibson, 1988).

Conclusion

In summary, some of the major obstacles to health for the African-American elderly include poverty or lack of financial resources, fragmented care or a lack of fair quality of care, unemployment, lack of qualified staff (indigenous and nonindigenous), current public policies (which should be restructured for more community-based care and for more effective use of formal as well as family caregivers), and access only to a "color-coded" health care system. In planning and evaluating care for black elders, it must be emphasized that the black elderly spent over half of their lives in a "separate but equal" health care system. Such a system did not foster positive attitudes for health promotion in old age. This observation must be considered when we note that the black elderly underutilize mental health and nursing home facilities and services. In some areas, such as Harlem, health care for the black elderly is worse than in some Third World countries (McCord & Freeman, 1990). It is imperative that corrective measures be instituted, particularly those that attack the underlying factor of poverty, if the health status of the black elderly is to improve.

Differentials in health and in effective access to health services cannot be considered apart from other dimensions of life, especially where public policy plays such a large role. In some areas, there has been progress, while in others, discontinuities and inequities prevail. The elimination of overt barriers of racial segregation has not ensured active inclusion and full participation for many black elderly. With respect to public strategy, a combined approach of consensus building, "universality," and efficient "targeting" seems especially promising.

Resources Available to the Black Elderly

Available resources for elderly populations differ depending on various factors, including geographical locales. Some resources available to the black elderly throughout the country include the following:

1. *Training in Self-Care for the Black Elderly with Chronic Diseases* is a manual by Lee Senott-Miller at the University of Arizona, Tucson, and K. S. Prezbinowski at the College of Mount St. Joseph, Cincinnati, Ohio. The program Positive Adults Taking Health Seriously (PATH) offers videos and manuals on issues pertinent to the elderly.
2. American Association for Retired Persons (AARP) — 601 E Street, N.W., Washington, DC 20049; phone (202) 434-2277.
3. National Caucus/Center on Black Aged (NCCBA) — 1424 K St., Suite 500, Washington, DC 20005.

4.   National Council on Aging (NCOA)—409 3rd St., N.W., 2nd Floor, Washington, DC 20201.
5.   National Commission for the Preservation of Social Security and Medicare—2000 K St., N.W., Suite 800, Washington, DC 20006.
6.   Self-Help for the Elderly—445 Grant Ave., 2nd Floor, San Francisco, CA 94108-3248.
7.   Washington Seniors Wellness Center—3857-A Pennsylvania Ave., S.E., Washington, DC 20020.
8.   National Council on Black Aging—Box 8522, Durham, NC 27707.
9.   National Black Women's Health Project—1237 Gordon St., S.W., Atlanta, GA 30310.
10.   American Cancer Society (national office)—1599 Clifton Rd., N.E., Atlanta, GA 30329 (or contact your local chapter).
11.   American Heart Association—7320 Greenville Ave., Dallas, TX 75231.
12.   National Resource Center on Minority Aging Populations—University Center on Aging, San Diego State University, San Diego, CA 92182-0273.

     Each state has one or more Area Agency on Aging offices, a state unit on aging, and an ombudsman (usually listed in the yellow and/or white pages of the telephone directory).

References

Adebimpe, V. R., Gigandet, J., & Harris, E. (1981). MMPD diagnosis of black psychiatric patients. *American Journal of Psychiatry, 13*(1), 85–87.

American Association of Retired Persons. (1988). *A portrait of older minorities.* Washington, DC: Author.

American Association of Retired Persons. (1990). *A profile of older Americans 1990.* Washington, DC: Author.

Anderson, W. F. (1966). The prevention of illness in the elderly: The Rutherglen experiment in medicine in old age. *Proceedings of a conference held at the Royal College of Physicians.* London: Pitman.

Barker, J. C., Mitteness, L. S., & Wood, S. J. (1988). Gatekeeping: Residential managers and elderly tenants. *Gerontologist, 28,* 610–619.

Bernstein, J. (1982). Who leaves, who stays? Residency policy in housing for the elderly. *Gerontologist, 22,* 305–313.

Besdine, R. W. (1980). Geriatric medicine: An overview. In C. Eisdorfer (Ed.), *Annual Review of Gerontology and Geriatrics* (Vol. 1, pp. 135–153). New York: Springer.

Brenner, M. H. (1977). Personal stability and economic security. *Social Policy, 8*(1), 2–4.

Butler, F. R. (1987). Minority wellness promotion: A behavioral self-management approach. *Journal of Gerontological Nursing, 13*(8), 23–28.

Butler, R. N., & Hyer, K. (1990). The aging populace. *Journal of Health Care for the Poor and the Underserved, 1*(1), 156–168.

Chen, Y. (1985). Economic status of aging. In B. Binstock and E. Shanas (Eds.), *Handbook of aging and the social sciences* (pp. 641–665). New York: Van Nostrand Reinhold.

Committee on an Aging Society. (1985). Aging and the age-dependent disease: Cognition and dementia. In R. Katzman (Ed.), *Health in an older society* (pp. 129–152). Washington, DC: National Academy Press.

Cooper, R., Steinhauer, M., Schatzkin, A., & Miller, W. (1981). Improved mortality among U.S. blacks, 1968–1978: The role of antiracist struggle. *International Journal of Health Services, 11,* 511–522.

Davis, K., Lillie-Blanton, B., Lyons, B., Mullan, F., Powe, N., & Rowland, D. (1987). Health care for black Americans: The public sector role. *Milbank Quarterly, 65* (Suppl.), 213–248.

Davis, K., Lillie-Blanton, M., Lyons, B., Mullan, F., Powe, N., & Rowland, D. (1989). Health care for black Americans: The public sector role. In D. P. Willis (Ed.), *Health policies and black Americans* (pp. 213–247). New Brunswick, NJ: Transaction.

Davis, K., & Schoen, C. (1978). *Health and the war on poverty: A ten year appraisal.* Washington, DC: Brookings Institution.

Egbert, L. D., & Rothman, I. L. (1977). Relationship between the race and economic status of patients and who performs their surgery. *New England Journal of Medicine, 297*(2), 90–91.

Gambert, S. R. (1990a). Atypical presentation of diabetes mellitus in the elderly. *Clinics in Geriatric Medicine, 6*(4), 721–729.

Gambert, S. R. (1990b). When to treat: Glucose intolerance versus diabetes mellitus. In S. R. Gambert (Ed.), *Diabetes in the elderly: A practical guide* (pp. 15–20). New York: Raven Press.

Gibson, R. C. (1988). The work, retirement, and disability of older black Americans. In J. S. Jackson (Ed.), *The American black elderly: Research on physical and mental health* (pp. 304–324). New York: Springer.

Gibson, R. C., & Jackson, J. S. (1987). The black aged. *Milbank Quarterly, 65* (Suppl. 2), 421–454.

Gibson, R. C., & Jackson, J. S. (1989). The health, physical functioning, and informal supports of the black elderly. In D. P. Willis (Ed.), *Health policies and black Americans* (pp. 421–453). New Brunswick, NJ: Transaction.

Harper, M. S. (1988). Behavioral, social, and mental health aspects of home care for older Americans. *Home Health Care Services Quarterly, 9*(4), 61–124.

Haywood, J. L. (1984). Coronary heart disease mortality/morbidity and risk in blacks: II. Access to medical care. *American Heart Journal, 108*(3), 794–796.

Howell, E. L., Corder, L., & Dobson, A. (1985). Out of pocket health expenses for Medicaid and other poor and near poor persons in 1980. *National Medical Care Utilization and Expenditure Survey* (Series B, Descriptive Report

No. 4, DHHS Publication No. 85-20204). Washington, DC: Office of Research and Demonstration, Health Care Financing Administration.

Jackson, J. (1981). Urban black Americans. In A. Harwood (Ed.), *Ethnicity and medical care* (pp. 37–129). Cambridge, MA: Harvard University Press.

James, S. A., Wagner, E. H., Strogatz, D. S., Geresford, S. A., Kleenbaum, D. G., Williams, L. M., Crutchin, L. M., & Ibrahim, M. A. (1984). The Edgecombe County (NC) High Blood Pressure Control Program: 2. Barriers to the use of care among hypertensives. *American Journal of Public Health*, *74*(2), 468–472.

Kitagawa, E. M., & Hauser, P. M. (1973). *Differential mortality in the United States*. Cambridge, MA: Harvard University Press.

Lang, N. M., Kraegel, J. M., Rontz, M. J., & Krejci, J. W. (1990). *Quality of health care for older people in America: A review of nursing studies*. Kansas City, MO: American Nurses Association.

Lawson, W. B. (1986). Racial and ethnic factors in psychiatric research. *Hospital and Community Psychiatry*, *37*(1), 50–54.

Manton, K. G., Poss, S. S., & Wing, S. (1979). The black/white mortality crossover: Investigations from the perspective of the components of aging. *Gerontologist*, *19*, 291–300.

Manton, K. G., & Saldo, B. J. (1985). Dynamics of health changes in the oldest old: New perspectives and evidence. *Milbank Memorial Fund Quarterly/Health and Society*, *63*(2), 206–285.

McCord, C., & Freeman, H. P. (1990). Excess mortality in Harlem. *New England Journal of Medicine*, *322*(3), 173–177.

Miller, S. M. (1989). Race in the health of America. In D. P. Willis (Ed.), *Health policies and black Americans* (pp. 500–531). New Brunswick, NJ: Transaction.

Mitchell, J. B., & Cromwell, J. (1980). Medicaid mills: Fact or fiction? *Health Care Financing Review*, *2*, 37.

Mitchell, J. B., & Cromwell, J. (1983). Access to private physicians for public patients: Participation in Medicaid and Medicare. In *Securing access to health care* (pp. 105–130). Washington, DC: President's Commission for the Study of Ethical Problems in Medicine and Biomedical and Behavioral Research.

Myers, H. F. (1984). Summary of Workshop III: Working Group on Socioeconomic and Sociocultural Influences. *American Heart Journal*, *108*, 706–710.

National Vital Statistics System and National Health Interview Survey. (1990, September). *Prevention Report*. Washington, DC: Office of Disease Prevention and Health Promotion.

O'Hare, W. P. (1989). Black demographic trends in the 1980's. In D. P. Willis (Ed.), *Health policies and black Americans* (pp. 35–55). New Brunswick, NJ: Transaction.

Okie, S. (1991, April 17). Study links cancer and poverty: Blacks' higher rates are tied to income. *Washington Post*, pp. A1, A6.

Parks, A. G. (1988). *Black elderly in rural America: A comprehensive study*. Bristol, IN: Wyndham Hall Press.

Pathy, M. S. (1967). Clinical presentation of myocardial infarction in the elderly. *British Heart Journal, 29*(2), 190–199.

Rabin, P. V., Fischer, P., & Shapiro, S. (1986, May). Mental disorders in elderly public housing sites. Paper presented at the annual meeting of the American Psychiatric Association, Washington, DC.

Regier, D. A., Boyd, J. H., & Burke, J. D. (1988). One month prevalence of mental disorders in the United States. *Archives of General Psychiatry, 25,* 977–986.

Riessman, C. K. (1974, May/June). The use of health services by the poor. *Social Policy, 5*(1), 41–49.

Robinson, B., Stewart, B., & Baker, F. M. (1990). Screening for cognitive impairment and depressive illness in African American elders. Unpublished manuscript.

Roca, R. P., Storer, D. J., Robbins, B. M., Tlasek, M. E., & Rabins, P. V. (1990). Psychogeriatric assessment and treatment in urban public housing. *Hospital and Community Psychiatry, 41*(8), 916–920.

Rosenfield, S. (1984). Racial differences in involuntary hospitalization: Psychiatric vs. labeling perspectives. *Journal of Health and Social Behavior, 25*(1), 13–23.

Rosenthal, E., & Carty, L. A. (1988). *Impediments to services and advocacy for black and Hispanic people with mental illness.* Washington, DC: Mental Health Law Project.

Rowe, J. W. (1983). Clinical research in aging strategies and directions. *New England Journal of Medicine, 309*(6), 1246–1248.

Rowe, J. W. (1985). Health care of the elderly. *New England Journal of Medicine, 312,* 827–835.

Rowe, J. W. (1989). The clinical impact of physiologic changes with aging. In E. W. Busse and D. G. Blazer (Eds.), *Geriatric psychiatry* (pp. 35–64). Washington, DC: American Psychiatric Press.

Rowe, J. W. (1991). Reducing the risk of usual aging. *Generations, 15*(1), 25–28.

Siegel, J., and Davidson, M. (1984). Demographic and socioeconomic aspects of aging in the United States. U.S. Bureau of the Census, *Current Population Reports* (Series P-23, No. 138). Washington, DC: U.S. Government Printing Office.

Sullivan, L. W. (1989, July). Keynote address and remarks presented at the AARP Minority Affairs Initiative conference, Washington, DC.

U.S. Congressional Budget Office. (1983). *Changing structure of Medicare benefits: Issues and options.* Washington, DC: U.S. Government Printing Office.

U.S. Department of Health and Human Services, Public Health Service. (1990). *Healthy People 2000: National health promotion and disease prevention objectives.* Washington, DC: U.S. Government Printing Office.

Wilson, L. A., Lawson, I. R., & Brass, W. (1962). Multiple disorders in the elderly: A clinical and statistical study. *Lancet, 2*(3), 841–843.

Wing, S., Manton, K. G., Stallard, E., Haines, C. G., & Tyroles, H. A. (1985). The black/white mortality crossover: Investigation in a community-based study. *Journal of Gerontology, 40*(2), 78–84.

Woolhandler, S., Himmelstein, R., Silber, M., Bader, M., Hornly, T., & Jones, A. (1985). Medical care and mortality: Racial differences in preventable deaths. *International Journal of Health Services, 15*(2), 1–22.

World Health Organization, Regional Office for Europe. (1959, July 28–August 2). *The public health aspects of the aging of the population* (Report of an Advisory Group, Oslo). Copenhagen: Author.

PART IV

Health Education and
Resource Development

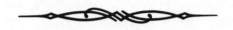

18

Health Education and
Black Health Status

Rueben C. Warren

This chapter addresses some of the important factors in health education as they pertain to the health status of African Americans. It covers salient issues related to the black experience in the United States, selected theories and practices of health education, evaluation of health education programs, application of health education principles, and outcome and significance of health education efforts.

Salient Issues Related to the Black Experience in the United States

Since the African slave trade and the landing of black people in America in 1619, much has happened to African Americans (Bennett, 1975). Yet by relative standards, little has changed. General improvements have occurred in income and standard of living and in the educational, occupational, political, and social well-being of the citizens of the United States as a whole. Measurable advances in health have also been made. However, in spite of the overall improvements in American society, there remain significant disparities in most social measures of well-being (Armor, 1980; Thomas, Alexander, & Ecland, 1979; Hill, 1986; Levy, 1966; Apostte, Glock, Piazza, & Suelyle, 1983; National Research Council, 1989; Woodlander et al., 1985; U.S. Department of Health and Human Services, 1985, 1990a, 1990b).

African Americans make up more than 12 percent of the population of the United States—some 30.2 million people. In 1988, 32 percent of the African-American population had incomes below the poverty level. In that same year, 44 percent of all African-American children were below the poverty level, and nearly 52 percent of all African-American households were headed by women (U.S. Department of Health and Human Services, 1990a, 1990b). In 1986, the unemployment rate for African Americans was 14.5 percent, more than twice that of whites. In April 1988, unemployment for whites had dropped to 4.6 percent, while the rate for African Americans fell only to 12.2 percent (Commission on Minority Participation in Education and American Life, 1988).

Educational attainment and income level are associated, because higher educational attainment usually results in a better standard of living. Between 1970 and 1975, the percentage of African-American high school graduates, twenty-four years or younger, who enrolled in or completed one or more years of college increased from 39 percent to 48 percent. Over the same period, the rate for whites remained at 53 percent. Between 1975 and 1985, the college participation rates for white youth climbed to 55 percent; the rate for African Americans dropped to 44 percent. In 1986, 20.1 percent of whites over twenty-five had completed four or more years of college. The rate for African Americans was 10.9 percent. African-American youths are graduating from high school at an increasing rate. Yet the number of these students in college is not increasing at the same rate (Commission on Minority Participation in Education and American Life, 1988). Between 1975 and 1985, the pool of African-American high school graduates was bigger and better. Nonetheless, African Americans' rate of college attendance remains low.

Low income and poor education have well-documented associations with health (Warren, 1990; Berk & Wilenksky, 1985; Egbert & Rothman, 1977; Egbuono & Starfield, 1982; Davis, 1983, 1986; Neighbors & Jackson, 1986; Rice, 1987). These two variables are statistically correlated with adverse health conditions in African Americans because they are disproportionately represented among the low-income and poorly educated. One must, therefore, consider income and educational factors in designing any strategy for health improvement among African Americans. It should be noted, however, that income and educational barriers do not fully explain the health gaps among this subgroup of the U. S. population (Otten, Teutsch, Williamson, & Marks, 1990).

Health statistics, while routinely recorded by state and local health agencies, often have not been appropriately used to improve health. The following quotation reflects the need for careful interpretation and use of scientific information about the health of African Americans.

> In considering the health statistics of [African Americans] we seek first to know their absolute condition rather than their relative status. We want to know what their death rate is, how it has varied and is varying, and what its tendencies seem to be. With these facts fixed we must then ask, what is the meaning of the death rate like that of [African Americans]? Is it, compared with other races, large, moderate, or small, and in the case of nations or groups with similar deaths, what has been the tendency and outcome? Finally, we must compare the death rate of [African Americans] with that of the communities in which they live and thus roughly measure the social difference between

> these neighboring groups. We must endeavor also to eliminate
> so far as possible from the problem disturbing elements which
> would make a difference in health among people of the same
> social advancement. Only in this way can we intelligently inter-
> pret statistics of [African-American] health [Du Bois, 1899,
> p. 148].

Fundamental issues that must guide research include intent of data collection, scientific rigor of methodology, and interpretation of descriptive and
inferential statistics. Additionally, data manipulation and analysis resulting
in more meaningful results and with greater capability for deriving practical
implications are needed. For African Americans, these factors are particularly important because of continuing health disparities on the basis of race
and ethnicity.

The *Report of the Secretary's Task Force on Black and Minority Health* (U.S.
Department of Health and Human Services, 1985) documented 60,000 excess deaths among African Americans. By 1990, these excess deaths had risen
to 75,000. (It should be noted that these figures represent conservative
estimates.) The concept of "excess" death uses the death rates of white
Americans as a baseline to measure expected deaths among other racial and
ethnic groups. The excess deaths in 1985 and 1990 among African Americans probably would not have occurred if those individuals were white.

The *Report of the Secretary's Task Force* identified six major causes of
excess deaths. Table 18.1 lists these excess deaths for selected causes of
mortality in blacks for the period 1979–1981. Subsequently, acquired immune deficiency syndrome (AIDS) has been added as a seventh cause of
death (see Table 18.2).

**Table 18.1. Average Annual Total and Excess Deaths in African Americans,
Selected Causes of Mortality, United States, 1979–1981.**

Causes of Excess Deaths	*Excess Deaths Males and Females Cumulative to Age 45*		*Excess Deaths Males and Females Cumulative to Age 70*	
	Number	*Percent*	*Number*	*Percent*
Heart disease and stroke	3,312	14.4	18,181	30.8
Homicide and accidents	8,041	35.1	10,909	18.5
Cancer	874	3.8	8,118	13.8
Infant mortality	6,178	26.9	6,178	10.5
Cirrhosis	1,121	4.9	2,154	3.7
Diabetes	223	1.0	1,850	3.1
Subtotal	19,749	86.1	47,390	80.4
All other causes	3,187	13.9	11,552	19.6
Total excess deaths	22,936	100.0	58,942	100.0
Total deaths, all causes	48,323		138,635	

Source: Adapted from U.S. Department of Health and Human Services, 1985, p. 5.

In 1985, the Secretary of Health and Human Services, Margaret Heckler, succinctly summarized the problem when she stated that "there was a continuing disparity in the burden of death and illness experienced by black and other minority Americans as compared to the nation's population as a whole. That disparity has existed ever since accurate federal record keeping began more than a generation ago. And although our health charts do itemize steady gains in the health status of minority Americans, the stubborn disparity remains an affront to our ideals and to the ongoing genius of American medicine" (U.S. Department of Health and Human Services, 1985, p. ix).

Secretary Heckler's statement had previously been documented by those involved in research, service, or education related to the health of African Americans. Nonetheless, the government's acknowledgment initiated a renewed national effort to address this problem. The *Report of the Secretary's Task Force* also used the expression *years of potential life lost* (YPLL) to quantify the needless deaths and years of productivity lost largely by African Americans compared to their white counterparts. The concept recognizes a national crisis among a subgroup of the American population. Moreover, YPLL emphasizes that the human loss not only impacts on the African-American population, but it adversely affects the entire nation.

The National Center for Health Statistics (NCHS) indicated that the excess deaths among African Americans between 1985 and 1990 were due to the six causes documented in the *Report of the Secretary's Task Force* plus AIDS and homicide. However, the Report of the Secretary's Task Force also acknowledged the importance of morbidity, finance and access, health data, and the need for more minority health professionals. These and other factors will need particular attention if the health of African Americans is to improve. There must also be more research related to understanding the relationships between health and health care, income, education, literacy, employment, and other social barriers such as poverty, discrimination, and racism. An Afrocentric theoretical framework for health must be proposed and tested if the well-being of African Americans is to be a high priority (Asante, 1990).

Current Health Disparities Among African Americans

The *Report of the Secretary's Task Force* documents the disparities in health between various racial and ethnic groups in the United States. Much work has been done since the report was published. However, according to a 1990 report by the National Center for Health Statistics, the disparity continues. In some instances, the health gap has widened. Figure 18.1 illustrates age-adjusted death rates for all causes for African Americans and whites for 1980–1988. Figure 18.2 shows the widening gap between African-American and white-American life expectancies for the period 1970–1988. These data strongly suggest the need for new strategies and targeted resources to reverse

Figure 18.1. Age-Adjusted Death Rates for All Causes Among African Americans and Whites, United States, 1980–1988.

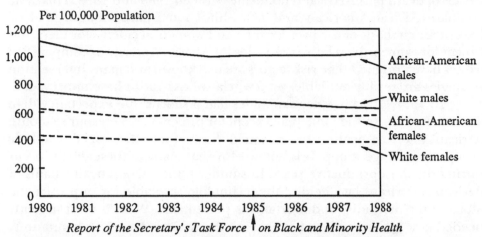

Report of the Secretary's Task Force ↑ on Black and Minority Health

Source: U.S. Department of Health and Human Services, 1990a, p. 12.

this trend. Also included are male and female death rates, which indicate that health problems exist both within and across gender categories.

Most major health indicators rank African Americans behind other racial and ethnic groups. Because of the high rates of health problems among low-income African Americans, federal health programs have targeted this group for many years. Nonetheless, their health continues to lag behind that of most segments of the U.S. population. What is needed is more scientific evaluation of the goals and methodologies of these programs to determine their efficacy.

Figure 18.2. Life Expectancy at Birth Among African Americans and Whites, United States, 1980–1988.

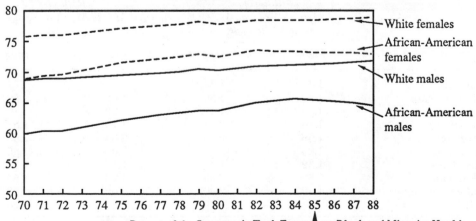

Report of the Secretary's Task Force ↑ on Black and Minority Health

Source: U.S. Department of Health and Human Services, 1990a, p. 76.

Table 18.2 lists the ratio of age-adjusted death rates for the six major causes of death plus AIDS and homicide between 1980 and 1988. This table compares African Americans and their white counterparts for both genders. Except for cirrhosis of the liver for men and women, accidents for men, and cancer for women, the relative risk ratios for African Americans compared to whites have worsened. The risk factors are well known and many intervention strategies are readily available, yet few relative risk ratios have improved.

In 1987, African-American males had a shorter life expectancy than any other group. In the same year, except for fifteen- to twenty-four-year-olds, African-American death rates exceeded those of all other racial or ethnic groups in each age group. It is noteworthy that many of these deaths occur during the most productive years. In summary, the current health status of African Americans lags behind the technology available for improvement. Much of the morbidity and mortality is preventable. What is most urgently needed now are methods to better reach the African-American community with well-tested preventive interventions. These methodologies are available. However, to be effective, the methodologies must be applied in a culturally appropriate manner.

Selected Theories and Practices of Health Education

Health education over the last twenty years has focused primarily on increasing the public's knowledge of health matters. This approach assumes that adequate knowledge will lead to effective behavioral change. Unfortunately, that change has not occurred. To explore some of the reasons for this failure, it will be useful to review some key issues in health education. This section

Table 18.2. Ratio of Age-Adjusted Death Rates Among Whites and African Americans for Selected Causes, United States, 1980a and 1988.

	Ratio of African-American Male to White Male		Ratio of African-American Female to White Female	
	1980	*1988*	*1980*	*1988*
All causes	1.49	1.56	1.54	1.54
Heart disease	1.18	1.30	1.49	1.59
Cancer	1.43	1.44	1.20	1.19
Stroke	1.86	1.93	1.75	1.83
Diabetes	1.86	2.06	2.54	2.63
Cirrhosis	1.95	1.71	2.06	1.86
Accidents	1.32	1.30	1.17	1.18
Homicide	6.60	7.56	4.28	4.54
Infant mortality	1.89	2.00	2.02	2.18
AIDS		3.19		8.86

a Data year of the *Report of the Secretary's Task Force on Black and Minority Health*, 1985.
Source: Adapted from U.S. Department of Health and Human Services, 1985, p. 5.

addresses aspects of the health education literature having particular rele-vance to the African-American health dilemma. These include (1) the scope and definition of health education; (2) the relationship between knowledge, attitudes, and behavior in health-related activities; (3) social science concepts related to health education; (4) studies of school health education; (5) a conceptual model of the health education process; and (6) evaluation of health education.

According to Young (1970, p. 3), "Health education includes all those experiences of an individual group or community that influence beliefs, attitudes, and behavior with respect to health, as well as processes and efforts of producing change when this is necessary for optimal health." She contin-ues, "This all inclusive concept of health education recognizes that many experiences, both positive and negative in nature, have an impact on what an individual, group, or community thinks, feels, and does about health, and it does not limit health education to those situations in which health activities are planned or formed. Young's definition of health education dates from 1970. Interestingly, in their text *Health Promotion Planning: An Educational and Environmental Approach* (1991), Green and Kreuter define health education in a similar way.

While Young's focus is correct, it is difficult to plan, implement, and evaluate health education interventions under this broad definition. Health education should be conceptualized in a manner that will lend itself to appropriate planning, implementation, and evaluation strategies, particu-larly for the African-American population. Thus, in this chapter, the term *health education* refers to planned or formal activities that stimulate and provide experiences leading to the development of health knowledge, at-titudes, and behaviors that are most conducive to the attainment of indi-vidual, group, or community health (Young, 1970; Green & Kreuter, 1991). Health education is not a single discipline, but a "field of interest" drawing on knowledge from the biomedical, biostatistical, and behavioral sciences as well as on various administrative, planning, and research skills (John E. Fogarty International Center, 1976, p. 11).

The foregoing definitions of health education emphasize three con-cepts—knowledge, attitudes, and behavior—and their interrelationships. But the classic linear model of knowledge, attitudes, and behavior that directs much of formal educational theory has limited applicability in the health setting. Most formal education is geared toward acquiring knowledge. Health education differs from formal education in that information getting and giving is not primary but secondary to behavioral change. This is because studies show that the distribution of accurate scientific information has limited influence on health and health behavior.

Influencing behavior, which is the goal of health education, is depen-dent on several psychosocial and cultural factors (Becker & Joseph, 1988). Ultimately, health education is concerned with the process of social change.

For this change to occur, human behavior has to be influenced by psychological, sociological, and cultural determinants. To understand these determinants, a firm foundation in behavioral and social science concepts is needed. Health educators and other health workers must familiarize themselves with the basic literature in the areas of learning theory, motivation, personality formation, values and value systems, perception, and communication. Several social science concepts have particular relevance to health behavior. These include the ideas of fear arousal and threat avoidance.

Fear Arousal

For many people, individual health and medical experiences are associated with pain and anxiety. Health workers have therefore used the fear-arousal approach to stimulate positive health behavior, However, it is doubtful whether there is any long-term change in health behavior once fear has been raised above some adequate threshold (Leventhal, 1965). A critical factor left to be determined is how fear threshold level relates to social class, race/ethnicity, personality structure, cultural factors, and the nature of the health issue (Russell & Robbins, 1964; Halfner, 1974; Berman & Wandersman,1990).

Threat Avoidance

The threat avoidance model represents an approach to understanding the parameters in which humans respond when confronted with conflicting stimuli in their environment. A person's perception of a health threat is based on two beliefs: perceived susceptibility and perceived severity. Kegeles (1968) has reported extensively on this subject. His work shows that variables in the threat-avoidance model are relevant but not sufficient to explain health behaviors. Rosenstock (1966) has concluded that this model has the following strengths: (1) it can account for more variations in behavior in groups of people studied in a variety of settings than other models can; (2) it appears to be applicable to a wide range of health actions and beliefs; and (3) it has the virtue of simplicity.

The threat-avoidance strategy has been applied primarily to preventive health behaviors. Further research is needed to clarify the influence this approach has on individuals seeking curative and emergency care. With the heavy influence of the behavioral sciences on health education, one would expect health care providers to be well versed in behavioral science concepts. However, this has not been the case. The curricula of schools in the health professions must be improved so that they equip students with the behavioral principles necessary for health education. Continuing medical education programs should be developed to accomplish the same goal. Health providers must not only acquire the behavioral skills necessary for health education, but they must also understand when these skills are most applicable.

For example, learning theory indicates that health education is most effective among young people. The school setting occupies many hours of a child's life. After age five, children are required by law to attend school. Therefore, school systems are ideal places for health education. The school provides, in theory, a captive audience for learning principles of healthful living. Life-style and nutrition are now emerging as major contributors to positive or negative health status (U.S. Department of Health and Human Services, 1990a, 1990b). With respect to preventable conditions, these two variables undoubtedly have great impact. Although there are still many unknown factors in health education, there is sufficient knowledge to develop workable health education programs, particularly in the school system.

However, data on which to plan sound health education programs are more limited than they should be. Thus, most programs in schools are developed based on personal preference, professional opinion, and experience (Sliepcevich, 1964). One cannot develop school health education programs effectively unless a definitive programmatic data base is available. For example, parents should play an important role in health education activities in the schools; however, there is little reported in the literature on how best to use parents in health education. It is agreed, though, that maternal influence has a definite impact on child preventive behavior (Derryberry, 1963). African-American families represent a disproportionate number of single-parent, female-headed households (U.S. Department of Health and Human Services, 1990a, 1990b). Thus, the single-parent familial structure among African Americans should be further studied to determine its effectiveness in health education. Parents must also be motivated to take preventive actions for themselves if they are ever expected to influence their children.

Many health educators assume that there is a linear relationship between their message and a change in the beliefs and/or behaviors of the learner. What they fail to realize is that there are other influences that may take precedence over health goals. Economic, social, and cultural factors are examples of other goals that may influence the learner.

Evaluation of Health Education Programs

Most evaluation studies of health education programs have been related to improvement in health knowledge. In the school setting, numerous studies have shown a significant improvement in what the students know about health. However, as with other health education programs, subsequent improvement in health behavior has not occurred (Fodor & Ziegler, 1966). The students know far more than they are putting into practice. For example one need only observe teenagers who refuse to use condoms, yet are fully aware of the risks of acquiring sexually transmitted diseases. This conclusion is supported by numerous studies of different health issues among various age groups throughout the world (Rhode Island Department of Health, 1968;

Holt, 1968). If the objective of health education is to influence health behavior, the overall results of health education activities must be evaluated in terms of behavioral change. Assessment of health knowledge and health attitudes is desirable. However, one must be very careful to clarify the importance of these two variables in improving overall health status.

The evaluation of health education programs is essential if school health programs are to succeed. Such evaluation must be conducted with respect to immediate, intermediate, and ultimate goals. To be most effective, it must be directly related to predetermined objectives. The concerns of health providers, teachers, school administrators, and consumers must be included so that continuity of the program will be enhanced. A report on health education and health promotion by the task force from the John E. Fogarty International Center for Advanced Study of the Health Sciences, the National Institutes of Health, and the American College of Preventive Medicine (1976) clarifies the direction for the future. The report indicates that data are unavailable on the exact effectiveness of most current health education and health promotion programs and practices. Substantial empirical research is needed to identify specific and long-term results if health education is to be most efficacious in the future.

Application of Health Education Principles

Health education is most effective when targeted specifically to the individual, group, or community. For the African-American population, the material must consider the historical and current psychosocial dynamic of the African-American experience.

In his book *The Souls of Black Folk*, W.E.B. Du Bois (1903, p. 215) wrote:

> After the Egyptian and Indian, the Greek and Roman, the Teuton and Mongolian, the Negro is a sort of seventh son, born with a veil and gifted with a second sight in this American world—a world which yields him no true self-consciousness, but only lets him see himself through the revelation of the other world. It is a peculiar sensation, this double consciousness, this sense of always looking at one's soul by the tape of a world that looks on in amused contempt and pity. One ever feels his twoness—an American, a Negro; two souls, two thoughts, two unreconciled strivings, two warring ideals in one dark body, whose dogged strength alone keeps it from being torn asunder.

This "double consciousness" has forced African Americans to carefully assess all messages to determine both the content of the message and the intent of the messenger. Health messages are no exception. A determination must be made early on concerning the value of these messages and one's trust in the messenger. Too often health messages are delivered in a culturally inappropriate manner, without properly considering many competing goals and social or behavioral barriers and enablers that may exist. Too often the messages conflict with more pressing priorities of food, clothing, and shelter. At times, because of prior negative health experiences, there is a lack of confidence in both the health educator and the health delivery system. Health educators are often of different ethnic or racial backgrounds than the learner. They may be either unaware of or indifferent to the background and experience of the individual they are trying to influence.

The limited utility of knowledge-focused health education has particular relevance to the African-American population. Due to the lack of support from the educational system, many African Americans are alienated by standard educational pedagogy. Years of segregation and discrimination in the public school system have led to distrust of educational institutions. Differences in fiscal and human resources at predominantly white schools reinforce this distrust, thus retarding African Americans' learning opportunities. This is particularly important among low-income inner-city children, who attend the most segregated schools. In short, what some view as a positive "captive" audience in the public schools is often perceived by African Americans as a "captured" audience. The effective health educator must be aware of this perception.

Conclusion

For health education to be most effective for African Americans, a holistic rather than a disease-specific approach is needed. Health education for African Americans must be comprehensive in scope. It must address issues of education, employment, housing, income, and racism as well as health status. The strategies must focus on broader psychological issues such as positive self-worth, self-concept, and human values. While some health successes have been recorded, poor self-esteem and the lack of positive self-images have, in many cases, led to poor responsiveness to health education messages. A health education pedagogy for African Americans that emphasizes a positive self-concept can make health education programs much more effective. Strategies and tactics must include correcting defective self-concepts resulting from individual and institutional racism (Jones, 1980). Health education for African Americans must emphasize the value of African-American life before addressing issues that improve the quality or quantity of that life. The value of health must evolve out of the value of life.

The seven leading causes of death among African Americans can be specifically addressed by generic changes in behavior. These behavioral changes relate primarily to nutrition and eating habits; tobacco, alcohol, and drug abuse; exercise; and conflict resolution. If basic changes occur in these areas, health risks will be substantially reduced. Knowledge of how to reduce these risk factors is widespread. Yet too few practice behaviors commensurate with this knowledge. An Afrocentric approach to reach the black community may appear simplistic. However, other strategies have only partial success in the African-American community. In particular, though bioscience has obvious importance, its effectiveness in dealing with the diseases most likely to strike this community is limited. Alternative approaches are not only appropriate and demand consideration; they may be the only realistic alternative.

It is clear that public health strategies can be useful, because they benefit large population groups at reduced cost. Because of the social, economic, and demographic character of the African-American population, effective public health interventions will be difficult. Nonetheless, these innovations can work for African Americans, if appropriately implemented. Strategic planning is an effective approach. Public health science is the correct methodology, and evaluation research is the most valid means to determine success. With a concentrated focus on these aspects of health and consistent planning with the Year 2000 Health Objectives, the next decade can witness appreciable health improvement in the African-American population.

References

Apostte, R. A., Glock, C. Y., Piazza, T., & Suelyle, M. (1983). *The anatomy of racial attitudes*. Berkeley: University of California Press.

Armor, D. J. (1980). White flight and the future of school desegregation. In W. G. Stephan and J. R. Feagin (Eds.), *School desegregation: Past, present, and future* (pp. 187–226). New York: Plenum.

Asante, M. (1990). *Kemet, Afrocentricity, and knowledge*. Trenton, NJ: African World Press.

Becker, M. H., & Joseph, J. (1988). AIDS and behavioral change to reduce risk: A review. *American Journal of Public Health, 78*, 394–410.

Bennett, L. (1975). *The shaping of black America*. Chicago: Johnson.

Berk, M. L., and Wilensky, G. R. (1985). Health care of the poor and elderly: Supplementing Medicare. *Gerontologist, 25*, 311–314.

Berman, S. H., & Wandersman, A. (1990). Fear of cancer and knowledge of cancer: A review and proposed relevance to hazardous waste sites. *Social Science and Medicine, 31*, 81–90.

Commission on Minority Participation in Education and American Life. (1988). *One-third of a nation*. Washington, DC: American Council on Education.

Davis, K. (1983). Uninsured and underserved: Inequities in health care in the United States. *Milbank Quarterly, 61*, 149–176.

Davis, K. (1986). Aging and the health-care system: Economic and structural issues. *Daedalus, 115*, 227–246.

Derryberry, M. (1963). Research procedures applicable to health education. *Journal of School Health, 33*(5), 215–220.

Du Bois, W.E.B. (1899). *The Philadelphia negro.* Milwood, NY: Kraus-Thomas.

Du Bois, W.E.B. (1903). *The souls of black folk.* Chicago: McClurg.

Egbert, L. D., & Rothman, I. L. (1977). Relationship between the race and economic status of patients and the doctors who perform their surgery. *New England Journal of Medicine, 297,* 90.

Egbuono, L., & Starfield, B. (1982). Child health and social status. *Pediatrics, 69,* 550–557.

Fodor, J. T., & Ziegler, J. E. (1966). A motivational study in dental health education. *Journal of the Southern California State Dental Hygiene Association, 34*(4), 203–216.

John E. Fogarty International Center for Advanced Study of the Health Sciences, National Institutes of Health, and American College of Preventive Medicine. (1976). *Preventive medicine U.S.A. — Health promotion and consumer education.* Prodist, NY: Author.

Green, L. W., & Kreuter, M. W. (1991). *Health promotion planning: An educational and environmental approach.* Mountain View, CA: Mayfield.

Halfner, D. P. (1974, October). *The use of fear in arousal in dental health education.* Paper presented at the annual meeting of the American Public Health Association, New York.

Hill, R. B. (1986). The black middle class: Past, present, and future. In James D. Williams (Ed.), *The state of black America* (pp. 43–64). Washington, DC: National Urban League.

Holt, B. (1968). A study among children in Ghana: The relationship of health, knowledge, and home background. *International Journal of Health Education, 11,* 2.

Jones, R. L. (1980). *Black psychology* (2nd ed.). New York: HarperCollins.

Kegeles, S. S. (1968). Some changes required to increase the public's utilization of preventive dentistry. *Journal of Health Dentistry, 28,* 1.

Leventhal, H. (1965). Fear communications in the acceptance of preventive health practice. *Bulletin of the New York Academy of Medicine, 41,* 11.

Levy, F. (1966). *Poverty and economic growth* (pp. 8–10). College Park: University of Maryland, School of Public Affairs.

National Research Council. (1989). *Memorandum to the Committee on the Status of Black Americans.* Washington, DC: Author.

Neighbors, H. W., & Jackson, J. S. (1986). Uninsured risk groups in a national survey of black Americans. *Journal of the National Medical Association, 78,* 275–282.

Otten, M. W., Jr., Teutsch, S. M., Williamson, D. F., & Marks, J. S. (1990). The effect of known risk factors on the excess mortality of black adults in the United States. *Journal of the American Medical Association, 263*(6), 845–850.

Rhode Island Department of Health. (1968). *The Rhode Island School Health Education Study.* Providence, RI: Author.

Rice, M. (1987). Inner city hospital closures/relocations: Race, income status, and legal issues. *Social Science Medicine, 11*, 889–896.

Rosenstock, I. M. (1966). Why people use health services (Pt. 2). *Milbank Memorial Fund Quarterly, 44*(3), 94–124.

Russell, R. D., & Robbins, P. R. (1964). Health education and the use of fear: A new look. *Journal of School Health, 34*, 6.

Sliepcevich, E. M. (1964). *School Health Education Study: A summary report*. New York: Samuel Bronfman Foundation.

Thomas, G. E., Alexander, K. L., & Ecland, B. K. (1979). Access to higher education: The importance of race, sex, social class, and academic credentials. *School Review, 87*, 133–156.

U.S. Department of Health and Human Services. (1985). *Report of the Secretary's Task Force on Black and Minority Health* (Vol. 1, Executive Summary). Washington, DC: U.S. Government Printing Office.

US. Department of Health and Human Services. (1990a). *Health United States, 1990*. (DHHS Publication No. PHS 91-1232). Washington, DC: U.S. Government Printing Office.

U.S. Department of Health and Human Services. (1990b). *Healthy people 2000: National health promotion and disease prevention objectives*. Washington, DC: U.S. Government Printing Office.

Warren, R. C. (1990). Oral health for the poor and underserved. *Journal of Health Care for the Poor and Underserved, 1*(1), 169–180.

Woodlander, S., Himmelstein, D. V., Siber, R., Bader, M., Hannly, T., & Jones, A. A. (1985). Medicare and mortality: Race differences in preventable deaths. *International Journal of Health Services, 15*, 1–22.

Young, M.A.C. (1970). Dental education: An overview of selected concepts and principles relevant to programme planning. *International Journal of Health Education, 13*(1), 1–26.

19

Indigenous
Community Health Workers
in the 1960s and Beyond

Doris Y. Wilkinson

Indigenous workers have assumed integral roles in community development throughout the world. In this country, the usefulness of neighborhood aides in preventive care and in self-help education was amply demonstrated during the community health movement of the 1960s. Since the impetus of the civil rights movement, increasing interest has been shown in community health work and especially in having residents of disadvantaged areas serve as health interventionists or physician-patient liaisons. A few studies have highlighted the formal and informal expectations for health aides as well as the norms associated with their organizational affiliations and roles. However, no systematic synthesis is available of the pertinent literature documenting their effectiveness in African-American communities as measured by patient outcomes (that is, positive health attitudes and behavioral changes).

Incorporating relevant literature from the 1960s and 1980s and a single case interview, this discussion is based on a recognition of the significance of the linkages between community-based health activities and patient education, especially in urban inner cities. The topic also has constructive implications for addressing high morbidity and mortality rates among blacks and whites in rural areas. Basically, the purpose of the chapter is to synthesize and review selected studies that offer insights into how community health workers have functioned in the United States and to suggest future roles and culturally sensitive models. Another objective is to assess training programs and the diversity of tasks that paraprofessional health aides have performed, despite similarities in expectations and in their responsibilities. Results from evaluation research provide valuable insights into the potential for more efficient use of indigenous helpers. The discussion is relevant to a broad focus on community health planning and development (Wilkinson, 1987) among the black elderly and low-income populations.

Who Is a Community Health Worker?

With its evolution and application in the United States, the label *community health worker* has served as a multipurpose one. The core role obligations and teaching-learning duties accompanying the position have had a long history. In an article on "Using Paraprofessionals in the Arkansas Health Education Programs," Fox (1978, p. 12) points out that "health aides are certainly not new, but aides who provide only education service to the people in their community have been less widely used. Usually, various types of health aides provide one or more health related services in addition to education."

The contemporary health education liaison is a product of the social consciousness and political activity that characterized the civil rights movement and the Peace Corps era. Reflecting major structural, ideological, and behavioral changes that evolved in the 1960s, modifications occurred in values and in the fundamental institutions: the family, politics, the economy, the educational sphere, and the health care delivery system. During that period of rapid social change, which continued until the mid 1970s, a principal concern was how to reach African Americans in inner cities and whites in "the other America" (Harrington, 1966) to provide needed health services. Families living in a poverty culture were the targets of innovative educational programming. Gradually, across the country, numerous experiments began to emerge. Some of the programs were designed specifically for migrant workers, particularly those in the rural South and Southwest. However, most projects were designed for urban and low-income African-American communities and relied on neighborhood representatives to assist in coping with escalating health care needs. Emphasis centered on involving volunteers or indigenous black community residents to provide educational services and basic health assistance. Over the years, various duties evolved to replace earlier ones. Not unexpectedly, the different job designations (for example, medical auxiliaries, social health workers), associated responsibilities, and expectations often depended on agency objectives, project goals, and in some cases the medical staff and other health professionals' preferences. Yet, taking into account the earlier difficulties, one can measure the success and future potential of nonprofessional health workers with low-income African Americans.

Unity and Diversity in Roles and Relationships

Earlier tasks of community health workers depended on the goals of local or state programs, research project plans, and the needs of clients to be served. Over the past twenty to twenty-five years in this country, primarily in metropolitan communities where large numbers of African Americans reside, responsibilities of health aides have been modified. Regardless of the changes and diversity in activities, at least two fundamental integrative dimensions have remained constant: acting as a resource to provide health information and assisting with patient education. Where families have traditionally relied on folk medical customs or home care, an indigenous worker has represented an extension of primary group networks (Wilkinson, 1987). This has been particularly characteristic of the backgrounds and experiences of African-American health education assistants.

In some community-based hypertension screening projects, health assistants have actually served as change agents. Such programs correspond with those that have proven successful using community workers for educational interventions. For example, in appraising the effectiveness of intervention in hypertension screening programs, an important aspect of performance evaluation has centered on the effectiveness of medical helpers in monitoring low-income inner-city residents identified as hypertensive. Although follow-up is difficult with dispersed populations that are screened at diverse locations such as libraries, schools, or shopping centers, door-to-door screening in a designated community offers a functional strategy that could enhance hypertension control efforts (Cooke & Meyers, 1983; Levine et al., 1979, 1982). This finding has important implications for work with black hypertensives.

Moreover, community health workers, also referred to as outreach assistants, have participated in preventive care with preschool children (Russo et al., 1982). For example, an outreach program in a neighborhood health center relied on women "indigenous to the poverty community" to serve as coordinators. Their practical and multiple health education and promotion tasks included the following: (1) recruiting poor families to participate in the experiment, (2) teaching the benefits that could be gained from exercise and proper diet, (3) motivating persons to obtain help when needed, (4) providing guidance in the use of local medical services, and (5) directing families to alternative resources when experiencing social and psychological problems linked to their poverty life-styles. Results of the health promotion activity confirmed that seeking assistance was influenced by the efforts of outreach workers (Colombo, Freeborn, Mullooly, & Burnham, 1979). Corroborating this finding, similar project outcomes have revealed substantial improvement in the use of preventive services and in the health status of adults and preschool children.

In the late 1960s, many politically active doctors volunteered to work in special projects targeted at the "ghetto poor," especially inner-city African-American youth. Young physicians were exposed to the mental and physical health consequences of poverty. Their experiences enabled them to develop an awareness of the shortage of medical personnel in low-income communities. As a result of acquiring an understanding of the health care needs of urban residents, the model of involving neighborhood or indigenous assistants was supported by socially conscious physicians. They ultimately grasped the fact that there are fewer doctors in poverty areas such as parts of rural Appalachia or the inner city (Mullan, 1978). On the other hand, physicians that are in these communities are less likely to have the time or surplus resources for volunteer health activities or to hire additional personnel.

Basically, use of health interventions has emanated from a value that is

deeply rooted in the American cultural system — individualism. This fundamental ethic has permeated the philosophy associated with reliance on
indigenous urban health workers. As a result of the ethos underlying the
seeking of authentic neighborhood representatives from among the economically disadvantaged, low-income residents have aspired to serve as
health aides. For some earlier experiments, homemakers were selected as
health workers. Regardless of the backgrounds of those serving in the role,
the principal objective has been to demonstrate how nonprofessionals from
the community could encourage positive health attitudes and behaviors.

During the 1960s, in a New York tuberculosis program, the Department of Health employed paraprofessionals for the first time in its history. A
basic objective was to involve indigenous helpers. The workers, mostly
females recruited from employment and welfare agencies, were residents of
the communities to which they were assigned. Supported by New York and
Brooklyn Tuberculosis and Health Associations as well as federal funding,
the project was an innovative one that established a rationale for neighborhood health aides. Reflecting the increased emphasis on including para-
medical staff at the time, the participation of urban assistants in the New York
tuberculosis program confirmed their usefulness in health promotion and
education. In fact, the success of the unique experiment and the subsequent
assessments of its effectiveness indicated that neighborhood workers could
make meaningful contributions to efforts to control a highly infectious
disease like tuberculosis (McFadden, Kirschenbaum, & Svigir, 1966). An
outcome such as this has significant implications for program development
in low-income urban black communities where a disease like tuberculosis is
presently increasing.

Further, the various health promotion efforts with Native American
populations have been especially enlightening in terms of their applicability
to health education among poor and inner-city blacks. In a model project,
interest centered on determining whether indigenous helpers would be able
to pursue several interrelated tasks: (1) interpret using their own language
and cultural experiences rudimentary information about health status,
(2) assume limited nursing responsibilities under the supervision of a public
health nurse, (3) collect health and demographic data, (4) maintain records
of instructions, and (5) determine emergencies and provide first aid. With the
exception of one participant, all had been hospitalized with pulmonary
tuberculosis. Based on their prior health status, each was instructed to
respond to and interpret patients' reactions to diagnosis and treatment. Also,
they were expected to convey their own experiences in recovering from
tuberculosis and to offer advice regarding medications and doctors' instructions (Deuschle, 1963, p. 464).

With respect to the professional hierarchy and the patient-physician
distance aspects of the Native American program, Navajo medical auxiliaries
occupied an intermediate rank. Since they shared the same ancestral lineage,
traditions, and ethnic perspectives as those with whom they were working,

they could identify and understand the social obstacles and strains in communicating with physicians. Being a product of the same cultural milieu permitted "taking the role of the other" and experiencing psychological empathy with patients' "needs" (Deuschle, 1963, pp. 468–469). This cultural dimension of health education was not unlike that observed in non-Indian communities; it has significant implications for similar programs in African-American communities.

Training Strategies for Interventions

Earlier health education programs across the country incorporated a variety of activities and training techniques. A number of these have the potential for interethnic and cross-cultural adoption. In fact, past experiments introduced a framework for cataloguing the array of duties carried out by neighborhood workers and for highlighting the kinds of social class, racial, and ethnically specific skills needed for effective health promotion and education.

Moreover, the training of community health workers has required special educational strategies and institutional models (Dalhaus, 1981; Fox, 1978; Knittel, Child, & Hobgood, 1971; Moodie & Rogers, 1970; Sterling, 1978). For example, an early West Coast project, designed to prepare economically disadvantaged persons as home health assistants, admitted participants with less than a high school education. At the same time, it was readily apparent that they could be "certified as home health aides" (Hoff, 1969b, p. 623). One of the interesting features of the unique experiment was its primary goal emphasizing the acquisition of basic home nursing care knowledge and skills. Results demonstrated that older unemployed men and women trainees performed successfully on a number of relevant performance identifiers: attitudes, professional behavior, interpersonal relations, and technical competencies. Findings from similar experiments were confirmed, namely, that "adults who are recruited from ghettos and other poverty areas can be trained in a relatively short time to become effective health workers" (Hoff, 1969b, pp. 617–622).

Complementing the results from special health education and promotion activities that embraced low-income persons as assistants, earlier programs often shifted their objectives from identifying medical care needs to analysis and eventually to problem solving. When this occurred, a dynamic cycle evolved that reflected the culturally specific experiences of indigenous community health liaisons. Also, when they acquired basic health knowledge and advanced to higher levels of problem resolution, reliance on professionals tended to decrease (Kent & Smith, 1967). In fact, in many projects, the workers exercised independence, thus attaining one of the desired outcomes for effective role performance. What is important with respect to the variety of experiments has been the emphasis on enabling neighborhood aides to pursue health education and promotion without constant surveillance (Galloway & Kelso, 1966; Oberlander, 1990). This finding is highly pertinent for the development of new programs to meet the increasing health needs of inner-city African Americans. Wherever neighborhood representatives have been members of the cultural group that they have served, essential "sub-culturally oriented communications skills" (Kent & Smith, 1967, p. 1000) have blended with the health promotion tasks. Thus, indigenous workers have been able to interact successfully with and speak the "language" of the people in their communities, a feature that remains essential for viable projects with urban and low-income African Americans. However, this constructive component has emerged as a politically explosive issue in health education initiatives. One reason for opposing perspectives has been that the criteria for selection and recruitment of workers often explicitly mandated that they not be members of "a group identifiably middle class" (Grosser, 1966). With the exclusion of middle-income persons, college-trained professionals felt that they were being denied an opportunity to take part in an important facet of the community health movement. Nevertheless, advocates of using local and low-income residents as interventionists insisted on neighborhood authenticity. The underlying philosophy was that "native" medical aides were necessary because they could relate more effectively and communicate more meaningfully with the residents in the areas to be served. Although a national debate ensued around the "insider-outsider" controversy, the indigenous community health worker concept embodied a value that merges with an Afrocentric perspective, as evidenced in the response to cultural styles that are authentic and representative of the customs and traditions of targeted populations.

An Urban High Blood Pressure Control Project

In a face-to-face interview conducted in a Johns Hopkins University East Baltimore hypertension project in 1985, a basic objective was to examine the role obligations, activities, and social placement of health aides within the professional status hierarchy. Interest centered on the effectiveness of a neighborhood worker who had been placed in a hospital environment. The East Baltimore Hypertension Control Program, in which a local health assistant was an integral participant at the time of my study, was located in the African-American community. Prior to the interview, the community health liaison had been with the project for one year. Her primary duty was blood pressure counseling. Other helpers, engaged in similar health education tasks, were located in churches and in urban neighborhood settings throughout the city.

Coinciding with the notion of the advantages of shared cultural backgrounds for effective blood pressure control with African-American populations, the health worker felt that she was in a better position than physicians or nurses to respond to the "why questions" asked by patients. She perceived herself as able to interpret their reluctance to comply with formal and impersonal medical care regimens. Noting that often doctors do not tell patients exactly what their problems are, she added that they also fail to inform them about unanticipated or adverse effects of prescribed medications for hypertension. In addition, neither the long-term importance of compliance nor the behavioral changes necessary to maintain one's health is stressed. Thus, she shared the view that health workers assumed responsible and practical roles in low-income African-American communities in a variety of contexts by supplementing the expectations of doctors and nurses. In the treatment process, they become "significant others": "We can ask questions doctors can't ask. [We] can get people's life-styles. Sometimes people come back. We act as information and referral sources."

Since neighborhood health workers in urban and rural areas have traditionally been nonprofessionals, questions were raised about their patterns of interaction and status relationships with professional staff. Although health education assistants are on the periphery of the medical occupational hierarchy, the worker I interviewed received support, encouragement, and "compliments from the staff." Her experience demonstrated that the professional employees appreciate the health aides. In appraising the purposes of her duties, the worker felt that she carried out essential health promotion functions. "It is an important role. Patients will tell us everything and practitioners nothing." Pride was conveyed in her comments about enjoying the medical care setting and being given an opportunity for personal growth. On the other hand, she pointed to the need to develop more diverse outlets and higher-level training for nonprofessional community health workers. Program expansion was defined as essential in order to meet the increasing multiple health problems facing poor African Americans in urban inner cities as well as the poor in rural Appalachia and the South.

Future Possibilities

During the past three decades, intervention projects have been designed to test the success of neighborhood assistants in health education and in disease prevention. Emphases have concentrated on health promotion, hygiene, exercise, breast self-examination, adequate nutrition, blood pressure control, and the use of health services. In one model experiment, community workers were instructed to offer basic information that could be readily understood and applied. They highlighted the following concerns and goals: (1) how daily habits affect health, (2) ways to modify life-styles and engage in preventive practices, (3) procedures for seeking help when needed, and (4) strategies for learning about local services and the medical care system. Following a six-month instruction period, the majority of the participants could specify risks associated with one of the leading health problems—coronary heart disease. Similarly, the ability to recognize cancer's seven warning signals increased, as did the use of monthly breast self-examinations. In addition, there was greater awareness of the available medical services and facilities for families needing them. Finally, the number of women who went for blood pressure readings as well as to dentists for regular checkups increased (Fox, 1978).

Since the 1960s, a principal emphasis of health education has been on devising techniques for appraising the patient behavioral outcomes and the usefulness of indigenous workers. In an exemplary infant immunization surveillance program, the impact of referrals on additional service contacts was assessed. The results demonstrated that local helpers influenced a significant number of the referrals reporting immunization (Moore, Morris, Burton, & Kilcrease, 1981). Those responding in the monitoring project observed that health aides assisted in two basic ways: in initiating the immunization or in seeking additional information. A case such as this further illustrates the potential for involving assistants in a wide range of health promotion and education activities in both low-income and working-class communities.

Finally, indigenous workers from African-American and other ethnic minority communities have served as connecting links by assisting in a diversity of health education and intervention activities (for example, cigarette smoking cessation, prevention of HIV infection, infant mortality reduction, reduction of intravenous drug use, obesity control, and high blood pressure prevention). This brief synopsis of pertinent literature, combined with a single case interview, has alluded to variations as well as continuity in the services provided. Confirming their immense value and ways they can be maintained in African-American communities, health liaisons have also been successfully utilized in Africa, China, Latin America, and the Middle East, and on American Indian reservations (Bastien, 1990; Christensen & Karlqvist, 1990; Conn, 1983; Galloway & Kelso, 1966; Gagnon, 1991; Hoff, 1969b; Jolly, 1982; Mathur & Kumar, 1978; Moodie & Rogers, 1970; Kent & Smith, 1967; Mashalaba, 1979; Gong & Chao, 1982; Orient, 1982; Rubin et al., 1983; Kesie, 1966; Shook, 1969; Long & Viau, 1974; Cooke & Meyers, 1983; Delano, 1980).

In spite of the variations in the roles assigned, health workers have had a significant impact on health education and promotion. One earlier representative project focused on providing services to an urban and poor community. A number of emphases were outlined as necessary for meaningful use of health assistants: (1) the criteria for selection and recruitment, (2) training content and objectives, (3) supervisory style and philosophy, and (4) role expectations and duties. Those programs that have worked highlighted these multiple components for preparing nonprofessional neighborhood residents as community health resources (Salber, 1979). Also, professional staff members have pointed to the uniqueness and cultural significance of the special abilities of indigenous workers in establishing rapport with patients (Galloway & Kelso, 1966; Kent & Smith, 1967).

Conclusion

From past and recent health education projects, useful information has been obtained regarding ways to use paraprofessional or nonprofessional community health workers more successfully. The importance of homogeneity in economic, cultural, and social characteristics between patients and the health liaison has been highlighted. Concern about role performance and identity among indigenous health education aides has revealed the potential for overidentification with professional staff who come from middle-class backgrounds (Moore & Stewart, 1972). Nevertheless, attempts have been made through training to avoid restrictive self-definitions (Kent & Smith, 1967; Knittel, Child, & Hobgood, 1971). These concerns are applicable to a variety of health education programs, whether designed to prevent teenage pregnancy, promote "safe sex," manage diabetes, or control cancer.

Moreover, enabling neighborhood health workers to feel as if they are active participants in a team is imperative for successful results. As this discussion has shown, feelings of autonomy, professional identity, and personal worth are basic expectations. Whatever the nature of the organizational context or the formal role requirements, community health workers or paramedical personnel represent "a new challenge to doctors" and to health promotion among low-income patients (Buerki, 1985). Given the nature of their responsibilities, their value in meeting the escalating health needs in low-income rural and urban African-American communities should receive the recognition it deserves (Artz, Cooke, Meyers, & Stalgaitis, 1981; Giblin, 1989; Grosser, 1966; Matomora, 1989).

As indicated earlier, indigenous health aides have served as valuable contributors to community health activities. Their tasks have been fundamental in tuberculosis control, school health education (Russo et al., 1982), and high blood pressure monitoring (Bone et al., 1989), for example. Not unexpectedly, women have served in the majority of the lay counseling and paraprofessional health education activities (Mejia & Varju, 1983; Salber, 1979). Older adults have also been trained as home care personnel (Heller, 1981). In view of the past successes with the involvement of local residents in health promotion and education, they should continue to be supported in the coming decades by government and the medical profession. In order to meet the multiple health care needs that are increasing in poor and working-class African-American communities and in a growing population of medically indigent families, numerous personnel and resources will be needed.

References

Artz, L., Cooke, C. J., Meyers, A., & Stalgaitis, S. (1981). Community change agents and health interventions: Hypertension screening. *American Journal of Community Psychology, 9*(3), 361–370.

Bastien, J. W. (1990). Community health workers in Bolivia: Adapting to traditional roles in the Andean community. *Social Science and Medicine, 30,* 281–287.

Bone, L. R., Mamon, J., Levine, D. M., Walrath, J. M., Nanda, J., Gurley, H. T., Noji, E. K., & Ward, E. (1989). Emergency department detection and follow-up of high blood pressure: Use and effectiveness of community health workers. *American Journal of Emergency Medicine, 7,* 16–20.

Buerki, R. C. (1985). The increasing role of para-medical personnel. *Journal of Medical Education, 40,* 850–855.

Christensen, P. B., & Karlqvist, S. (1990). Community health workers in a Peruvian slum area: An evaluation of their impact on health behavior. *Bulletin of the Pan American Health Organization, 24,* 183–196.

Colombo, T. J., Freeborn, D. K., Mullooly, J. P., & Burnham, V. R. (1979). The effect of outreach workers' educational efforts on disadvantaged preschool children's use of preventive services. *American Journal of Public Health, 69,* 465–468.

Conn, R. H. (1983). Using health education aides in counseling pregnant women. *Public Health Reports, 11,* 979–982.

Cooke, C. J., and Meyers, A. (1983). The role of community volunteers in health interventions: A hypertension screening and follow-up program. *American Journal of Public Health, 73,* 193–194.

Dalhaus, A. A. (1981). Training of community health aides by means of a self-instruction package. *Educación Medica y Salud, 15,* 124–133.

Delano, B. G. (1980). Paid aides in home hemodialysis: No panacea. *Procedures in Clinical Dialysis Transplant Forum, 10,* 138–140.

Derian, P. S. (1968). The creation of the medical therapist. *Journal of the American Medical Association, 266,* 2524–2525.

Deuschle, K. W. (1963). Training and use of the medical therapist. *Public Health Reports, 78,* 461–469.

Fox, E. L. (1978). Using paraprofessionals in the Arkansas health education programs. *Health Education, 9,* 12–13.

Gagnon, A. J. (1991). The training and integration of village health workers. *Bulletin of the Pan American Health Organization, 25,* 127–138.

Galloway, J. R., & Kelso, R. R. (1966). Don't handcuff the aide. *Rehabilitation Record, 7,* 1–3.

Giblin, P. T. (1989). Effective utilization and evaluation of indigenous health care workers. *Public Health Reports, 104,* 361–368.

Gong, Y. L., & Chao, L. M. (1982). The role of the barefoot doctors. *American Journal of Public Health, 72,* 59–61.

Grosser, C. F. (1966). Local residents as mediators between middle-class professional workers and lower-class clients. *Social Service Review, 40,* 56–63.

Harrington, M. (1966). *The other America.* Baltimore, MD: Penguin Books.

Heller, B. R. (1981). Seniors helping seniors: Training older adults as new personnel resources in home health care. *Journal of Gerontological Nursing, 7,* 552–555.

Hoff, W. (1969a). Role of the community health aide in public health programs. *Public Health Reports*, *84*(11), 998–1002.

Hoff, W. (1969b). Training the disadvantaged as home health aides. *Public Health Reports*, *84*(11), 617–623.

Jolly, P. W. (1982, May). Health technician in Turkey. *World Health*, 5–7.

Kent, J., & Smith, C. H. (1967). Involving the urban poor in health services through accommodation—The employment of neighborhood representatives. *American Journal of Public Health*, *57*, 997–1002.

Kesie, B. (1966). Training and use of auxiliary public health personnel in Latin America. *Bolletini Oficina Sanitaria Panamericana*, *60*, 469–485.

Knittel, R. E., Child, R. C., & Hobgood, J. (1971). Role of training of health education aides. *American Journal of Public Health*, *61*, 1571–1580.

Levine, D. M., Green, L. W., Deeds, S. G., Chwalow, J., Russell, R. P., & Finley, J. (1979). Health education for hypertensive patients. *Journal of the American Medical Association*, *241*, 1700–1703.

Levine, D. M., Morisky, L. R., Bone, L. R., Lewis, C., Ward, W. B., & Green, L. W. (1982). Data-based planning for educational interventions through hypertension control programs for urban and rural populations in Maryland. *Public Health Reports*, *97*, 107–112.

Long, E. C., & Viau, A. (1974). Health care extension using medical auxiliaries in Guatemala. *Lancet*, *1*, 127–130.

Mashalaba, N. N. (1979, March). Contact with the community: Family welfare educators in Botswana. *World Health*, 28–31.

Mathur, Y. C., & Kumar, A. (1978). Role of village health worker in health problems of developing countries. *Journal of the Tropical Pediatrician*, *24*, 133–134.

Matomora, M. K. (1989). Mass produced village health workers and the promise of primary health care. *Social Science and Medicine*, *28*, 1081–1084.

McFadden, G. M., Kirschenbaum, S., & Svigir, M. (1966). Employment of health aides in a tuberculosis program. *Public Health Reports*, *81*, 43–48.

Mejia, A., & Varju, L. (1983, September). Women as health providers. *World Health*, 10–12.

Moodie, A. S., & Rogers, G. (1970). Baltimore uses inner city aides in a tuberculosis control program. *Public Health Reports*, *85*(11), 955–963.

Moore, B. J., Morris, D. W., Burton, B., & Kilcrease, D. T. (1981). Measuring effectiveness of service aides in infant immunization surveillance program in north central Texas. *American Journal of Public Health*, *71*, 634–636.

Moore, F. I., & Stewart, J. C. (1972). Important variables influencing successful use of aides. *Health Service Reports*, *87*, 555–561.

Mullan, F. (1978). City ghettos suffer from MD shortage. *Health Care Week*, *1*, 14.

Oberlander, L. B. (1990). Work satisfaction among community-based mental health service providers: The association between work environment and work satisfaction. *Community Mental Health Journal*, *26*, 517–532.

Orient, J. M. (1982). Medicine in China as reflected in a barefoot doctor's manual. *Arizona Medicine, 39,* 185–189.

Rubin, G., Chen, C., de Herra, Y., de Aparicio, V., Massey, J., & Morris, L. (1983). Primary health care workers: The rural health aide program in El Salvador. *Bulletin of the Pan American Health Organization, 17,* 42–50.

Russo, R. M., Harvey, B., Kukafka, R., Supino, P., Freis, P. C., & Hamilton, P. (1982). *Journal of School Health, 52,* 425–478.

Salber, E. J. (1979). The lay advisor as a community health resource. *Journal of Health Politics, Policy, and Law, 3,* 469–478.

Shook, D. C. (1969). Alaska Native community health aide training. *Alaska Medicine, 11,* 62–63.

Sterling, M. (1978). Visiting aides training program. *Health Social Work, 3,* 155–164.

Wilkinson, D. (1987). Traditional medicine in American families: Reliance on the wisdom of elders. In D. Wilkinson and M. Sussman (Eds.), *Alternative health maintenance and healing systems* (pp. 65–76). New York: Haworth Press.

20

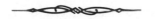

Health Promotion and Disease Prevention Strategies for African Americans: A Conceptual Model

Collins O. Airhihenbuwa

Increasing numbers of health professionals, including researchers, have become concerned with the poor health status of ethnic minorities in the United States, particularly African Americans. This new wave of concern was, in part, triggered by the *Report of the Secretary's Task Force on Black and Minority Health* (U.S. Department of Health and Human Services, 1985), which depicts smoking, alcohol, diet, and obesity as being clearly linked to higher rates of cancer, cirrhosis, infant mortality, cardiovascular and other diseases afflicting minorities. The report recommended that it will take health education and behavioral change to close the gap between the health status of whites and African Americans and other ethnic minorities. The report also cites six health problems as major threats to the health status of African Americans. These health problems—cardiovascular disease and stroke, homicide and accidents, cancer, infant mortality, cirrhosis, and diabetes—are responsible for approximately 80 percent of excess deaths in the African-American population. According to Sullivan (1989, p. 127), "Better control of fewer than 10 risk factors—such as poor diet, infrequent exercise, the use of tobacco, and alcohol and drug abuse—could prevent between 40 and 70 percent of all premature deaths, a third of all cases of acute disability, and two thirds of all cases of chronic disability." As a result, health educators must continue to target these six conditions and AIDS (approximately 28 percent of those affected are black) for morbidity and mortality reduction.

It has been suggested that an aggressive campaign will increase the level of health knowledge within the African-American population, particularly for the diseases and conditions identified above. Assuming this to be the case, a problem still exists to the extent that frameworks are not readily available to guide the issues of cultural sensitivity for such educational

Note: Special thanks to Aaron Gresson, Angele Kingue, Catherine Lyons, and Richard Smith for their comments and suggestions during the preparation of this chapter.

interventions. Existing health promotion strategies for the minority population tend to be based on the theory and framework of the nonminority white population (Green & Kreuter, 1991; Glanz, Lewis, & Rimer, 1990). Researchers have offered alternative theories for examining those neglected but pivotal cultural factors related to understanding the individual and family psychology of African Americans. Useful as these theories are, they do not provide needed programmatic frameworks for planning, implementing, and evaluating health promotion and disease prevention programs for African-American communities. In this chapter, a conceptual model (the PEN-3 model) that was originally developed for use in African countries (Airhihenbuwa, 1989a, 1990–1991) has been modified for the planning and development of culturally appropriate health promotion interventions for the African-American community. The adaptation is both useful and pragmatic due to the shared cultural heritage of Africans and African Americans. However, a modification was necessary to account for the adaptive and maladaptive behaviors of African Americans that have resulted from the experience of oppression in America.

Health Status of African Americans

The failure to devise a health intervention model appropriate to the cultural values of African Americans is directly related to the health crises in African-American communities. An African-American baby is about three times as likely as a white baby to be born to a mother who has had no prenatal care, and more than twice as likely as a white infant to die before the first birthday (Edelman, 1989). A third of all African Americans are poor; an even larger percentage fits this description if one uses a measurement of poverty that is closer to the income needs required to meet minimally decent living standards. The current poverty index is based on a formula designed to determine the minimum necessary for short-term survival (Jacob, 1989).

The poor and the near poor are the hardest hit by rising medical costs. Although government entitlement programs (Medicaid) are available to protect the medically indigent, none of the states in this country provides coverage for individuals up to the federal poverty level. In 1982, the income cutoff limit for Medicaid in twenty-nine states was less than 50 percent of the federal poverty level. Overall, Medicaid reported coverage for only 39.1 percent of the population below the poverty level (Cafferats, 1983). However, even when financial barriers are not a problem, the opportunity cost associated with adoption of a healthful practice, such as participation in an exercise program, is often ignored.

Opportunity cost, which represents the synergy of time and money required to access available health services, is a major barrier for economically disadvantaged health consumers. For example, the cost and convenience of hiring a babysitter will determine if and how long a poor mother participates in a supposedly "free health risk reduction workshop." Since this population's daily activities are not always quantifiable in dollars, their time is often less valued. Thus, the opportunity cost for a poor health consumer to access the same health services is higher than that of a middle- or upper-class consumer. This factor must be seriously considered when exploring why poor African Americans may not utilize available services or tend to delay treatment until the problem becomes critical.

Although socioeconomic status influences health outcome, racial and cultural differences are associated with the low health status of African Americans (Airhihenbuwa, 1989a). A position paper adopted by the American Public Health Association's (APHA) Governing Council in 1974 referred to racism as an established characteristic of the health care delivery system (Muller, 1985). The impact of health service accessibility problems on the African-American family is a reflection of the poor quality of care received. When choices for available services are limited or nonexistent, the quality of services is hardly ever questioned by public policy makers. The underrepresentation of African Americans in the health and medical profession has complicated this problem. African Americans constitute 12.1 percent of the U.S. population but account for only 6.6 percent of the total entering medical school, 2.6 percent of practicing physicians, 1.7 percent of medical school faculty (Hanft, Fishma, & Evans, 1983), and 5.8 percent of doctorates in health education (Airhihenbuwa, Olsen, St. Pierre, & Wang, 1989). It is very important to have African-American health providers who understand and respect the culture, history, and social status of their clients and community. Proctor and Rosen (1981) found that African Americans may not always express racial preference or expectation in their health care provider, but when preference and expectation are expressed, it was a desire to be seen by an African-American health care provider. Even if a patient is not seen by an African-American physician in a medical facility, the knowledge of the presence of an African-American physician in a particular facility does help to alleviate some apprehensions an African-American patient may have about its services. People who share similar cultural patterns, values, experiences, and problems are more likely to feel comfortable with and understand each other (Levy, 1985).

Various scholars have proposed psychological theories and models to provide cultural insights into the understanding of the personality and behaviors of the African-American individual and family. These models help to provide a holistic approach toward enhanced health.

Cultural Basis for Program Development for African Americans

Afrocentric scholars are increasingly challenging the application of traditional models based on the white culture for treatment and disease prevention among African Americans. Past research corroborates the lack of congruence of these practices with the African-American experience, lifestyle, and culture (Akbar, 1977; Leonard & Jones, 1980; Jackson, 1983a,

1983b). In response to these deficits, some researchers have proposed African- and African-American-based personality and treatment models (Baldwin, 1981; Baldwin & Bell, 1982; Parham & Helms, 1985; Nobles, 1980). Consequently, new approaches for educational and behavioral change models have been advanced. "Cultural theories in Black psychology are characterized generally by an emphasis on 'wellness' or normality instead of psychopathology. The focus on normality in turn is based on an African value system" (Jackson, 1983a, 1983b, p. 20). Theoretical formulations are relevant only to the extent that cultural values are recognized and incorporated (Hall, 1977). Since health behaviors are culture bound, primary prevention efforts that address preventable disease and illness must emerge from a knowledge and an understanding of the target culture so that health interventions are culturally sensitive and linguistically appropriate (Braithwaite & Lythcott, 1989).

It has been suggested by some professionals that there is no authentic African-American culture, and therefore that alternative theories and perspectives on health seeking behavior are unnecessary. Seemingly, some of those who believe that there is a different African-American culture and family only view them as a deviant variation of the majority culture (Aldous, 1969; Parker & Kleiner, 1969). However, some in the health profession have argued that African-American culture is different from white culture (the salad bowl paradigm), and thus health promotion activities in African-American communities should be designed to recognize such differences in order to promote strength in cultural diversity (Airhihenbuwa & Pineiro, 1988).

Given the faulty premise that African-American culture is not different from white culture, it has been easy for white psychologists, health professionals, and laypeople to delude themselves into thinking that they are familiar with African-American culture in all of its aspects (Jackson, 1983b). The consequences of such a mind-set are health programs for African-American communities that may have been conceived out of genuine concern for the communities but that are methodologically and theoretically flawed. There is no doubt that the failure to recognize the cultural inadequacies of traditional models, so as to promote and educate people to use an alternative model, has contributed significantly to the profound disparity between the health status of African Americans and that of the white population.

Afrocentric scholars tend to agree that African-American values are a confluence of the African heritage and the American experience (Nobles, 1980; Baldwin, 1981; Jackson, 1983b). Although the focus for many years has been on the American experience (Jackson, 1983b), scholars such as Baldwin (1981) and Asante (1988) have emphasized the retained African values and behavioral patterns. Examples include the extended family, the belief that all the aunts and uncles are responsible parents of all their nieces and nephews, the belief in collectivism as opposed to individualism, respect for age, and so on (Allen, 1978). A life-style of acquiescence to nature rather than challenging it and an emphasis on oral tradition are hallmarks of African values.

Akbar (1977) characterizes the African American as having an innate humaneness with emphasis on religiosity. These qualities are manifested in caring, sensitivity, and concern for the welfare of others. Stewart (1989) has called for the development and prioritizing of a grand theory of Africology based on a full understanding of the nature of history, time, space, and technology in Afrocentric terms. He argues that political and intellectual efforts should be devoted to restructuring community ties and translating the language of African-American intellectual elites into the language of African-American popular culture. Such a framework will capture the belief of Africans and African Americans in postmodern history (Asante, 1988).

In spite of these efforts to understand cultural values as they relate to personal behaviors, little attention has been given to the development of a culturally appropriate paradigm for health promotion in the African-American community. Currently, culturally sensitive educational and behavioral change models for health promotion in the African-American communities tend to be based primarily on the Caucasian experience. Attempts to make these programs culturally appropriate tend to rely on the individual and family psychology of African Americans. The outcome is that these approaches offer no models for translating these known cultural and psychological realities into a working framework that could guide the development of culturally appropriate health promotion and disease prevention programs in the African-American community. Myers and King (1983) presented a dialectic crisis-conflict model for understanding the mental health outcome in the development of the African-American child. This model is unique in that it not only recognizes the significance and depth of the personal crisis faced by the African-American child, but it also emphasizes the etiological significance of the undeveloped consciousness in the victim of the fundamental social contradictions that he or she faces. Based on these established foundations for an understanding of the personality and behaviors of the African American, a model is proposed in this chapter to translate what is known about the African-American individual and family into effective, culturally sensitive health programs for the African-American community. Thus, this model as applied to the African-American community health program is a confluence of existing health education theory, African values, and African-American experience.

The PEN-3 Model

A conceptual model for health education programs in the African-American community must address cultural sensitivity and cultural appropriateness in program development. This model, known as *PEN-3*, was originally developed to be used as a framework for health promotion and disease prevention

in African countries (Airhihenbuwa, 1989b, 1990–1991) and has been successfully applied for child survival interventions in African countries (Airhihenbuwa, in press). The model consists of three dimensions of health
beliefs and behavior that are dynamically interrelated and interdependent
(health education, educational diagnosis of health behavior, and cultural
appropriateness of health behavior). It is illustrated in categories that form
the acronym PEN for each of the three dimensions (see Figure 20.1). The first
dimension of the PEN-3 model is health education. The following explains
each letter in the acronym:

   P—Person. Health education is committed to improving the health of
everyone. To this end, individuals should be empowered to make informed
health decisions, appropriate to their roles in their family and community.

   E—Extended Family. Health education should be targeted not only
toward the immediate family but also toward extended kinships. However,
when a program is designed to target a particular member of the family (for
example, the mother), the individual should become the focus of the study
and must be so recognized. Such recognition must be noted within the
context of the individual's environment.

   N—Neighborhood. Health education is committed to promoting health
and preventing disease in neighborhoods and communities. Involvement of
community members and their leaders becomes critical in providing culturally appropriate health programs. In fact, since community leadership often
defines community boundaries, it is critical for African Americans to define
what comprises their community or neighborhood at the beginning of a
project (see Figure 20.1).

   The second dimension of the PEN-3 model is the educational diagnosis of health behavior. Educational diagnosis has been utilized by researchers to attempt to determine what factors influence individual, family,

Figure 20.1. The PEN-3 Model.

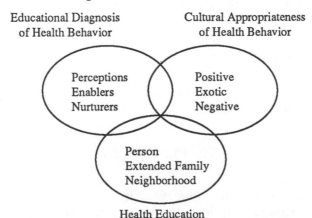

Source: Airhihenbuwa, 1989b, p. 61. Reprinted with the permission of Guilford
Publications, Inc.

and/or community health actions. The three models or frameworks that have predominantly been used to understand and predict healthy and health related behaviors are the Health Belief Model, Fishbein/Ajzen's (1975) theory of reasoned action, and the PRECEDE framework (Mullen, Hersey, & Iverson, 1987). Influenced by Kurt Lewin's "life space" notion, the Health Belief Model (Rosenstock, 1974) focuses on people's perceptions of their susceptibility to a disease and the severity of the disease as predictors of their health actions. Fishbein/Ajzen's theory of reasoned action postulates that the behavior intention is a function of attitude toward performance of an impending behavior reinforced by feedback from significant others. The PRECEDE framework (Green, Kreuter, Deeds, & Partridge, 1980) dealt with how to identify which behaviors (both health related and non–health related) are most important and changeable. Thus, this dimension of PEN-3 has evolved from the confluence of the three models in health education just discussed. However, in adapting this model for Afrocentric utilization in the United States, it should be noted that African Americans do confront and operate in a social order in which the rules appear to be stacked against them. "The degree to which they perceive the 'odds against them' as manageable or overwhelming will depend to a significant degree on the transactional competency and success of their parents, the competence of the role models in their primary community of competency, and, finally, on the availability and accessibility of resources and supports to help them in their coping efforts" (Myers & King, 1983, p. 294). The following are the factors in the second dimension:

P—Perceptions. These are knowledge, attitudes, values, and beliefs that may facilitate or hinder personal motivation to maintain or change health beliefs and/or practices. For example, when African Americans answer yes to the question "can someone get AIDS from donating blood," some researchers misinterpret this to always mean low AIDS knowledge. In fact, this response sometimes indicates a strong distrust of white health care providers, reflecting a belief that white health providers may intentionally infect blacks with the AIDS virus—a legacy of the "Tuskegee syphilis experiment." Regarding differing perceptions of body weight between African Americans and whites, several researchers (Kumanyika & Wilson, 1987; National Center for Health Statistics, 1988; Dawson, 1988; Desmond, Price, Hallinan, & Smith, 1989) reported that being overweight is not necessarily associated with a negative body image for many African Americans. According to these researchers, African Americans who are heavy or of normal weight are more likely to perceive themselves as thinner than their white counterparts. In fact, one study shows that 40 percent of African-American women who were classified as overweight considered their figures attractive or very attractive (Desmond, Price, Hallinan, & Smith, 1989). However, the perceptions about body image should not compromise the seriousness of obesity as a predisposing factor to chronic degenerative conditions such as type II diabetes and heart disease. Another example of differing perceptions is the notion that all teenage pregnancies are unwanted pregnancies. An increasing number of teenage pregnancies among African Americans are wanted pregnancies. Thus, appropriate health interventions for teenage pregnancy should begin with individual perceived needs and desires rather than those needs and expectations that are defined by program planners as perpetuated by the dominant groups in the society.

E—Enablers. These are societal, systematic, or structural influences or forces that may enhance or create barriers to maintain or change health beliefs and/or practices. These include availability of resources, accessibility, referrals, skills, and types of services (for example, folk medicine). As indicated earlier, opportunity cost is always an important factor to be considered in planning and implementing health intervention programs for the African-American community.

N—Nurturers. These are reinforcing factors that a person may receive from significant others. Examples include attitudes and behavior of health personnel, peers, feedback from extended family, kin, employers, government officials, and religious leaders. Here again, it is very important and necessary to significantly increase the number of African Americans in the health professions who understand and respect the culture and community. It is also important to promote an understanding of cultural beliefs and practices among non–African Americans. For example, due to the disproportionately high level of cardiovascular disease in the African-American population, special emphasis has been placed on eating practices and weight control. Since food is a cultural symbol, and eating is a symbolic act through which people communicate, perpetuate, and develop their knowledge and attitudes toward life, an understanding of cultural influences on eating habits is essential to provide realistic educational interventions designed to positively modify dietary practice (Kaufman-Kurzrock, 1989).

The third and most critical dimension of this model is the cultural appropriateness of health beliefs. This dimension is pivotal to developing a culturally sensitive health education program for ethnic minority cultures. This final dimension of the PEN-3 model follows:

P—Positive. These are perceptions, enablers, and nurturers that may lead persons, families, and/or neighborhoods to engage in health practices that contribute to improved health status and that must be encouraged. These positive health practices are critical in the empowerment of persons, extended families, and neighborhoods. These practices are also very critical to program success and sustainability. An example is the promotion of the traditional practice of eating green vegetables. There is a tendency on the part of upwardly mobile African-American professionals to slowly disengage in eating green vegetables, as was done traditionally, since it is not believed to be associated with progress and affluence.

E—Exotic. These are unfamiliar practices that have no harmful health consequences, and thus need not be changed. The programmatic thrust of public health should address "what is" in terms of matching intervention with current health practices such as sexual activities among teenagers, rather than "what ought to be," such as abstinence. Therefore, we should refrain from moralizing over behaviors that are unfamiliar or maybe familiar but ill-understood. Understanding these exotic beliefs is where African-American theoreticians have made significant contributions. For example, these researchers link African-American life-styles with African values such as a holistic worldview as opposed to an abstract view. Health educators should also refrain from assessing personality in terms of "normality" and from viewing the individual as pathological.

N—Negative. These are perceptions, enablers, and nurturers that may lead persons, families, and neighborhoods to engage in health practices that are harmful to their health. An example would be unprotected sexual intercourse. Health providers must therefore attempt to change these practices.

Health education programs involve health beliefs and behaviors. Thus, they must reflect the cultural perspectives of the people for whom the programs are designed. Health educators should focus on both positive (empowerment process) and negative behaviors in a health program. Very often, too much attention is focused on negative behavior, with little or no reward for positive behavior. In some instances, the failure to change negative behavior is mistakenly blamed on the presence of exotic behavior.

This process affords the health educator the level of sensitivity required to properly select the most culturally appropriate educational intervention strategy for a community. Questions to be considered at the planning phase include whether the intervention should be person to person or media based, and how and when to use community leaders as change agents.

Application of the Model

When developing programs to fit in with a community's existing beliefs and practices, the PEN-3 model can be utilized as follows: In the first phase, the program planners must determine if the emphasis of the program will be on persons, on the extended family, or on the neighborhood (health education), realizing that these are not mutually exclusive. In the second phase, the planners should explore (through surveys and/or interviews) the beliefs and practices related to perceptions, enablers, and nurturers (education diagnosis of health behavior). Such examinations will relate to a particular health problem in different segments of the family or community. For example, if the project is weight reduction in the community, how effective is an educational campaign that features skinny persons if a significant segment of the population considers slight overweight as normal? In such an instance, it might be useful to highlight the negative health consequences of being overweight rather than the presumed appeal of being skinny. Research efforts designed for African Americans must be based on the assumption that the African-American individual is an entity independent of the Caucasian individual, and not an entity to be known mainly by comparison (Myers & King, 1983).

Based on the information generated, the third phase involves categorizing the different beliefs and practices as positive, exotic, or negative beliefs (cultural appropriateness of health behavior). Finally the planners, with assistance and guidance from community health workers and community leaders, will classify all the health beliefs into two groups. The first category will comprise all the identified health beliefs that are historically rooted in the cultural patterns and life-styles of the target community. The second group will comprise all the identified health beliefs that are newly formulated and have only superficial ties with the cultural patterns and life-styles of the target community.

The results of the interview and the information generated by the participants in their respective groups prior to the interview should be categorized into positive, exotic, and negative health beliefs and practices. The third phase of the model—cultural appropriateness of health behavior—involves positive and negative health beliefs, including perceptions/beliefs related to knowledge, attitudes, and practices; enablers/skills and resources necessary for health actions; and nurturers/reinforcement for health beliefs and actions.

In this phase, a scheme is developed to identify the perceptions, enablers, and nurturers that are rooted in the culture, as opposed to those that are not rooted in cultural patterns and life-styles. Hence, cultural ties include health beliefs and practices that are historically grounded in cultural patterns and life-styles, while noncultural ties involve health beliefs and practices that are recent and only superficially tied to cultural patterns.

The challenge for health educators is to identify which positive beliefs and practices are supportive of the person, extended family, and neighborhood. How are these influenced by perceptions, enablers, and nurturers? How do these health beliefs and practices influence negative health practices of persons and their extended families? What role do exotic beliefs and practices play in health promotion and disease prevention? What role can they play? Such information is used to develop health promotion strategies for maintaining and promoting positive health practices and changing negative health practices. The health educator, therefore, must understand the rationale behind stated beliefs and practices. This is necessary for appropriate classification and the selection of health education strategies. The next step will be to decide on the most effective strategy for educating the community.

When selecting appropriate interventions, one should address reinforcing or changing cultural beliefs within the context of the African-American culture and not against standards developed to assess the behavior of whites (Myers & King, 1983). One must not assume that the substance and meaning of concepts, images, and behavior are "essentially the same" across cultures simply because they are similar in form (King, 1978). Furthermore, the selection of an appropriate health education strategy must respond to the degree to which the health practices are grounded in cultural beliefs. An

Afrocentric interventionist must employ health education in the home (home visits) or person-to-person contact in the community, making sure that community members representing different segments of the community are involved with the selection of positive practices to be reinforced and negative practices to be changed. According to Fuglesang (1973), face-to-face communication is effective because it allows the communicator to use all the senses (sight, hearing, touch, smell, taste), as opposed to media. On the other hand, mass media are most effective in increasing knowledge, reinforcing previously held attitudes, and changing behaviors that were recently established or behaviors that were predisposed to change, as opposed to those that are tied to cultural values or are contrary to the attitudes and values expressed in the mass media (Griffiths & Knutson, 1960; Green et al., 1980). Simply put, the most effective medium through which beliefs and practices can be unlearned is the same medium through which they were learned.

Conclusion

The need to examine the personal or cultural health beliefs of African Americans is critical and is increasingly becoming an area for analysis. For example, teenage pregnancy is an issue that has received increased public attention in the past decade. For purposes of developing health interventions for this social issue, the assumption is usually made that all teenage pregnancies are unwanted. Consequently, birth control methods are recommended to all teenagers. This may be an acceptable intervention for those whose pregnancies are unwanted and unplanned, but it is totally irrelevant to those teenagers whose pregnancies are wanted and planned, an increasing number of whom are African American. Thus, the need to be culturally sensitive when addressing the health needs of African-American communities is crucially important. Health and social practices are usually the manifestations of cultural beliefs and individual life experiences.

Cultural beliefs and experiences, when properly understood, can be used to promote the success of health education programs in African-American communities. The PEN-3 model offers the health educator the opportunity to consider varied health beliefs and behaviors in terms of (1) the positive, which promotes good health and should be encouraged, (2) the exotic, which is indifferent to health and should not be targeted for change, and (3) the negative, which threatens health and should be targeted for change. While the extent of this model's utility has yet to be systematically tested with African-American populations, it has been successfully applied to child survival in Africa (Airhihenbuwa, in press). The involvement of community members is strongly recommended in order to adequately assess culturally relevant health beliefs and practices and to plan appropriate interventions.

References

Airhihenbuwa, C. O. (1989a). Health education for African-Americans: A neglected task. *Health Education, 20*(5), 9–14.

Airhihenbuwa, C. O. (1989b). Perspectives on AIDS in Africa: Strategies for prevention and control. *AIDS Education and Prevention, 1*(1), 57–69.

Airhihenbuwa, C. O. (1990–1991). A conceptual model for health education program in developing countries. *International Quarterly of Community Health Education, 11*(1), 53–62.

Airhihenbuwa, C. O., Olsen, L. K., St. Pierre, R. W., & Wang, M. Q. (1989). Race and gender: Analysis of the granting of doctoral degrees. *Health Education, 20*(3), 4–7.

Airhihenbuwa, C. O., & Pineiro, O. (1988). Cross-cultural health education: A pedagogical challenge. *Journal of School Health, 58*(6), 240–242.

Airhihenbuwa, C. O. (in press). The application of a culturally appropriate health intervention model for child survival in Africa. *African Journal of Mental Health and Society.*

Akbar, N. (1977). *Natural psychology and human transformation.* Chicago: World Community of Islam.

Aldous, J. (1969). Wives' employment status and lower-class men as husband-fathers: Support for the Moynihan thesis. *Journal of Marriage and the Family, 31*, 469–476.

Allen, W. (1978). The search for applicable theories of black family life. *Journal of Marriage and the Family, 40*(1), 117–129.

Asante, M. K. (1988). *Africentricity.* Trenton, NJ: African World Press.

Baldwin, J. A. (1981). Notes on an Africentric theory of black personality testing. *Western Journal of Black Studies, 5*(3), 172–179.

Baldwin, J. A., & Bell, Y. R. (1982). *The African self-consciousness scale manual.* Unpublished manuscript, Florida A&M University, Department of Psychology.

Braithwaite, R. L., & Lythcott, N. (1989). Community empowerment as a strategy for health promotion for black and other minority populations. *Journal of the American Medical Association, 261*(2), 282–283.

Cafferats, G. L. (1983). *Private health insurance: Premium expenditures and sources of payment* (Data Preview 17, National Health Care Research, DHHS Publication No. 84-8364). Washington, DC: U.S. Government Printing Office.

Dawson, D. (1988). Ethnic differences in female overweight: Data from the 1985 National Health Interview Survey. *American Journal of Public Health, 78*, 1326–1329.

Desmond, S. M., Price, J. H., Hallinan, C., & Smith, D. (1989). Black and white perception of their weight. *Journal of School Health, 59*(8), 353–358.

Edelman, M. R. (1989). Black children in America. In J. Dewart (Ed.), *The State of Black America 1989.* New York: National Urban League.

Fishbein, M., & Ajzen, I. (1975). *Belief, attitude, intention, and behavior.* Reading, MA: Addison-Wesley.

Fuglesang, A. (1973). *Applied communication in developing countries: Ideas and observations*. Uppsala, Sweden: Dag Hammarskjöld Foundation.

Glanz, K., Lewis, F. M., & Rimer, B. K. (Eds.). (1990). *Health behavior and health education*. San Francisco: Jossey-Bass.

Green, L. W., & Kreuter, M. W. (1991). *Health promotion planning: An educational and environmental approach* (2nd ed.). Mountain View, CA: Mayfield.

Green, L. W., Kreuter, M. W., Deeds, S. A., & Partridge, K. B. (1980). *Health education planning: A diagnostic approach*. Mountain View, CA: Mayfield.

Griffiths, W., & Knutson, A. L. (1960). The role of mass media in public health. *American Journal of Public Health, 50*, 515–523.

Hall, E. T. (1977). *Beyond culture*. New York: Doubleday.

Hanft, R. S., Fishma, L. E., & Evans, W. J. (1983). *Blacks and the health professions in the 80s: A national crisis and a time for action*. Washington, DC: Association of Minority Health Profession Schools.

Jackson, A. M. (1983a). The black patient and traditional psychotherapy: Implications and possible extensions. *Journal of Community Psychology, 11*, 303–307.

Jackson, A. M. (1983b). A theoretical model for the practice of psychotherapy with black populations. *Journal of Black Psychology, 10*(1), 19–27.

Jacob, J. E. (1989). Black America, 1988: An overview. In J. Dewart (Ed.), *The State of Black America 1989* (pp. 1–7). New York: National Urban League.

Kaufman-Kurzrock, R. D. (1989). Cultural aspects of nutrition. *Topics in Clinical Nutrition, 4*(2), 1–6.

King, L. M. (1978). Social and cultural influences on psychopathology. *Annual Review of Psychology, 29*, 405–433.

Kumanyika, S., & Wilson, J. F. (1987, October). *Attitudinal and behavioral influences on black female obesity*. Paper presented at the 115th annual meeting of the American Public Health Association, Washington, DC.

Leonard, P., & Jones, A. C. (1980). Theoretical considerations for psychotherapy with black clients. In R. C. Jones (Ed.), *Black psychology* (2nd ed., pp. 429–438). New York: HarperCollins.

Levy, D. R. (1985). White doctors and black patients: Influence of race on the doctor-patient relationship. *Pediatrics, 75*(4), 639–643.

Mullen, P. D., Hersey, J. C., & Iverson, D. C. (1987). Health models compared. *Social Science and Medicine, 24*(11), 973–981.

Muller, C. (1985). A window of the past: The position of the client in twentieth century public health thought and practice. *American Journal of Public Health, 75*(5), 470–476.

Myers, H. F., & King, L. M. (1983). Mental health issues in the development of the black American child. In E. G. Powell (Ed.), *The psychosocial development of minority group children*. New York: Brunner/Mazel.

National Center for Health Statistics. (1988). Health promotion and disease prevention, United States, 1985. *Vital and Health Statistics* (Series 10, No. 163) (DHHS Publication No. PHS 88-1591). Washington, DC: U.S. Government Printing Office.

Nobles, W. W. (1980). African philosophy: Foundations for black psychology. In R. L. Jones (Ed.), *Black psychology* (2nd ed.). New York: HarperCollins.

Parham, T. A., & Helms, J. E. (1985). Relation of racial identity attitudes to self-actualization and affective states of black students. *Journal of Counseling Psychology, 32*(3), 431–440.

Parker, S., & Kleiner, R. (1969). Social psychological dimensions of the family role performance of the Negro male. *Journal of Marriage and the Family, 33,* 500–506.

Proctor, E., & Rosen, A. (1981). Expectations and preferences for counselor race and their relation to intermediate treatment outcomes. *Journal of Counseling Psychology, 28*(1), 40–46.

Rosenstock, I. M. (1974). Historical origins of the Health Belief Model. *Health Education Monographs, 2*(4), 328–335.

Stewart, J. B. (1989, July). *The state of black studies: Perspectives from the first NCBS Summer Faculty Institute and implications of the NRC report "A Common Destiny."* Paper presented at Temple University, African American Studies Department.

Sullivan, L. W. (1989). Shattuck lecture: The health care priorities of the Bush administration. *New England Journal of Medicine, 321*(2), 125–128.

U.S. Department of Health and Human Services. (1985). *Report of the Secretary's Task Force on Black and Minority Health* (Vol. 1, Executive Summary). Washington, DC: U.S. Government Printing Office.

21

Effective Intervention Strategies for Producing Black Health Care Providers

Moses K. Woode
Kathleen Bodisch Lynch

The underrepresentation of blacks and other minorities in the field of medicine has been a long-standing problem for this country. The diversity of racial and ethnic groups in the general population is not reflected in the population of health care providers. Statistics on blacks are illustrative: the National Science Foundation reports that while blacks make up approximately 12 percent of the national population, less than 3 percent of U.S. physicians, less than 3 percent of dentists, and less than 2 percent of biomedical scientists are black (Gunby, 1989). In 1985, while there were an estimated fifty-four black physicians for every 100,000 blacks in the population, the physician-to-population ratio for the United States as a whole was 220 for every 100,000 (U.S. Department of Health and Human Services, 1986). Compounding the problem, the number of black physicians in practice suffered a 27 percent decline from 1984 to 1987, dropping from 26,000 to 19,018, according to the Bureau of Labor Statistics (Raymond, 1989). The insufficient presence of minorities in medicine manifests itself at all points on the medical education pathway. Their disproportionately low representation in the pool of medical school applicants can be predicted as early as the third grade where, for example, black and Hispanic students have already fallen well below whites in mathematics and reading achievement; by the completion of high school, they are less likely to be prepared to take college-

Note: The University of Virginia School of Medicine's minority medical education programs have been supported in part by the U.S. Department of Health and Human Services Bureau of Disadvantaged Assistance Health Careers Opportunity Program Grant 2-D18-MBO1000-06, the Robert Wood Johnson Foundation, the State Council of Higher Education for Virginia, the National Institutes of Health, the Charlottesville City Public Schools, Abbott Laboratories, the Charlottesville-Albemarle Foundation, the Commonwealth Fund, the Charles C. Dana Foundation, the Pew Charitable Trusts, and the W. Alton Jones Foundation.

　　We gratefully acknowledge the support of Robert M. Carey, dean of the School of Medicine, and the members of the Advisory Committee for Minority Medical Education Programs.

level science courses or to be premed majors (Simpson & Aronoff, 1988). Although blacks constitute more than 12 percent of this country's population, in 1989 only 5.7 percent of the baccalaureate degrees awarded were received by blacks (Petersdorf, Turner, Nickens, & Ready, 1990). Between 1980 and 1988, blacks made up approximately 7.5 percent of the medical school applicant pool; first-year enrollment of blacks in medical school hovered around the 7 percent mark, and total enrollment of blacks in medical school averaged approximately 6 percent (Association of American Medical Colleges, 1989). Exacerbating the problem, during this same period, there was a 16.7 percent drop-off in medical school applications from blacks. Other minority groups who show similar patterns of underrepresentation in medicine are Mexican-Americans, mainland Puerto Ricans, Native Americans, and Alaskan natives (Petersdorf, Turner, Nickens, & Ready, 1990).

In addition to the problem of disproportionately fewer applications to medical school, blacks and other minorities also lag behind whites in their scores on the quantitative academic criteria typically given heavy weight by medical schools in making admissions decisions (for example, science grade-point average and Medical College Admission [MCAT] scores). For example, in 1986 the mean MCAT subtest score for white applicants to medical school was 8.9 (on a scale of 1 to 15), while for blacks it was 6.0. Moreover, despite improvements in minorities' scores during the past decade, and despite conflicting evidence regarding the relationships between quantitative academic criteria and minority students' admissions to medical school (Lynch & Woode, 1990), the rate of acceptance of minorities into medical school has not increased at the same pace as that for all applicants — rising from 39 to 49 percent for minorities versus 30 to 61 percent for all applicants during the years 1977 to 1987 (Lloyd & Miller, 1989).

Once they are in medical school, retention of minority students is also a concern (Woode & Lynch, 1990b). With only about 1,000 blacks being accepted into medical school each year, "any attrition is significant" (Lloyd & Miller, 1989, p. 272). For the medical school class graduating in 1988, for example, the retention rate of blacks, while high (89 percent), was still lower than the 97 percent retention rate for all medical students (Association of American Medical Colleges, 1989).

Perhaps even more disturbing than the underrepresentation of blacks and other minorities in the medical profession, however, is their overrepresentation in many health problem areas. Unconscionable disparities exist between the health status of blacks and other minorities and that of the U.S. population as a whole. Robert E. Windom, Assistant Secretary for Health, reported in a 1989 issue of the *Journal of the American Medical Association* that blacks and members of other minority groups suffer "excess deaths" from a number of specific causes, far above the levels experienced by whites. These causes include cancer, cardiovascular disease and stroke, diabetes, homicide and injuries, maternal and infant mortality, and acquired immune deficiency syndrome (AIDS). In 1988, the overall age-adjusted mortality rate for blacks exceeded that of the white population by 50 percent, and the average life expectancy for blacks, which has been declining since 1984, was 69.2 years compared with 75.6 years for whites, according to the National Center for Health Statistics ("Experts Find," 1990).

It is vitally important, therefore, to increase the number of minority physicians and other health care providers, because they can have a direct impact on the health status of less advantaged persons through the improved access to medical care that their presence brings about. For example, a study published in the *New England Journal of Medicine* revealed that black physicians are more likely than others to choose primary care specialties and set up practices in underserved inner-city areas (Keith, Bell, Swanson, & Williams, 1985). More recently, the Association of American Medical Colleges (AAMC) (1989) reported that in response to its 1988 Medical Student Graduation Questionnaire, 48.9 percent of black medical students said they intend to practice in underserved communities, compared with 13.6 percent of whites. Again in 1989, minority medical school graduates were more likely than their majority counterparts to indicate plans to practice in large cities and in rural areas, and were far more likely to indicate that their career plans included location in a socioeconomically deprived area. In addition, compared with majority physicians, in graduate medical education and in practice, minority physicians choose primary care specialties more often (Petersdorf et al., 1990).

Because of the complex factors operating to inhibit minorities' pursuit of and attainment of medical careers (such as inadequate academic preparation, particularly in the sciences; insufficient academic and career counseling; the substantial costs of medical education; decreasing availability of grants and scholarships; and increased opportunities in other career areas), the trend toward inadequate production of minority health care providers is not likely to reverse itself without sound intervention programs. Such programs must attract blacks and other minority students to the fields of medicine and allied health; facilitate their entry into health professions schools by enhancing their competitiveness for admission; and ensure that once enrolled, these students complete their education.

Historically, several events converged that established conditions favorable to the development of programs aimed at increasing the representation of minorities in medicine. In 1970, the Association of American Medical Colleges made a policy decision to advocate for parity between representation in medicine and representation in the overall population (Petersdorf et al., 1990). In 1971, federal legislation was enacted specifically to address the underrepresentation of minorities and other disadvantaged persons in the health fields. Important efforts have occurred under the aegis of the Health Careers Opportunity Program (HCOP), administered by the Bureau of Health Professions, Division of Disadvantaged Assistance, in the Health Resources and Services Administration. Since 1972, funds have been awarded to health professions schools and other public and nonprofit private institutions that operate programs aimed at increasing the number of persons from disadvantaged backgrounds who enter the health professions. Between 1972 and 1978, almost 400 such programs for students aspiring to be physicians, dentists, optometrists, pharmacists, podiatrists, chiropractors, veterinarians, public health administrators, and allied health workers were funded (U.S. Department of Health and Human Services, 1989). In 1990, there were 165 HCOP programs in operation throughout the country, meeting the five HCOP legislative purposes: to identify and recruit minorities and other disadvantaged persons for education in the health professions, provide preliminary educational experiences for undergraduates interested in careers in health, facilitate their entry into health professions schools, provide counseling and other retention services, and distribute financial aid information. Complementing the federal government's initiatives are programs funded by philanthropic organizations and private foundations, such as the Robert Wood Johnson Foundation and the Josiah Macy Foundation (Simpson & Aronoff, 1988).

In the next section, strategies employed by the University of Virginia School of Medicine to increase the production of black and other minority and disadvantaged health care providers are described. The School of Medicine has developed a comprehensive approach, which includes elements common to other existing minority medical education programs, as well as incorporating innovative features that have proven to be successful.

University of Virginia Minority Medical Education Programs

The University of Virginia School of Medicine has had a strong record of initiating, developing, operating, and expanding highly successful academic enrichment programs for blacks and other minority and disadvantaged students interested in careers in medicine and the health professions, since 1984. In that year, the School of Medicine funded a pilot residential six-week summer academic enrichment program designed to enhance the opportunities for minority and disadvantaged students to be accepted into, and successfully graduate from, medical school.

Each year since the pilot program was conducted, the School of Medicine has operated an array of academic enrichment programs for minority and disadvantaged students, at the high school, undergraduate, postbaccalaureate, and medical school levels. These programs have been supported with a combination of funds from the School of Medicine, the U.S. Department of Health and Human Services Bureau of Disadvantaged Assistance Health Careers Opportunity Program (HCOP), the National Institutes of Health, the State Council of Higher Education for Virginia, the Charlottesville City Public Schools, and several private foundations. The latter include the Robert Wood Johnson Foundation, Abbott Laboratories, the W. Alton Jones Foundation, the Commonwealth Fund, the Charles C.

Dana Foundation, the Charlottesville-Albemarle Foundation, and the Pew Charitable Trusts. Between 1984 and 1991, minority academic enrichment programs conducted by the University of Virginia School of Medicine served over 1,800 blacks and other minority and disadvantaged students interested in careers in the health professions. (Specific data on these programs are available from the chapter authors.)

Students who have participated in the School of Medicine's academic enrichment programs have enjoyed a high rate of success in their pursuit of medical education. Follow-up data show that twenty-nine past participants have received M.D. degrees, three students an M.P.H., and one an associate degree in allied health; in the 1991–92 academic year, 150 students were enrolled in medical or allied health professions schools. Moreover, the retention rate for all past program participants, most recently documented at 99 percent, exceeds the national minority medical student retention rate (Association of American Medical Colleges, 1989).

The operation of two summer residential Medical Academic Advancement Programs (MAAP-I and MAAP-II) serves as the cornerstone of a comprehensive plan for increasing the number of blacks and other minorities in medicine. Through MAAP-I and MAAP-II, the School of Medicine identifies undergraduate and postbaccalaureate students interested in careers in medicine and provides them with academic enrichment, exposure to the practice of clinical medicine, and personal and academic guidance and support. Other School of Medicine programs, at the high school and medical school levels, complement MAAP-I and MAAP-II and enhance their effectiveness. Following is a description of these programs.

Medical Academic Advancement Program-I

The primary purposes of the Medical Academic Advancement Program-I (MAAP-I) are to identify and recruit talented minority students into the field of medicine and to enhance their competitiveness for entry into medical and allied health professions schools. Students who are eligible to participate in MAAP-I are sophomores, juniors, seniors, and recent graduates who have not yet taken the MCAT or who have taken the MCAT but have not achieved scores that are competitive for admission into medical school. The MAAP-I, a six-week residential program held during the summer, has several components.

MCAT Preparation Course

The major component of the MAAP-I is a rigorous MCAT preparation course. MAAP-I participants attend MCAT classes five days a week throughout the six weeks of the program. Experienced instructors provide four hours per week of intensive focused review in each content area covered by the

MCAT (biology, chemistry, physics, quantitative relationships, reading, science problem solving, and essay writing). Problem-solving techniques relevant to the content area under study are incorporated into the lecture sessions. Students take simulated MCAT exams at the beginning and end of the program to get exposure to MCAT-like questions and testing conditions, to help reduce anxiety about the MCAT, and to measure gains in test scores over the course of the program. Students are also regularly given instructor-developed quizzes and homework assignments designed to provide practice in analyzing and responding to a variety of test item types. Minority medical students, graduate students, and course instructors are all available after class hours to provide tutoring assistance as needed.

Faculty Mentorships

In order to provide students with a more in-depth and personalized look at the world of medicine, each MAAP-I participant is assigned to a faculty mentor. Mentors are School of Medicine faculty members who have volunteered their time to work with minority students interested in medicine. At the outset of the program, all students are polled to determine areas of interest, and whenever possible, students are given their first choice in the area of clinical medicine or biomedical research that interests them. Students meet with their mentors on a regular basis during the course of the MAAP-I. Faculty from the following clinical and research areas have served as mentors for MAAP-I participants: ambulatory care, anatomy, cardiology, craniofacial surgery, endocrinology, gastroenterology, general medicine, geographic medicine, geriatrics, hematology/oncology, immunology, internal medicine, liver physiology, medical genetics, microbiology, neurology, obstetrics/gynecology, pediatric pharmacology, pediatrics, physical medicine and rehabilitation, physiology, psychiatry, pulmonary and critical care, radiology, sports medicine, student health, surgery, and urology.

Clinical Medicine Lecture Series

Organized by the chairman of the Department of Internal Medicine, the Clinical Medicine Lecture Series is designed to give MAAP-I participants exposure to, and an experiential appreciation of, the "real" world of medicine. This component of the MAAP-I presents students with the opportunity, for example, to observe open heart surgery or an autopsy, to accompany physicians on their hospital rounds, and to visit patient care areas such as the emergency room or the renal dialysis unit. Presentations are given on a broad range of medical specialties, techniques, and problem areas, including alcohol and drug abuse, sexually transmitted diseases including HIV and AIDS, cardiology, chemotherapy, dermatology, geriatrics, hematology, obstetrics, oncology, pediatrics, and the physician's ethical responsibilities. In addition, MAAP-I participants receive tours of clinical and research facilities of the

Health Sciences Center and get exposure to state-of-the-art equipment such as the Gamma Knife, an instrument that promises to revolutionize neurovascular surgery, and the Lithotripter, an instrument for the nonsurgical removal of kidney stones. Each year, MAAP-I participants report that the Clinical Medicine Lecture Series stimulates their interest in areas of medicine with which they were previously unfamiliar and reinforces their motivation for wanting to become a physician.

Introduction to Biomedical Research Lecture Series

In order to acquaint students with topics and methods in biomedical research, lectures are given by eminent scientists on the faculty of the University of Virginia School of Medicine and other institutions. Presentations include research topics of particular interest to blacks and other minorities — such as sickle cell anemia, hypertension, diabetes, cancer, and cardiovascular diseases — as well as current developments in the biomedical field, basic research methodology, and quantitative methods and data analysis.

Special Lecture Series

The Special Lecture Series is designed as a means of presenting information about the medical school application and admissions process and other topics of interest to students pursuing careers in medicine. Many of the lecturers are renowned minority physicians, biomedical researchers, educational administrators, and other minority professionals who serve as excellent role models and speak on issues of particular relevance to minority students. Topics have included the following: research opportunities for minorities in the biomedical field, minorities in medicine (past, present, and future), minority physicians' contributions and responsibilities, psychosocial variables related to academic success for minority students, admission to medical school, overview of the medical school curriculum, time management, stress management, interviewing skills, financial aid, the role of premedical advising in the admissions process, test-taking skills, and life as a medical student (discussed by a panel of minority medical students and graduates from the University of Virginia School of Medicine). A Minority Leadership Forum is also conducted; it is composed of a panel of successful black professionals from a variety of fields who present their personal maxims for success. Panelists have included the associate provost for policy and assistant to the president of the University of Virginia, the assistant vice president for administration, the associate provost for student academic support, the dean of Afro-American Affairs, a professor of architecture, the affirmative action officer/equal opportunity officer and special assistant to the president, and the first black School of Medicine graduate. Each summer a symposium and reception are also held during which a minority physician or biomedical researcher of national prominence serves as guest lecturer and motivational speaker.

Support Services

Students who participate in MAAP-I are housed in air-conditioned university dormitory rooms with kitchen facilities located within walking distance of the School of Medicine. Each student receives a stipend to help cover daily living expenses and receives assistance with the cost of travel to the program site. All MAAP-I courses and activities take place in the School of Medicine or Health Sciences Center facilities. Resident advisors who are University of Virginia minority medical students, and several of whom are former MAAP participants, are employed to provide on-site assistance with living arrangements and to act as role models and firsthand sources of information about life as a medical student. Tutors come to the dormitory each night to assist students with their studies.

MAAP-I students are provided with a variety of other support services to enhance their participation in the program and to strengthen skills that they will use throughout their academic and professional careers. A day-long study skills session is offered during the first weekend of the MAAP-I. Students learn techniques for increasing the effectiveness of the time they spend studying, for developing study skills that best match their personal learning styles, for organizing large amounts of course material, and for analyzing and responding to test questions. Participants in MAAP-I also receive individualized academic and personal guidance and counseling. After the program is completed, students who have participated in MAAP-I continue to receive support from program staff on a year-round basis through follow-up correspondence, telephone calls, and personal visits. In addition, each year the MAAP-I director visits many of the undergraduate institutions from which MAAP-I students come, and meets with former participants and their fellow students, to provide encouragement, support, and information about opportunities for minorities as health care providers.

Medical Academic Advancement Program-II

While the MAAP-I is aimed at increasing the number of minority students who enter medical school, the Medical Academic Advancement Program-II (or MAAP-II) is aimed at increasing the number of minority students who are retained in and graduate from medical school. Thus, eligible students are those who have been accepted into medical school but have not yet matriculated ("prematriculants"), or undergraduate students who have taken the MCAT and have achieved scores that are highly competitive for admission into medical school. Like the MAAP-I, the MAAP-II is a six-week residential program held during the summer and has several components.

Academic Schedule

The academic offerings of the MAAP-II are designed to give prematriculants advanced instruction in the basic sciences as well as realistic exposure to the pace, volume, and content of medical school courses that have traditionally caused the greatest academic difficulties for entering medical students. MAAP-II participants have an intensive schedule, attending classroom lectures five days a week. Each course meets two hours daily for two weeks. During the first two weeks of the MAAP-II, "bridging" courses are conducted to develop concepts and principles that mediate between undergraduate and medical school basic science courses. These courses include biostatistics, chemistry-in-medicine, and structure and function. During the remaining four weeks of the program, the MAAP-II participants receive instruction in selected portions of actual School of Medicine courses, taught by School of Medicine faculty in the same format that they use with medical students. The medical school courses include biochemistry, cell physiology, genetics, gross anatomy laboratory, introduction to clinical medicine, microbiology, and pathology. Students are given required readings taken from medical school textbooks and instructors' handouts, are assigned daily homework, and are given medical school–type examinations to help them assess their performance at the conclusion of each course. In the gross anatomy laboratory, MAAP-II participants study anatomy using human cadavers and perform dissection on parts of the human body. Minority medical students act as laboratory assistants for this course. Throughout the six weeks of the program, MAAP-II faculty offer individual and group tutorial sessions as determined by student needs.

Through their participation in MAAP-II, students acquire introductory-level knowledge in several areas of the medical school curriculum and experience the type of demands typically made on medical students. Former MAAP-II participants have reported that, as a result, their adjustment to the medical school life-style was made somewhat easier.

Support Services

MAAP-II students live in the same dormitory and receive the same amenities and supportive services as described for the MAAP-I students, including participation in the study skills workshop, attendance at relevant sessions of the various lecture series, individualized academic and personal counseling and guidance, and follow-up contacts. Those students who enroll in the University of Virginia School of Medicine are also eligible to participate in all retention services provided, as described later.

Postbaccalaureate Program

In 1990, the School of Medicine received a grant from the federal government's Health Careers Opportunity Program to initiate the Medical Academic Advancement Postbaccalaureate Program (MAAP POSTBACC). The purposes of this program are the following: (1) to identify minority and disadvantaged students who have completed an undergraduate prehealth professions program and have applied to but were not accepted into a health professions school, or who made a late decision to enter a health profession; (2) to select ten eligible students each year and provide them with a full-year rigorous educational experience, including participation in MAAP-I, completion of an individualized academic-year curriculum, and participation in MAAP-II; (3) to guarantee enrollment in the University of Virginia School of Medicine to each selected student who successfully completes the full-year academic program, and to provide each student scholarship assistance; (4) to provide a continuum of retention services to enhance students' successful completion of the medical school requirements for graduation. Through this program, the University of Virginia plans to build on its past successful minority medical education programs and to make great strides in increasing the presence of blacks and other minorities in the School of Medicine, and ultimately, in the health professions.

School of Medicine Support Programs for Retention

The University of Virginia School of Medicine realizes that, if the representation of minorities in medicine is to begin to approach parity with their representation in the general population, it is not enough merely to increase enrollment of minorities in health professions schools; their rate of retention in and graduation from such schools must also be increased. Indeed, improving the retention rates for minorities already enrolled in health professions schools has been singled out as "probably the most effective means for increasing the number of underrepresented minority health care professionals in a relatively short time span" (U.S. Department of Health and Human Services, 1990, p. IV-H-5). Besides the MAAP-II—the retention-oriented program offered each summer that is available to prematriculants accepted into any medical school—the School of Medicine also offers academic-year retention services for its own medical students. Among these are a peer tutorial program in which fourth-year medical students are employed as tutors to assist their first- and second-year classmates; workshops for the improvement of study skills, learning habits, test-taking strategies, and National Board of Medical Examiners (NBME) preparation; and referral services for students with specialized needs, such as support groups for spouses, programs for students with special learning needs, and counseling for students with serious emotional or psychiatric problems. The director of the Office of Student Academic Support, a black faculty member, is also the director of all the School of Medicine's minority medical education programs. His appointment as associate dean has lent additional credibility and support to the institutional goal of increasing the numbers of minority students entering and graduating from the School of Medicine (Carey, 1989).

The Student Affairs Office in the School of Medicine also provides ongoing support to minority and disadvantaged students. The associate dean for minority affairs and director of the Division of Ethnic Studies in the School of Medicine, another black faculty member, was trained as a child and adolescent psychoanalyst by Anna Freud. He meets regularly with the minority medical students to ensure that their cognitive, emotional, and social needs are met, and provides year-round academic and personal counseling through a variety of methods. These include group and individual counseling sessions, micro-counseling sessions, lecture, discussion, and simulation exercises. In addition, the associate dean of student affairs meets individually with medical students to provide academic and personal guidance and assists them in the process of applying for residency programs.

The medical students at the University of Virginia are also involved with minority concerns. The student governing body has organized a Minority Affairs Committee concerned with increasing the number of minority students applying to, matriculating at, and graduating from the University of Virginia School of Medicine. The local branch of the Student National Medical Association, of which all minority medical students are members, is very active at the University of Virginia. It provides an atmosphere of mutual support and encouragement that is conducive to the continuing academic progress of its members.

High School Academic Enrichment Programs

Since 1985, the School of Medicine has operated nonresidential summer and year-round academic enrichment programs for minority high school students. The Summer High School Academic Reach-up Program (SHARP) was designed in response to problems identified by high school guidance counselors and parents, who were concerned about an apparent tendency for talented black students to drift away from college preparatory courses. Inadequate academic preparation at the high school level, particularly in mathematics and the sciences, has been identified as one of the leading causes of the insufficient numbers of minorities entering health professions schools (Simpson & Aronoff, 1988). The SHARP is a six-week academic enrichment program open to college-bound minority students who have expressed an interest in careers in the health professions. Held on the grounds of the University of Virginia, SHARP offers courses in mathematics, sciences, writing and communication skills, and computer skills. Students also attend a Minority Lecture Series covering medical topics at a level appropriate to a high school audience, as well as presentations on educational issues such as how to apply to college, academic requirements for the health professions, financial assistance, and interviewing skills.

Another summer program that the School of Medicine has offered since 1986 is the National Institutes of Health Minority High School Student Research Apprentice Program. Every year minority high school students are placed with faculty members from the School of Medicine who volunteer to provide a six- to ten-week supervised research experience in the setting of the Health Sciences Center. Students receive a stipend from NIH and prepare reports on their work at the conclusion of their apprenticeships.

Finally, the School of Medicine also works with guidance counselors, science teachers, parents, and black and other minority students from the local high schools throughout the school year. Minority medical students from the University of Virginia, who serve as excellent role models, offer tutoring services for the students. They and the staff of the School of Medicine minority medical education programs also meet with the minority high school students and their parents to provide support and encouragement for, and practical information about, pursuing the goal of a medical education.

In the course of offering a wide range of minority medical education programs over the past several years, the University of Virginia School of Medicine has identified several strategies that facilitate accomplishment of program objectives (Woode & Lynch, 1990a). Medical or other health professions schools interested in launching or expanding minority medical education programs may be able to profit from the University of Virginia experience by adopting those strategies that are relevant to their institutions. Some of the key elements of an effective approach to increasing the representation of minorities in medicine are delineated below.

Institutional Support for Minority Medical Education

In order for educational innovations to have the greatest probability of success, key institutional administrators must publicly lend their support. At the University of Virginia, minority concerns have been made a priority. The Board of Visitors has called on the entire university community to take all possible steps to increase the meaningful participation of minorities in all aspects of university life, as faculty, students, and staff members. Through the leadership of the Office of the President, the Schools within the university have undertaken institutional changes supportive of the enrollment, retention, and graduation of minority students. Evidence that such changes are indeed taking place can be seen in the 1990 entering class—the most ethnically and racially diverse in the university's history to date. In addition, graduation rates for black students at the University of Virginia averaged more than 75 percent from 1987 through 1989, nearly double that of many comparable institutions ("More Blacks," 1989).

The University of Virginia School of Medicine has a strong record of commitment to the goal of increasing the representation of minorities in medicine. Key administrators, from the vice president for health sciences and the dean of the School of Medicine on down, have consistently provided both material and philosophical support for the objectives of the minority medical education programs. For example, members of the Advisory Committee for Minority Medical Education Programs, which is chaired by the dean of the School of Medicine, include, among others, the senior associate vice president for health sciences; the assistant to the president of the university and associate provost for policy; the university's associate provost for student academic support; the School of Medicine associate deans for admissions, academic affairs, student affairs, finance, and educational program development; the chairmen of the departments of internal medicine and pharmacology; the assistant vice president for allied health sciences; and the assistant vice president for development and community relations. School of Medicine faculty act as instructors for the summer Medical Academic Advancement Programs, and many faculty members and administrators, including the vice president for health sciences, the dean of the School of Medicine, and the chairmen of the departments of anesthesiology, dentistry, family practice, internal medicine, obstetrics/gynecology, pediatrics, and pharmacology, volunteer their time to serve as mentors and guest lecturers. Another factor that has contributed to the effectiveness and stability of the minority medical education programs is that key program personnel have regular faculty status and receive salary support from the School of Medicine. In addition, the School of Medicine routinely contributes classroom, laboratory, and office facilities; faculty and staff time; equipment and supplies; and supplemental funding. Far from being considered peripheral or fringe activities, then, the minority medical education programs are integral to the short- and long-term goals of the institution, and, in the dean's own words, are "of paramount importance to the School of Medicine" (R. M. Carey, personal communication, November 2, 1989).

Establishment of a Consortium

In 1987, having been awarded major grants from the U.S. Department of Health and Human Services Bureau of Disadvantaged Assistance Health Careers Opportunity Program (HCOP) and the Robert Wood Johnson Foundation, the School of Medicine had the opportunity to increase by almost tenfold the number of minority students served by its Medical Academic Advancement Program-I (MAAP-I). In order to develop a large enough MAAP-I applicant pool, the School of Medicine undertook a creative approach to the concept of a consortium. Formal subcontracts were established, primarily with historically black and predominantly minority institutions, to help the School of Medicine identify and recruit minority students interested in medicine and to encourage their application to participate in MAAP-I. (As of January 1992, the following historically black institutions have joined the consortium: Bennett College, Hampton University, Langston University, Norfolk State University, Oakwood College, St. Paul's College, Virginia State University, and Virginia Union University; the majority institutions include Brown University, Queens College of the City University of New York, Southern Illinois University, Stanford University, University of Rochester, and the University of Virginia.) Each institution selected a representative who had specific responsibilities regarding MAAP-I, including attending an orientation session at the University of Virginia, publicizing the availability of MAAP-I through a variety of methods, identifying and referring to MAAP-I minority students interested in medicine, helping to ensure that MAAP-I applicants filed completed applications, and assisting MAAP-I staff in monitoring the progress of past participants from each institution in regard to application to, acceptance to, and matriculation in medical and allied health professions schools. The success of this approach is demonstrated in that, from 1988 through 1990, almost 40 percent of the MAAP-I participants were from consortium institutions. These institutions are partners with the University of Virginia School of Medicine in the training of minorities in medicine (Woode & Lynch, 1988).

Multiple Funding Sources

Minority medical education programs at the University of Virginia School of Medicine have been funded through a variety of sources. Several programs were initiated as pilot projects with School of Medicine funding. After demonstrating the feasibility and success of the programs, the School of Medicine applied to external funding sources to expand existing programs and to develop new ones. Funds have been obtained from the federal government, the state, the locality, and a number of private foundations, as described earlier. As a result, the loss of any one source of funding does not have catastrophic consequences for maintaining minority medical education programs.

Continuum of Educational Programs

The University of Virginia School of Medicine has developed a continuum of innovative enrichment activities and other educational and support programs for minority students, spanning the high school, undergraduate, postgraduate, and medical school years. Working at the high school level allows program staff to identify students who might be interested in careers in medicine, to nurture their interest, and to provide academic guidance specifically related to preparing for future pursuit of medical education. At the undergraduate level, students are provided with academic enrichment, as well as specialized instruction to help them achieve competitive scores on the MCAT to facilitate their entry into medical school. At the postbaccalaureate level, talented minority students who have made a late decision to enter the field of medicine are identified and given the opportunity to complete a sequenced educational program designed specifically to meet their individual needs prior to enrolling in medical school. Prematriculating medical students receive an advance look at the content, pace, and volume of the medical school curriculum, along with clinical experiences, thus easing their future adjustment to the actual medical school environment. And finally, minority medical students at the University of Virginia receive academic support services and academic and personal counseling as needed to ensure their successful completion of the medical school curriculum. Through these diverse programs, the School of Medicine has assisted literally hundreds of minority students interested in medicine.

Student Tracking System

It is essential to maintain an efficient system for tracking past program participants. This makes it possible to assess the effectiveness of minority medical education programs in increasing the number of minority students who enter and graduate from medical and allied health professions schools. At the University of Virginia School of Medicine, a computerized student tracking system has been in place for several years (Lynch, Lynch, & Woode, 1990). A follow-up survey of past participants is mailed annually to students and to institutional representatives in order to obtain the most up-to-date information about each student. In addition, many students maintain personal contact with program staff through letters, telephone calls, and visits.

Community Support

The University of Virginia School of Medicine enjoys a great deal of community support for its programs for minority and disadvantaged students. Many community leaders, including the mayor, the assistant city manager, a coalition of black ministers, and the chairman of the board of the Charlottesville Public Schools, have taken a personal interest in the School of Medicine's minority medical education programs. Their support has been instrumental in securing supplemental funding and in mobilizing parent and teacher involvement, particularly in the high school programs.

Conclusion

In order to increase the representation of blacks and other minorities in medicine, medical schools must aggressively recruit talented minority students to the field and provide them with the academic and personal support they might need to sustain their commitment and successfully pursue their professional education. Strategies that the University of Virginia School of Medicine has found to be effective in addressing these objectives include the following: securing institutional support; establishing a consortium of other institutions, particularly historically black institutions, as partners in the training of minority health care providers; operating programs with the aid of multiple funding sources; offering a continuum of educational enrichment programs from high school through medical school; maintaining an effective student tracking system; and enlisting community support. Through this multifaceted approach, the University of Virginia School of

Medicine has served over 1,800 minority and disadvantaged students interested in careers in the health professions during the years 1984 through 1991, and has seen the retention rate of minority medical students who have participated in its programs exceed the national level. Programs like those at the University of Virginia School of Medicine offer the means of increasing blacks' and other minorities' access to health professions training, and, eventually, of leading to improved access to health care for the minority and disadvantaged members of our society.

References

Association of American Medical Colleges. (1989). *Minority students in medical education: Facts and figures* (Vol. 5). Washington, DC: Author.

Carey, R. M. (1989). *The biennial evaluation (1986–1987) and long range planning report (1988–2000).* Unpublished manuscript, University of Virginia School of Medicine, Office of the Dean, Charlottesville.

Experts find life expectancy for blacks continues decline. (1990, November 29). *Richmond Times-Dispatch,* p. A-8.

Gunby, P. (1989). Minority physician training: Critical for improving overall health of nation. *Journal of the American Medical Association, 261*(2), 187–189.

Keith, S. N., Bell, R. M., Swanson, A. G., & Williams, A. P. (1985). Effects of affirmative action in medical schools: A study of the class of 1975. *New England Journal of Medicine, 313,* 1519–1525.

Lloyd, S. M., & Miller, R. L. (1989). Black student enrollment in US medical schools. *Journal of the American Medical Association, 261,* 272–274.

Lynch, K. B., Lynch, R. R., & Woode, M. K. (1990, October). *Use of a computerized student tracking system in research and evaluation: Examples from a minority medical education program.* Paper presented at the eleventh annual Conference for Generalists in Medical Education, San Francisco.

Lynch, K. B., & Woode, M. K. (1990). The relationship of minority students' MCAT scores and grade point averages to their acceptance into medical school. *Academic Medicine, 65,* 480–482.

More blacks remain at U. Va. for degrees. (1989, December 28). *Richmond Times-Dispatch,* p. D-2.

Petersdorf, R. G., Turner, K. S., Nickens, H. W., & Ready, T. (1990). Minorities in medicine: Past, present, and future. *Academic Medicine, 65,* 663–670.

Raymond, C. (1989). Preventing twists, turns on road to medical education from becoming permanent detours. *Journal of the American Medical Association, 261,* 189–193.

Simpson, C., & Aronoff, R. (1988). Factors affecting the supply of minority physicians in 2000. *Public Health Reports, 103,* 178–184.

U.S. Department of Health and Human Services. (1986). *Estimates and projections of black and Hispanic physicians, dentists, and pharmacists to 2010* (DHHS Publication No. HRS-P-DV-86-1). Washington, DC: U.S. Government Printing Office.

U.S. Department of Health and Human Services. (1989). *HCOP Digest* (DHHS Publication No. 1989-241-280/05319). Washington, DC: U.S. Government Printing Office.

U.S. Department of Health and Human Services. (1990). *Seventh report to the President and Congress on the status of health personnel in the United States* (DHHS Publication No. HRS-P-OD-90-1). Washington, DC: U.S. Government Printing Office.

Windom, R. E. (1989). From the Assistant Secretary for Health. *Journal of the American Medical Association, 261*, 196.

Woode, M. K., & Lynch, K. B. (1988, February). *Strategies for increasing minority representation in medicine*. Paper presented at the sixteenth annual symposium of the Sixteen Institutions Health Sciences Consortium, Norfolk, VA.

Woode, M. K., & Lynch, K. B. (1990a, April). *Effective intervention strategies for producing more minority health care providers*. Paper presented at the thirteenth annual Southern Regional Conference of the National Association of Medical Minority Educators, Birmingham, AL.

Woode, M. K., & Lynch, K. B. (1990b, October). *Effective strategies for the retention of minority medical students*. Paper presented at the eleventh annual Conference for Generalists in Medical Education, San Francisco.

PART V

The Future of Health
for African Americans

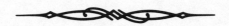

22

Reproductive Rights and the Challenge for African Americans

Faye Wattleton

Women and African Americans stand at a remarkable moment in history. As the bicentennial of the Bill of Rights is celebrated along with the hard-won expansion of those rights in recent decades, a most fundamental freedom— our right to make private decisions about childbearing—is being gravely threatened. This right is essential to human dignity and self-determination. It is the key to sexual and social equality, and for African Americans in particular, it is a life or death issue.

African-American women suffer the triple jeopardy of sexism, racism, and classism. Nowhere is this more deeply felt than in the realm of reproductive health care. As women, we are victimized by a society that treats us as secondary and seeks to control us by controlling our sexuality and reproduction. As African Americans, we face truncated educational and vocational opportunities, resulting in extreme economic disparity: 56 percent of African-American women aged fifteen to forty-four have family incomes below 200 percent of the official poverty level; for black females aged fifteen to nineteen, that figure is 69 percent (Forrest & Singh, 1990b). Thus, African Americans are uniquely burdened by society's systemic classism, which effectively bars poor people from adequate health care.

This triple threat adds up to extraordinary barriers between African Americans and contraceptive services—which lead in turn to disproportionately high rates of teen pregnancy, unwanted pregnancy among adult women, AIDS, and infant morbidity and mortality. Inadequate preventive care also renders African-American women disproportionately reliant on abortion and uniquely vulnerable to health risks when access to safe, legal abortion is curtailed.

Historically, the African-American community has recognized that reproductive autonomy is essential to our empowerment. As early as 1919, W.E.B. Du Bois wrote that "the future woman must have . . . the right of motherhood at her own discretion" (Du Bois, 1920, pp. 164–165). Martin Luther King, Jr. (1966, p. 4) affirmed voluntary family planning as "a special and urgent concern" for African Americans, "a profoundly important ingredient in [our] quest for security and a decent life." And in 1966, on the heels of the Supreme Court decision that legalized birth control, the National Association for the Advancement of Colored People (NAACP) (1966) adopted a policy statement on family planning: "Mindful of problems of family health and of economic stability, we support the dissemination of information and materials concerning family health and family planning to all those who desire it."

Today, virtually every major African-American and civil rights organization supports the right to contraception and safe, legal abortion. The African-American public, too, recognizes that restricting access to these voluntary options is tantamount to coercing women to bear children — much as the enslaved foremothers of African Americans were forced to do. Recent polls show that 79 percent of African Americans favor government spending to develop better birth control methods (Louis Harris & Associates, 1988), and 73 percent agree that a woman should be able to choose abortion in consultation with her doctor (Media General/Associated Press, 1989).

Today, the reproductive choices that determine a woman's autonomy are under escalating attacks. It is the self-interest of the African-American community to defend these choices, not just for African-American women, but for all Americans. To ignore the threats to basic fundamental rights and to neglect the need to preserve responsible, compassionate, noncoercive policies on family planning and abortion is to neglect the future.

Reproductive Freedom: The Health Impact on Black Women

In 1965, the U.S. Supreme Court in *Griswold v. Connecticut* struck down state laws that had banned the use of contraceptives by married couples. The ability of individuals to control their fertility soon led to profound public health benefits for all Americans. Maternal deaths declined almost 80 percent between 1965 and 1987 (National Center for Health Statistics, 1967, 1990). By 1988, infant deaths had dropped more than 60 percent from 1965 levels. Births defined by the mother as unwanted fell from 20 percent in 1965 to 12 percent in 1988, and mistimed births declined from 45 percent in 1965 to 28 percent in 1988 (Mosher, 1988; Forrest & Singh, 1990b).

Further health benefits accrued after 1973, when the Supreme Court in *Roe v. Wade* legalized abortion nationwide. Deaths from illegal abortion plummeted 80 percent between 1972 and 1974 (Cates & Rochat, 1976). In 1965 illegal abortion caused nearly 17 percent of pregnancy-related deaths (National Center for Health Statistics, 1967); today illegal abortion is virtually unknown and deaths from legal abortion are extremely rare. One death occurred in 1985, representing less than 0.3 percent of all pregnancy-related deaths (Tietze & Henshaw, 1986). The risk of death from childbirth is eleven times the risk for abortion in all trimesters (Gold, 1990).

These health benefits have profoundly affected African Americans.

When contraception and abortion were illegal, affluent women — which usually meant Caucasian women — were better able to circumvent the law. They
could obtain "black market" contraceptives; they could find physicians willing to certify a medical indication that would permit a safe, clean abortion;
or they could fly to other states or countries where contraception and
abortion were legal. Few African-American women had the economic means
to exercise these options, and they paid with their lives. From 1972 to 1974,
80 percent of U.S. deaths from illegal abortion occurred to nonwhite women;
the mortality rate from illegal abortion for minority women was twelve times
the rate for white women (Cates & Rochat, 1976).

Even legalization of birth control and abortion has not guaranteed
access to these services (and to the attendant health benefits) for less affluent
African Americans. Because of inadequate contraceptive care, minority
women are twice as likely as white women to experience unplanned pregnancy and to seek abortions: in 1983 the abortion rate was 23.3 per 1,000 for
white women, 55.8 per 1,000 for nonwhite women (Henshaw, 1987).

Further, inadequate government funding effectively blocks poorer
African-American women from exercising their right to abortion. Federal
Medicaid funding of poor women's abortions has been prohibited since
1978 — a policy that has been only partly mitigated by the continuation of
funding by some state governments. All but twelve states (Alaska, California,
Connecticut, Hawaii, Maryland, Massachusetts, New Jersey, New York, North
Carolina, Oregon, Vermont, and Washington) prohibit Medicaid coverage of
abortions in almost all circumstances (Alan Guttmacher Institute, 1989). In
states where public funds are not available, 20 to 25 percent of low-income
women who want an abortion cannot pay for it and are forced to bear
children they cannot afford to care for (Trussell, 1980). A small number
attempt illegal or self-induced abortions instead (Torres, Donovan, Dittes, &
Forrest, 1986), and the rest endure hardship in order to save up the money for
an abortion (Henshaw & Wallisch, 1984). Scraping together the necessary
sum may take considerable time (Henshaw & Wallisch, 1984), often delaying
the procedure into the second trimester — when it is significantly riskier.
(While legal abortion is an extremely safe procedure, after the first eight
weeks of pregnancy the risk of major complications increases 15 to 30
percent for each week of delay [Cates & Grimes, 1981].)

Recent Attacks on Reproductive Health

Despite the manifest health benefits of expanded access to reproductive
health care, for ten years the Reagan and Bush administrations have waged
war on both legal abortion and the family planning programs that help avert
abortion. They have failed to eliminate either, but both administrations have
successfully whittled away access to contraception and abortion services and
have set the stage for future encroachments. These inroads pose a special

threat to African-American women, who will again be the first victims of the
back alley if contraception and abortion are again restricted.

Supreme Court Curbs on Abortion Access

The most profound impact of these attacks has come from the U.S. Supreme
Court, which President Reagan reshaped along narrow, conservative lines.

In July 1989 the Supreme Court ruled in *Webster v. Reproductive Health
Services* that the state of Missouri could: bar public employees from performing abortions unless the woman's life is endangered; prohibit public facilities
from performing abortions, even if no public funds are involved; and require
fetal viability tests after twenty weeks' gestation, even though most physicians
agree that such tests are risky and inconclusive before the twenty-eighth week.

The crack in the foundation of reproductive freedom was deepened a
year later. In *Hodgson v. Minnesota* (1990) and *Ohio v. Akron Center for Reproductive Health* (1990), the Supreme Court sharply curtailed access to abortion for
teenagers.

The Ohio law requires physicians to personally notify a minor's parent
or guardian twenty-four hours before performing an abortion. The law
provides the option of a "judicial bypass," whereby a minor may petition a
court for a waiver of the notice requirement. Lower courts in the Ohio case
found that the bypass scheme caused unreasonable delays, breached the
minor's anonymity, and required her to present unusually burdensome proof
of her entitlement to a waiver. The Supreme Court, however, rejected these
arguments.

Hodgson requires notification of *both* the teenager's biological parents—
even noncustodial, nonresident, or abusive parents, and even when biological parents are divorced or never were married. The law also mandates a
forty-eight-hour waiting period before the abortion may be performed. Like
the Ohio law, the Minnesota statute provides a judicial bypass procedure
through which the minor may attempt to convince a judge to waive the
notification requirement.

In addition to the specific restrictions they permit, all three cases have
broad and disturbing ramifications. First, they invite *every* state to attempt to
curb reproductive rights, following the lead of Missouri, Ohio, and Minnesota. Second, they effectively change the standard of judicial review for
future abortion cases from a very stringent standard to a far more lenient
one. This new standard may support highly restrictive requirements that
have previously been found unconstitutional, such as waiting periods and
spousal notification.

Finally, these rulings mark a dramatic step back from the constitutional protection of privacy. This right was recognized by the Supreme Court
as early as 1923 (*Meyer v. Nebraska*), was enunciated most clearly in the 1965
Griswold ruling that legalized contraception, and was expressly upheld in *Roe
v. Wade*. In *Hodgson*, the Bush administration filed a brief challenging the very

concept of a constitutional right to privacy; we anticipate future attempts to undermine the settled doctrine that allows couples to make their own child-bearing choices.

The Far-Right Crackdown on Family Planning

Well aware of the adage that "knowledge is power," extremists are seeking to limit not only women's access to abortion *services*, but also their access to *information*. Ironically, this censorship is linked to a crackdown on the family planning services that prevent the need for abortion. This crusade, too, targets the women least capable of fighting back and least equipped with other options—the young and the poor, who are disproportionately African American.

Title X of the Public Health Service Act, the nation's family planning program, provides a broad range of health care services—primarily contraception and family planning education—to lower-income women and teenagers. In 1983, the last year for which data are available, 4.5 million women received family planning services and other health care from federally funded sources (Forrest & Singh, 1990a). Eighty-three percent had incomes below 150 percent of the official poverty level, 37 percent were women of color, and 33 percent were women under twenty (Forrest, 1988). For many lower-income women, Title X and other federal programs are their primary or sole source of health care.

The Title X program has been remarkably effective. Recent research (Forrest & Singh, 1990b) projects that, without government support for family planning services, an average 1.2 million additional unintended pregnancies would occur each year to women of reproductive age in the United States. Of that number, an estimated 516,000 would end in abortion.

For a decade after its enactment in 1970, Title X enjoyed broad bipartisan support in Congress. But in 1981 the Reagan administration launched an annual call to repeal the program. Congress refused to eliminate Title X, but it did slash its funding from $162 million in 1980 to $136 million in 1990—a decrease of 47 percent if adjusted for inflation (Planned Parenthood Federation of America, 1990; Gold & Guardado, 1988). In 1988 a stymied President Reagan proposed crippling regulatory changes (U.S. Department of Health and Human Services, 1988). President Bush, in turn, called for elimination of Title X and backed the new rules. For three years a lawsuit brought by Planned Parenthood (*PPFA v. Bowen*, 1988) blocked enforcement of these regulations pending Supreme Court review, but in May 1991, the High Court upheld these dangerous and unfair restrictions (*Rust v. Sullivan* and *New York v. Sullivan*, 1991).

The regulations bar any family planning clinic receiving Title X funds from providing referral for abortion services—even if a patient requests such assistance, and even if her health is endangered by continuing the pregnancy.

The regulations also bar nonphysicians (who provide nearly all counseling in most Title X facilities) from answering clients' questions about abortion.

Title X has never funded abortions but has always mandated counseling on all options for pregnant women. The legislative authors of Title X recognized that withholding such information would constitute medical malpractice and would threaten women's health.

The new regulations comprise a "gag rule" that is medically and morally unconscionable. Further, the gag rule violates the intent of Congress and interferes with the constitutional right to free speech. Above all, by penalizing ethical health care providers, the regulations are counterproductive in the extreme.

In response to vociferous outcry from the public and the American medical establishment, Congress has twice voted overwhelmingly to overturn the gag rule. In November 1991, President Bush vetoed the first of these legislative attempts, and the House of Representatives narrowly failed to muster the two-thirds majority needed to override the veto. As of May 1992, a second legislative effort to overturn the gag rule is under way, as are new federal lawsuits to enjoin enforcement of the regulations (*National Family Planning and Reproductive Health Association et al. v. Sullivan*, 1992; *Planned Parenthood Federation of America v. United States Department of Health and Human Services*, 1992).

Meanwhile, the Department of Health and Human Services has implemented the gag rule, forcing thousands of health care facilities to make an agonizing choice: gag their clinicians and endanger their patients' welfare, or forgo funding and curtail services to low-income clients.

It is clear that the Title X program—which provides the very services that best reduce the need for abortion—is being held hostage to the abortion controversy. If this cynical manipulation is allowed to continue, millions of nonaffluent women and teenagers will pay the price.

Teenagers: Black America's Future in Peril

Young African Americans bear the brunt of curbs on access to family planning and abortion. All teens face extraordinary barriers to reproductive health care. However, black teenagers are especially victimized because, like their adult counterparts, they are more likely than their white peers to be burdened by poverty. The problem is particularly acute for female African-American teens, 69 percent of whom are poor (Forrest & Singh, 1990b).

In addition to the threat to teenagers posed by restrictions on publicly funded family planning (discussed in the previous section), attacks on legal abortion pose special dangers to young people.

Researchers project that, if legal abortion were banned, adolescent childbearing—and childbearing by minority adolescents in particular—would increase significantly, reflecting the many young women who would not have access to abortion, legal or illegal. In the two years following legalization of abortion in New York State, births to African-American adolescents in New York City decreased by 18.7 percent, while births to white teens dropped 14 percent (Joyce & Mocan, 1990). The same study projects that if abortion had been banned in 1988, an additional 2,618 births would have occurred to black teenagers in New York City within two years.

While all abortion restrictions harm young people, those that target teens specifically — such as those upheld in the *Ohio* and *Hodgson* cases — have catastrophic impact. Coercing parental involvement in a minor's abortion decision does a great deal more harm than good. At best, mandatory notice or consent laws are ineffective or unnecessary. Most teenagers who seek abortions (55 percent of those aged eighteen and under and 75 percent of those aged fifteen and under) do so with their parents' knowledge (Torres, Forrest, & Eisman, 1980). Moreover, evidence suggests that such laws do not influence more teens to involve their parents. In a study comparing notification patterns of adolescents in Minnesota (which has a parental notification requirement) and Wisconsin (which has none), no significant difference was found in the proportion of teens who notified one or both parents (Blum, Resnick, & Stark, 1987).

At worst, these laws can devastate young people and their families. Pregnant teens who choose not to involve their parents have very compelling reasons. They often come from dysfunctional families, where one or both parents are alcoholic, drug-addicted, abusive, or absent altogether. The Children's Defense Fund (1989) reports that, in 1986, 2.2 million children and adolescents were reported victims of abuse, neglect, or both — and that in families where physical abuse is present, the incidence of violence escalates when a family member is pregnant.

Two-parent notification or consent laws (like that upheld in *Hodgson*) undermine the authority of the custodial parent and can throw the entire family into turmoil, especially when the absent parent's whereabouts are unknown. Such laws are particularly damaging to African-American minors, only 39 percent of whom live with both parents — compared to 79 percent of white minors (U.S. Bureau of the Census, 1989).

Forced parental involvement also wreaks damage on the healthiest and most intact families, where teenagers simply may not want to disappoint their parents (Blum, Resnick, & Stark, 1990). This fear may drive teens to travel out of state, to delay the procedure, to bear children they are incapable of rearing, or to risk their young lives to dangerous illegal methods.

An analysis of the parental consent law in Massachusetts (Cartoof & Klerman, 1986) found that the statute's major impact was to increase by 300 percent the number of teenagers who crossed state lines to obtain abortions. This travel delayed their abortions by an average of 4.2 days, and in some cases by nearly six weeks (Yates & Pliner, 1988). In Missouri, during the first three years a parental consent law was in effect, the percentage of abortions among Missouri minors that were obtained in Kansas rose by 62 percent (Missouri Department of Health, 1990).

Whether they leave their home state or not, teens who fear confronting their parents may delay seeking an abortion until the second trimester of pregnancy, when the procedure is not only riskier but more difficult to obtain and more costly. In Minnesota, the parental notification law increased by 26.5 percent the percentage of minors' abortions performed in the second trimester (*Hodgson v. Minnesota*, Plaintiff's Exhibit 122, 1986).

Still other teens, tragically, are driven by family intrusion laws to bear children they do not want, or to seek unsafe, illegal abortions. One study (Torres et al., 1980) estimated that if parental notification requirements were adopted by all abortion providers, 23 percent of adolescent abortion seekers would not obtain legal abortions. Of these, about 45 percent would give birth to an unwanted child, about 45 percent would attempt illegal or self-induced abortion, and about 10 percent would run away from home—either to give birth to an unwanted child or to seek an illegal abortion. Based on the latest available data—183,370 abortions were performed on minors in 1987 (Henshaw, Koonin, & Smith, 1991)—those estimates translate into an *annual average* of 19,000 additional unwanted births, 19,000 teens risking illegal abortion, and 4,200 runaways.

Since the central issue in mandatory involvement laws is the parent's cognizance of the minor's pregnancy—and her fear of the consequences of that knowledge—such laws are equally damaging whether they mandate consent or merely notification. Some proponents of parental involvement laws argue that the judicial bypass alternative protects minors from abusive parents and provides them with the adult guidance they need. Many teens do elect the judicial bypass alternative—43 percent of Minnesota teens, for example (Blum et al., 1987). But research suggests (Blum et al., 1990) that minors from less affluent families are far less likely to avail themselves of this option. They may be unaware that it exists, or they may lack the resources to tackle "the system."

But the cruel reality for *all* teens and parents is that the judicial bypass option serves no one's best interests. First, it does not protect the teenager. In requiring that she justify her personal decision to one or more strangers, judicial bypass fosters humiliation and, often, breach of confidentiality (*Hodgson v. Minnesota*, Transcript of Record, 1985; Planned Parenthood Federation of America, 1989). Worse, the complex legal proceedings necessary to obtain the bypass often dangerously delay the abortion procedure. Second, the bypass option places judges in an untenable position: they must rule either that a young woman is mature enough to make her own decision, or that she is too immature to decide for herself on abortion—yet somehow mature enough to become a mother. (Significantly, no state requires parental permission for a minor to continue the pregnancy and have a child.) Finally, judicial bypass provisions do nothing to improve family communication or to provide parents with increased control over their children's behavior.

Laws that mandate parental consent, then, present a Hobson's choice: In the absence of a judicial bypass alternative, they are dangerous—even deadly — intrusions into a young woman's life. With a bypass mechanism, they present a new set of obstacles that can have health-threatening consequences. In either case, there is no evidence that the laws promote their stated aims of fostering family communication and protecting the welfare of vulnerable teenagers.

Access to abortion services can, in fact, be beneficial to young women's lives. A two-year study of 334 urban African-American teens (Zabin, Hirsch, & Emerson, 1990) showed that, in comparison with a group who opted to carry a pregnancy to term, young women who chose to terminate a pregnancy were more likely to have stayed in school, economically better off, less likely to experience psychological problems, less likely to have subsequent pregnancies, and more likely to practice contraception consistently.

There are many steps we can take to protect the health of young people and the integrity of families. Comprehensive sexuality education — starting in early childhood — can foster sexual responsibility. So can better family communication on sexual issues, including contraception and abortion. Young people can be helped to seek the guidance of trusted adults when making sexual decisions. But when teens cannot turn to their parents, family intrusion laws are not the answer. We must allow the widest possible range for private, voluntary resolution of these very private matters.

Exporting Indifference: International Family Planning

Not content to endanger the health of its own citizens, the U.S. government has exported its anti–family planning, antiabortion, and anti–free speech policies far beyond our shores. After decades of U.S. leadership in aid to foreign family planning projects, in 1984 the Reagan administration bowed to antichoice extremists and announced the "Mexico City policy," an international precursor to the gag rule on the domestic family planning program. The policy forbids most foreign, nongovernmental agencies from receiving U.S. government family planning funds if they engage in abortion-related activities. Such activities include not only performing abortions, but also advocacy, referral, or counseling for abortion — even if these activities are legal in the countries involved and are financed entirely by non–U.S. government funds.

Just as no Title X funds are used for abortion activities in the United States, the Helms Amendment of 1973 prohibits the use of U.S. funds for abortion activities overseas. And, like the Title X gag rule, the Mexico City policy denies the free speech of grantees and prohibits them from using their non-U.S. funds as they see fit — even in countries where abortion is legal.

In 1987 Planned Parenthood initiated a lawsuit to block implementation of the Mexico City policy (*Planned Parenthood Federation of America v. Agency for International Development*, 1990). Federal district courts and appeals courts upheld the policy, and in June 1991 the Supreme Court refused to hear Planned Parenthood's appeal of these rulings.

Despite the success of international family planning programs, more than 250 million people in the developing world still lack access to contraception (Population Crisis Committee, 1987). Each year, an estimated 500,000 women die from pregnancy-related causes; 200,000 of these deaths result from illegal, unsafe abortions (World Health Organization, 1987). Yet these entirely preventable deaths — 548 each day — are completely ignored by American media and government leaders. Can it be that human lives are considered expendable when they belong to women of color — the poorest women in the world, living thousands of miles away, who have no constitutional protections and who cannot vote?

The Mexico City policy is especially devastating to African nations, where access to contraception is already more deficient than in any other region (Population Crisis Committee, 1987). While significant population increases are imminent in many parts of the world, the largest relative increases are predicted for Sub-Saharan Africa (Family Health International, 1990). African Americans, who have a unique stake in Africa's social and economic development, must recognize that voluntary family planning is crucial to that development. African Americans must pool political clout to protest foreign policy that is designed not to promote public health, but to pacify antiabortion extremists.

Defending Reproductive Rights: The New Battleground

Across the ocean and across America, one can witness an all-out attack on reproductive health and rights — with the most disenfranchised individuals serving as primary targets. Here in the United States, the Supreme Court's decisions in *Webster*, *Ohio*, *Hodgson*, and *Rust*, as well as the White House attacks on legal abortion and on the national family planning program, provide a bitter lesson for Americans who believed women's reproductive freedom was firmly secured on those fronts. Courts and presidents have proven to be unreliable guarantors of these fundamental freedoms. Instead, legislators and the vagaries of politics in fifty states now wield the power to determine when, where, why, and to whom contraception and abortion will be accessible.

When one of the most cherished principles of democracy — the right to conduct our personal lives free from governmental interference — is imperiled, a dangerous era has clearly begun. Other human rights and civil liberties as well as reproductive rights are threatened. Now that the fight for these rights has shifted to legislative and electoral arenas, African Americans must bring voting and lobbying power to bear. African Americans must elect officials who are committed to returning reproductive matters to their proper arena — the private lives of individuals. Endless political struggle over issues of fundamental rights is morally unacceptable. In the face of recent setbacks, a national solution is needed. An amendment to the Constitution is one option. Another is federal legislation like the Freedom of Choice Act, a bill introduced in both houses of Congress in 1991, which would protect the rights enunciated in *Roe v. Wade.*

Until the freedom to individually determine childbearing is secured, the ability to exercise all other rights will remain severely weakened. The antiabortion, anti–family planning, anti–woman agenda can be thwarted. African Americans have an unusually great stake in doing so.

Conclusion

Choice is the very essence of empowerment and is at the heart of the struggle for equality. It is not surprising that reproductive freedom has always enjoyed strong support in the African-American community, both at the grassroots level and among key leaders and organizations.

Nevertheless, some of the zealous few who oppose reproductive rights seek to divide the African-American community with the spurious argument that "abortion is genocide"— a weapon of the white majority, aimed at exterminating people of color. It is demeaning not only to black women, but indeed to *all* women, to suggest that women are susceptible to manipulation and are incapable of making informed, moral decisions about themselves and their fertility. The argument is particularly ugly in light of the forced childbearing that so many African-American women endured in the dark days of slavery.

The struggle for uncompromised reproductive rights is about liberation, not enslavement— choice, not coercion. Those who would rob women of these choices today are no less racist and evil than those who held African Americans in bondage 150 years ago. It is no coincidence that such extremists do nothing to advance educational and economic opportunities for women, or to ensure decent lives for the children they want to coerce women to bear. Therein lies the true threat of genocide to our community— more unwanted children born into poverty, hunger, and neglect— more families shackled by the intergenerational chains of dependence and oppression.

There will always be those who try to stand in the way of African-American empowerment. But a people who have known tyranny and oppression must protect their self-interest by preserving reproductive rights. Until the complex inequities of this society are righted— until African Americans are no longer disproportionately victimized by poverty, ill-health, crime, joblessness, and homelessness— the need for reproductive freedom will be uniquely great. So must be the struggle to achieve it.

References

Alan Guttmacher Institute. (1989, January 12). Analysis of 1988 state laws and trends. *Washington Memo* (No. W-2). Washington, DC: Author.

Blum, R. W., Resnick, M. D., & Stark, T. (1987). The impact of a parental consent notification law on adolescent abortion decision-making. *American Journal of Public Health, 77,* 619–620.

Blum, R. W., Resnick, M. D., & Stark, T. (1990). Factors associated with the use of court bypass by minors to obtain abortions. *Family Planning Perspectives, 22,* 158–160.

Cartoof, V. G., & Klerman, L. V. (1986). Parental consent for abortion: Impact of the Massachusetts law. *American Journal of Public Health, 76,* 397–400.

Cates, W., & Grimes, D. (1981). Deaths from second trimester abortion by dilation and evacuation: Causes, prevention, and facilities. *Obstetrics and Gynecology, 58,* 401–408.

Cates, W., & Rochat, R. W. (1976). Illegal abortions in the United States: 1972–1974. *Family Planning Perspectives, 8,* 83–92.

Children's Defense Fund. (1989). *A children's defense budget, FY '89.* Washington, DC: Author.

Du Bois, W.E.B. (1920). *Darkwater: Voices from within the veil.* New York: Harcourt, Brace, Jovanovich.

Family Health International. (1990). *A penny a day.* Research Triangle Park, NC: Author.

Forrest, J. D. (1988). The delivery of family planning services in the United States. *Family Planning Perspectives, 20,* 88–98.

Forrest, J. D., & Singh, S. (1990a). Public-sector savings resulting from expenditures for contraceptive services. *Family Planning Perspectives, 22,* 6–15.

Forrest, J. D., & Singh, S. (1990b). The sexual and reproductive behavior of American women, 1982–1988. *Family Planning Perspectives, 22,* 206–214.

Freedom of Choice Act. (1991). H.R. 25, introduced January 3. S.R. 25, introduced January 14.

Gold, R. B. (1990). *Abortion and women's health: A turning point for America?* New York: Alan Guttmacher Institute.

Gold, R. B., & Guardado, S. (1988). Public funding of family planning, sterilization, and abortion services, 1987. *Family Planning Perspectives, 20,* 228–233.

Griswold v. Connecticut, 381 U.S. 479 (1965).

Helms Amendment to the Foreign Assistance Act. (1973). Pub. L. No. 93-189, December 17. S1443, Sec. 114.

Henshaw, S. K. (1987). Characteristics of U.S. women having abortions, 1982–1983. *Family Planning Perspectives, 19,* 5–9.

Henshaw, S. K., Koonin, L. M., & Smith, J. C. (1991). Characteristics of U.S. women having abortions, 1987. *Family Planning Perspectives, 23,* 75–81.

Henshaw, S. K., & Wallisch, L. S. (1984). The Medicaid cutoff and abortion services for the poor. *Family Planning Perspectives, 16,* 170–180.

Hodgson v. Minnesota, Nos. 88-1125 and 88-1309, 58 U.S.L.W., 4957 (1990).

Hodgson v. Minnesota, Plaintiff's Exhibit 122, 648 F. Supp. 756 (D. Minn. 1986).

Hodgson v. Minnesota, Transcript of Record, Civ. No. 3-81538 (D. Minn. January 23, 1985).

Joyce, T. J., & Mocan, N. H. (1990). The impact of legalized abortion on adolescent childbearing in New York City. *American Journal of Public Health, 80,* 273–278.

King, M. L., Jr. (1966). *Family planning—A special and urgent concern.* New York: Planned Parenthood–World Population.

Louis Harris and Associates. (1988). *Public attitudes toward teenage pregnancy, sex education, and birth control.* New York: Planned Parenthood Federation of America.

Media General/Associated Press. (1989, July 7–16). *Poll No. 27.* Richmond, VA: Author.

Meyer v. Nebraska. (1923). 262 U.S. 390.

Missouri Department of Health. (1990). *Focus: Missouri abortions 1980–1988.* Jefferson City, MO: Author.

Missouri Monthly Vital Statistics, (1990) *23*(11), 1–4. Jefferson City, MO: State Center for Health Statistics, Missouri Department of Health.

Mosher, W. (1988). Fertility and family planning in the United States: Insights from the National Survey of Family Growth. *Family Planning Perspectives, 20*(5), 209–217.

National Association for the Advancement of Colored People. (1966). *Policy statement on family planning.* Adopted July 1966, 57th Convention, Los Angeles.

National Center for Health Statistics. (1967). *Vital statistics of the United States, 1965: Vol. 2—Mortality, Part A.* Washington, DC: U.S. Government Printing Office.

National Center for Health Statistics. (1990, September). Advance report of final mortality statistics, 1988. *Monthly Vital Statistics Report, 38*(5) (Suppl.). Hyattsville, MD: Public Health Service.

National Family Planning and Reproductive Health Association et al. v. Sullivan, CA No. 03 0035 D. D.C. 1992.

New York v. Sullivan, Secretary of Health and Human Services, 89-1392 (1991).

Ohio v. Akron Center for Reproductive Health. (1990). No. 88-805, 58 U.S.L.W. 4979.

Planned Parenthood Federation of America. (1989). *Akron Center for Reproductive Health v. Ohio* (Fact Sheet). New York: Author.

Planned Parenthood Federation of America. (1990). *Celebrating Title X family planning funding: Yesterday, today, tomorrow.* Washington, DC: Author.

Planned Parenthood Federation of America v. Agency for International Development et al., 915 F.2d. 59 (2nd. Circuit 1990).

Planned Parenthood Federation of America v. Bowen, 687 F.Supp. 540 (D. Colo. 1988).

Planned Parenthood Federation of America v. United States Department of Health and Human Services, CA No. 92-714 (D. Co. 1992).

Population Crisis Committee. (1987). *Access to birth control: A world assessment* (Briefing Paper No. 19). Washington, DC: Author.

Roe v. Wade, 410 U.S. 113 (1973).

Rust v. Sullivan, Secretary of Health and Human Services, 89-1391 (1991).

Tietze, C., & Henshaw, S. K. (1986). *Induced abortion: A world review*. New York: Alan Guttmacher Institute.

Torres, A., Donovan, P., Dittes, N., & Forrest, J. D. (1986). Public benefits and costs of government funding for abortion. *Family Planning Perspectives, 18*, 111–118.

Torres, A., Forrest, J. D., & Eisman, S. (1980). Telling parents: Clinic policies and adolescents' use of family planning and abortion services. *Family Planning Perspectives, 12*, 284–292.

Trussell, J. T. (1980). The impact of restricting Medicaid financing for abortion. *Family Planning Perspectives, 12*, 120–130.

U.S. Bureau of the Census. (1989). Studies in marriage and the family. *Current Population Reports* (Series P-23, No. 162). Washington, DC: U.S. Government Printing Office.

U.S. Department of Health and Human Services. (1988). *Statutory prohibition on use of appropriated funds in programs where abortion is a method of family planning; Standard of compliance for family planning services projects; Final rule* (42 CFR Part 59). Washington, DC: Federal Register.

Webster v. Reproductive Health Services, 109 S.Ct. 3040 (1989).

World Health Organization. (1987). *Preventing the tragedy of maternal deaths*. Concluding statement to report on the International Safe Motherhood Conference, Nairobi, Kenya. New York: Author.

Yates, S., & Pliner, A. J. (1988). Judging maturity in the courts: The Massachusetts consent statute. *American Journal of Public Health, 78*, 646–649.

Zabin, L., Hirsch, M. B., & Emerson, M. R. (1990). When urban adolescents choose abortion: Effects on education, psychological status, and subsequent pregnancy. *Family Planning Perspectives, 17*, 25–30.

23

Health Policies and
the Black Community

Bailus Walker, Jr.

The persistent health problems of African Americans pose a dramatic chal-lenge to medical investigators, clinicians, social and behavioral scientists, and policy makers. These problems have ranged from infant mortality to large morbidity and mortality gaps between black and white adults. Many health policy issues arising from the black-white disparities in health have yet to be resolved. These include access to health services, cost of care, organiza-tion of care, and health care providers. Although it would be useful to address all of these issues, the purpose here is to examine those specifically related to access to health care.

When the history of the 1980s is written, the health status and access to health care of African Americans in the nation's large urban centers will appear repeatedly in many chronicles. And, along with the pictures of the homeless, the charts and tables of acute and chronic disease rates will illustrate many texts. They will underscore the fact that after decades of gradual improvement, the health of African Americans took a turn for the worse in the late 1980s and reached a critical condition in the early 1990s.

In the last three years of the 1980s, public health officials were report-ing increases among African Americans in the incidence of tuberculosis, hepatitis A, measles, mumps, whooping cough complicated by ear infec-tions, and AIDS. The number of cases was often small, but many of these diseases were considered on the verge of eradication less than a decade ago, after steadily declining since the beginning of the century. Many of them are virtually unknown in middle-class or wealthy neighborhoods (Centers for Disease Control, 1990).

Yet statistics, which at best count death and disease reportable by law, capture only a glimpse of the larger picture. They do not tally unnecessary suffering or lifelong handicaps that result when treatable conditions such as asthma go unrecognized or neglected. Nor do health statistics alone convey the concentration of urban poverty that is undermining faith in government

as an instrument of policy development and of implementation. This concentration of the poor also produces evidence of governmental breakdown
exhibited by overcrowded and inadequately supplied health clinics, lack of
adequate drug abuse treatment programs, substandard hospital physical
plants, and overburdened or neglected social services necessary to cope with
the social determinants of disease and premature death among African
Americans.

Access to Care

For many poor African Americans, the lack of access to comprehensive
health care is a critical health problem with a broad range of social and
economic ramifications. These include community disorder that lacerates
the civic fabric and drives people from shared institutions such as subways,
buses, parks, schools, and neighborhoods. These problems should not be
interpreted as the result of U.S. policy makers enacting legislation specifically denying access to effective health care based on race or socioeconomic
status. Such an overt bias would not be permitted by the citizenry or by the
courts. Ironically, however, the lack of a national health plan is bringing about
precisely that result.

The problem of access to comprehensive health care takes many forms.
For example, the Community Service Society of New York polled 248 primary care physicians in poor neighborhoods in the Bronx as to whether they
offered twenty-four-hour coverage, had twenty or more regular office hours a
week, accepted Medicare, and had admitting privileges at a hospital—what
society defined as a decent medical practice. Of this number, only six met the
criteria (Community Services Society of New York, 1990). As "managed care"
has become part of the strategies to control cost and encourage competition
among providers, it has also generated access issues. Many health maintenance organizations (HMOs) have begun charging copayments when an
enrollee makes an office visit as a way to discourage care for relatively "minor"
problems.

Recent surveys of HMOs show that when the cost of an office visit was
$15.00 or less, about half of the enrollees with minor problems saw their
physician. The number dropped to about one-third of enrollees when an
office visit cost $30.00 or more. One third of the enrollees refused to pay an
office visit fee of $15.00 or less even though they had more serious symptoms
such as fainting and chest pains during exercise. More than half of the
enrollees did not see a physician for such symptoms when the office copayment was $30.00 or more, the surveys found. There was also evidence that
office copayments discourage lower-income enrollees in poorer health from
seeking need care—care that may prevent the progression of disease or
dysfunction (Sudman, 1990).

Often overlooked in discussions of access issues are children. As this
group goes through developmental changes, they are vulnerable to a range of

social and behavior problems, to unintentional injuries, and to chronic illnesses, and they require access to care-preventive and outpatient care for acute illness. Yet ten to twelve million children are without health coverage, and even more are underinsured. African-American children are 63 percent more likely than white children to be uninsured (Children's Defense Fund, 1989). To address this problem, the American Academy of Pediatrics has proposed a detailed plan for congressional consideration to provide access to health care for all children up to twenty-one (Birt, 1990). Another dimension of the access problem was revealed in a 1991 study that shows that Americans without health insurance are less likely to be given routine diagnostic tests, less likely to undergo key surgical procedures, and more likely to die during their stay in a hospital than those with private medical insurance.

The difficulty people without health insurance have in obtaining physicians' care and related services has been much discussed. Much discussion has also focused on the observation that the insurance status of patients also makes a significant difference in how well they are treated by physicians after they have been admitted to the hospital. These findings provide a powerful condemnation of the ways in which financial considerations have intruded on the delivery of health care.

Medicaid

The developments reviewed above have occurred despite the fact that Congress created Medicaid in 1965 to provide health care to the poor; the federal and state government would share its costs and operations. However, millions of Americans do not qualify because each state sets its own eligibility policy, adjusting it annually to match its budget. Alabama currently has the most stringent standards: a family of two qualifies only if it earns less than $88.00 a month or 13 percent of the federal poverty level of $700.00 a month for one parent and one child. In Oregon, a family is eligible if it earns less than 58 percent of the federal level or approximately $400.00 a month. Because eligibility requirements can be raised, a family can be supported by Medicaid one year and dropped the next—subjecting citizens to a devastating medical roller coaster (Morrell, 1990). In summary, "Medicaid is generally underfunded, politically manipulated, unevenly administered, and thought of as a welfare system (which, in fact, it is, but should not be). It most resembles a giant national Rube Goldberg machine" (Davies & Felder, 1990; Thorpe, Siegal, & Dailey, 1989; Tallon, 1989). This situation provides unlimited opportunities for medical intrusions and disregard for financial considerations in relation to health care decisions.

Health Policy Reform Proposals

As intrusions intensify and as the number of African Americans who are denied financial access to health care continues to grow, the need for a national health plan is made more apparent. Ranging from superficial recommendations to a total revamping of the health care system, proposals for reform have been working their way to public light in increasing numbers. No less than eight proposals surfaced during 1989–1990 to address the issue of the uninsured. Although the eight proposals take a different tactic to "fix" the problem of the uninsured, their authors are motivated by a common problem and agree on a common set of goals (Russell, 1989).

A number of proposals for national health care call for employers to provide health insurance for their employees. On the surface, this would appear to be sound national health care policy. But as the U.S. economy continues to move from being manufacturing to service oriented, there is no indication that the number of uninsured will decrease. Service industries typically hire part-time or low-wage full-time employees—many of whom are African Americans—without offering benefits such as health insurance. Similarly, the growing number of small employers forgo health insurance as a benefit because of their inability to negotiate a reasonable premium. Moreover, group coverage tied to place of employment is not suited for coverage of those regularly outside the labor force, including mothers who stay home to care for young children and many African-American men, who are clustered disproportionately in the inner-city areas. Then, too, continuity of coverage may be affected by changing employers, unemployment, retirement, and disability—all changes in status that affect not only the African-American worker, but also members of his or her family (Ball, 1978).

Guiding Principles

Some professionals as well as laypersons contend that only a national health plan can ensure that everyone receives adequate health care—preventive as well as curative—at an affordable price and without regard to changes in status. What then are some of the elements that should be taken into account in establishing a national health plan? The following remarks illuminate the situation but should not be viewed as exhaustive.

1. All economic barriers to care should be removed. The plan must provide a single universal national health program covering the entire population, regardless of race, income, and employment or unemployment status.
2. The system should be unified (as opposed to the present fragmented approach) and should provide comprehensive services that include hospital care and prescription medications, as well as physician and other medical services.
3. Incentives should be built in to make possible the delivery of efficient, high-quality services, including services aimed at the prevention and early detection of disease.

4. Financing of health services should be simple and equitable. Strict budgeting and cost-control measures should be implemented.
5. Effective health planning and allocation of resources must be tied to a financing mechanism that provides the necessary leverage and support to bring about reform. Consolidation of hospital services and high-cost medical technologies would make better use of existing resources, reduce waste and excessive profits, and save literally billions of dollars.
6. Scrutiny of quality of care must be an integral part of national health policy; it should include monitoring programs to eliminate unnecessary surgery and laboratory tests and the inappropriate utilization of esoteric medical technologies, which are permitted by the present system and which are used with alarming frequency.
7. Consumers must be assured a role in every level of administrative decision making. Health care policies only become meaningful and relevant when those who pay for and use services play a role in determining the policies.

Conclusion

Although the above principles have been incorporated in various proposals over the years and have been repeated with monotonous regularity, it is highly doubtful that decisive action will be taken on universal access to health care before the year 2000. A number of reasons exist for the probable continuation of the current pluralistic system. First, there is a long history of unsuccessful proposals for national health care insurance, and the recent experience with the Medicare catastrophic-illness amendment has left many policy makers reluctant to pursue additional major reforms in health care.

Another potential obstacle to further development of a national health policy or related federal intervention in the health care system is that removing all barriers to health care would require unprecedented cooperation among consumers, providers, insurers, business leaders, and government officials. Such cooperation is unlikely to be easily obtained, due to the varying self-interests of these groups and their disparate objectives.

Federal action is inhibited by the power of these special interest groups in American political life and by the reluctance of policy makers to counteract their demands. A lack of consensus exists on a workable solution to the problem of universal access because it is difficult, if not impossible, to design a system that does not threaten one of the significant parties now involved in the national health care system (O'Connor & Combes, 1991). The likelihood appears very low for a complete government takeover of health care financing or the development of a comprehensive government-owned and government-operated system, similar to those used in many European countries. Such an extension of access would mean more taxes and higher cost—a serious concern among policy makers at the state and federal levels of government already faced with budget deficits. These concerns are relevant, since in the final analysis, the services included in a national health program will depend in large part on the resources available and on the alternatives for use of those resources (O'Connor & Combes, 1991).

Given these and numerous other considerations, the scope of which is beyond this chapter, it seems most likely that there will be continuing debate about practical and desirable approaches to a comprehensive national health plan. Despite the problems with employer-based health care, federal and state governments will be more aggressive in pressing employers to purchase health care for their employees — an approach that will not benefit many African Americans. At the same time, more proposals will emerge that narrow the focus of national policy on the health care needs of those with no insurance — a group that is rapidly expanding. The final years of the twentieth century may well be the most challenging ever for health policy development, as policy makers, health service planners, and health care economists confront the task of making up the omissions of earlier periods.

References

Ball, R. M. (1978). National health insurance: Comments on selected issues. *Science, 200,* 864–870.

Birt, B. (1990). A proposal to provide health insurance to all children and all pregnant women. *New England Journal of Medicine, 323,* 1216–1220.

Centers for Disease Control. (1990). Cases of selected notifiable disease. *Morbidity and Mortality Weekly Report, 39,* 704–707.

Children's Defense Fund. (1989). *Lack of health insurance makes a difference.* Washington, DC: Author.

Community Services Society of New York. (1990). Building primary health care in New York City's low-income communities. *CSS Working Papers.* New York: Author.

Davies, N. E., & Felder, L. H. (1990). Applying brakes to the runaway American health care system. *Journal of the American Medical Association, 263*(1), 73–76.

Morrell, V. (1990). Oregon puts bold health plan on ice. *Science, 249,* 468–471.

O'Connor, E., & Combes, J. (1991). *Universal health insurance: Much ado about nothing?* In S. Parker (Ed.), *Environmental assessment* (pp. 13–14). Farmington, MI: Mercy Health Services.

Russell, L. (1989). Proposed: A comprehensive health care system for the poor. *Brookings Review, 7,* 13–20.

Sudman, J. R. (1990). Access to health care. *Medical News, 29,* 207–209.

Tallon, J. R. (1989). A health policy agenda proposal including the poor. *Journal of the American Medical Association, 261*(7), 1044.

Thorpe, K. E., Siegal, J. E., & Dailey, T. (1989). Including the poor: The fiscal impacts of Medicaid expansion. *Journal of the American Medical Association, 261*(1), 1003–1007.

24

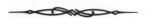

Coalition Partnerships
for Health Promotion and
Empowerment

Ronald L. Braithwaite

Most citizens, irrespective of ethnicity or class, have visions of a "quality of life" free of disease and disability. However, the disparities in the health status of African Americans and white Americans have been amply documented in other chapters of this book and in several published reports (Polednak, 1989; U.S. Department of Health and Human Services, 1985; National Research Council, 1989). These disparities are intertwined with issues of structural poverty, lack of control over one's political environment, powerlessness and hopelessness, racism, self-defeating behaviors, cultural values counter-productive to healthful living, and a lack of adequate health insurance, to name a few.

The purpose of this chapter is to discuss the conceptual knowledge base on community organization and development (COD) as an approach to engaging African-American communities, particularly low-income African-American communities, in health education and health promotion programming. Philosophically and pragmatically, the goal of such efforts is designed to foster community control and empowerment. A secondary purpose of this chapter is to advance the COD approach and to identify anticipated strengths and constraints of building community-based coalition partnerships. Toward these ends, a review of pertinent literature will elucidate concepts of a community organization and development model that embraces community control and empowerment as integral components.

Community Empowerment and Control

During the 1960s, the concept of *community empowerment* grew from its roots in social action ideology. The term was popularized in the mid 1970s to describe both traditional and innovative social work practices and interventions (Solomon, 1976; Gray, Hartman, & Saalberg, 1985). Rappaport (1984, p. 3), a leading authority who has addressed community empowerment through a program of ongoing research and development, maintains that "empowerment is easy to define in its absence: powerlessness, real or imagined; learned helplessness; alienation; loss of a sense of control over one's life. It is more difficult to define positively only because it takes on a different form in different people and contexts." Moreover, the engagement of African-American communities in community-based empowerment initiatives requires a deliberate cultural sensitivity to the "community way" by those in a facilitation role.

In the context of low-income African-American communities, residents are encouraged to become genuinely involved in making decisions and addressing policy issues that affect their quality of life. Increasing local residents' participation in community activities typically leads to improved neighborhoods, a stronger sense of community, and personal and political efficacy (Florin & Wandersman, 1990; Chavis & Wandersman, 1990). However, recent studies suggest that political empowerment for impacting the health status within African-American communities is more complex than some of these processes (LaVeist, 1992).

Powerlessness is a structural problem embedded in the fabric of our social institutions. Community empowerment and self-reliance are valuable strategies that need to be promoted on a large scale for poor communities (Braithwaite & Lythcott, 1989). Freire (1989) has effectively applied community-empowerment principles to address the illiteracy problem in Brazil. Freire defines community powerlessness as a pervading state of mind in which the individual assumes the role of "object," controlled by the random impulses of the environment, as opposed to "subject," exerting significant influence on factors that affect one's life and community. In the context of this definition, the individual is thus alienated from genuine participation in the construction of social reality.

For Freire, powerlessness results from the passive acceptance of oppressive cultures. Powerlessness further combines an attitude of self-blame, a sense of generalized distrust, a feeling of alienation from sources of social influence, an experience of disenfranchisement and economic vulnerability, and a sense of hopelessness in the sociopolitical struggle. Other authors (Swift, 1984; Russel-Erlich & Rivera, 1986) characterize empowerment as a process rather than a product or an event. Consequently, empowerment is often viewed as a political process, suggesting a societal redistribution of power and advancement of equity among community stakeholders.

In regard to addressing equity among community stakeholders, progressive social scientists and health professionals agree that "victim blaming" and "deficit model" approaches are no longer acceptable explanations for the ills that plague low-income African-American communities (Ryan, 1971). The question of what will motivate low-income African Americans to become more attuned to the "wellness movement" that gained momentum in the 1980s is a question that the African-American community will need to answer for itself. The problem of self-defeating life-style behaviors is one that will require both intracommunity and geopolitical analyses to derive viable solutions. Notions that low-income African Americans are necessarily "external" along a locus of control continuum (Rotter, 1976) and their classification with a "learned helplessness" label must be forthrightly addressed by debunking such myths (Taylor, 1988). To accept either myth is to relegate black communities to a state of diminished community control.

Braithwaite and Lythcott (1989) have advocated a community organization and development approach as an antecedent to community empowerment. They emphasize that poverty of the spirit and of resources remains the antecedent risk factor of preventable disease. Poverty and powerlessness create circumstances in people's lives that predispose them to high levels of social dysfunction, the highest indices of morbidity and mortality, the lowest access to primary care, and little or no access to primary prevention programs.

Community empowerment and its relationship to civil rights, justice, political and social structures, and quality-of-life issues have been the focus of study in such disciplines as philosophy (Rawls, 1971), religion (Cone, 1975; Garrow, 1986; Cleage, 1989), political science (Banfield, 1961; Dewart, 1990), sociology (Warren, 1977), education (Freire, 1970; Hilliard, Payton-Stewart, & Obedele-Williams, 1990; Hale-Benson, 1987) and psychology (Jones, 1991; Ryan, 1971; Akbar, 1985). Evolving from these areas of study, Wallerstein and Bernstein (1988) argue that empowerment education is an effective health education and prevention model for personal and social change. While considerable research documents the effects of lack of control or powerlessness in disease causation or, conversely, of empowerment in health enhancement; the literature in social epidemiology and social psychology examines lack of control over one's life as a risk factor stemming from an overburden of life demands without adequate resources to meet such demands (Syme, 1986). This literature points out the need for communities defined as "powerless" to affiliate with those external groups or organizations that can access resources in a meaningful manner consistent with the empowerment imperative.

A primary method of bringing about empowerment involves organizing community coalitions in the Saul Alinsky (1969) tradition of mobilizing groups around pressing social and economic issues. The genesis of such a movement dates back to the 1960s with the federal Model Cities legislation that targeted social problems in economically depressed cities. This movement gave birth to the *citizen participation* rhetoric, which, despite the implications of the term, seldom involved genuine participation by grassroots individuals and organizations. Though several top-heavy agency-represented coalition boards came into existence during this era, few of them are still active as sustained community action partnerships. Such coalition-building initiatives are rarely systematic; thus replication and validation of successful approaches become extremely difficult. Documentation of effective approaches to building coalition partnerships is a challenge to those who research COD models.

Community Empowerment and Health Promotion

Community empowerment has been defined as the process through which groups increase their control over consequences that are important to their members and to others in the broader community (Fawcett et al., 1984). For example, by organizing a tenants' rights organization, individual residents of a public housing complex may increase their ability to negotiate with management for housing repairs and improvements. Coalitions are formed to seek common solutions to common problems. They mobilize around territorial and proxemic issues (Sommer, 1961), social justice and economic issues (Bennett, 1975), minority-group issues (Cruse, 1987), and health and disease issues (Polednak, 1989). The April 1992 verdict in the California indictment against the videotaped police beating of Rodney King represents a social justice issue of great proportion that will certainly rejuvenate coalition building for social justice across the United States.

Labonte (1989) offers a definition of empowerment, suggesting that "it is the ability to choose or increase one's capacity to define, analyze and act upon one's problems." Inherent in this definition is that health professionals do not empower individuals or communities, but rather that individuals and communities (choose to) empower themselves. Couto (1990) advances a definition of empowerment similar to that of Labonte (1989), where empowerment is viewed as the transfer of information, skills, and resources that improve the decision-making power of individuals or groups.

Embedded in most definitions of community empowerment is a philosophy that members of a community are their own best resources for effecting change in the community. This idea is rooted in the notion that community members can participate in the process of shaping the conditions that affect their lives. This approach promotes a sense of ownership and a vested interest in seeing to it that change is achieved and maintained. Disease prevention research points to the need for reestablishing community linkages in order to counteract the effects of isolation and loneliness and to build "psychologically" healthy communities that empower people to acquire control over their lives (Bernard, 1986). A study by Resnick (1980) concerning minority populations suggests that human service needs of underserved minority populations in low-income communities are best met by empowering the community to carry out its own prevention programs. Wallerstein (1992, p. 198) has aptly stated the dilemma: "The most common use of the term empowerment in public health has unfortunately focused on only one level, that of individual change. Individual empowerment is often viewed as separate from the social system, similar to self-esteem, individual competency, or self-efficacy. Political conservatives have adopted this usage, calling for empowerment through increased individual skill training or coping skills instead of through changing the conditions that created the problems."

Health promotion programs targeted at low-income minority populations are more likely to be successful in such populations when the community at risk identifies its own prevention and intervention programs and forms a coalition board to make policy decisions and identify resources for program implementation (Braithwaite & Lythcott, 1989). The importance of a cultural perspective must also be noted, and health care providers need to develop comprehensive and culturally sensitive approaches to address the complex and multifaceted issues of minority health and wellness (Braithwaite & Lythcott, 1989).

Katz (1984) defines empowerment as access to and control of valued resources. This definition implies that there are people who are oppressed or disempowered—that is, they have limited or no access to valued resources. Since access and control of resources are associated with power, it is reasonable to consider those persons without access or control to be "power poor." McKnight (1985) discusses the impossibility of enhancing the health status of the power poor until the power imbalance has been corrected. More specifically, resources such as control over budgets and decision making must be transferred to the "power poor," enabling them to become "power equals." This group is then enabled to play a central role in identifying its problems, creating workable solutions, and monitoring and controlling resources. Such an outcome can be identified as a "bottom-up" approach, typical of an inverted triangle with the base, rather than the peak, at the top.

Coalition Building for Health Empowerment

For African Americans, poor health has historically been linked to powerlessness. The traditional social and political structure of the inner cities and the South, where the majority of African Americans reside, has dictated that state and local institutions—governments, schools, health departments, hospitals—would be controlled by white middle- and upper-class groups. While African Americans have gained political power in recent years, members of most low-income minority communities (urban and rural) still interface largely with commercial services or charity institutions that seem to be controlled by distant forces.

Hence, at least two psychological barriers must be overcome if health promotion programs are to succeed in a low-income African-American community: (1) the notion that one's health can only be improved by an outside agent such as a doctor (a notion that is shared by much of the population) and (2) the perception that one has no control over any important aspect of one's life, including health. Organization is a primary goal in building community coalitions for health empowerment. Often such organization results in a greater sense of control for community stakeholders. Various agencies and organizations have initiated coalition-building efforts for community health empowerment, including the Centers for Disease Control's (CDC) Planned Approach to Community Health (PATCH) program that was originally developed by Kreuter, Nelson, Stoddard, and Watkins (1985). Further coalition building efforts for community health empowerment include the National Cancer Institute's America Stop Smoking Intervention Study (ASSIST) (1991), designed to address smoking cessation at the community level, and programs of several philanthropic foundations (W. K. Kellogg Foundation, Robert Wood Johnson Foundation, and the Henry J. Kaiser Family Foundation).

Low-income African Americans are typically identified as medically underserved or lacking access to health care. Lack of access is the result of several interrelated barriers. One barrier to access is obviously financial; low-income African Americans with no health insurance have great difficulty obtaining health care. African Americans are about two-thirds more likely than whites to be uninsured. Although the rates among poor African Americans and poor whites are similar and are estimated to be approximately 35 percent, the lack of health insurance is an increasing social challenge (Short, Cornelius, & Goldstone, 1990). A second barrier is accessibility. For example, in the state of Georgia there are 159 counties. In 1989, forty counties had no physician who would provide treatment for Medicaid patients, and 78 counties had no obstetrical and gynecological care for any patient (Georgia Council on Maternal and Infant Health, 1989). Even in Atlanta, a city with more hospital beds and more physicians than can be justified by the size of the population, many of the poor still face accessibility barriers in which the only source of health care is typically a single large public hospital. A third barrier to access may be termed "lack of acceptability." This barrier is particularly relevant for low-income people who may be easily intimidated by middle-class health professionals. These low-income people often find the staff at public facilities unsympathetic or hostile. They are often unable to establish relationships with personal physicians that middle-class people take for granted. This barrier, indeed, is another manifestation of the aforementioned lack of empowerment.

During the late 1980s, the Kaiser Family Foundation advocated an approach to coalition building. The approach was also characterized as a social reconnaissance process for assessing the health status of communities as described by Sanders (1989) and Williams (1990). The Kaiser Family Foundation sought to facilitate community health problem solving in substance abuse, teen pregnancy, cancer prevention, cardiovascular disease prevention, nutrition, and intentional and unintentional injury. In 1988, the Health Promotion Resource Center (HPRC) at the Morehouse School of Medicine replicated the social reconnaissance process and developed a COD application for low-income African-American communities within the state of Georgia. This approach goes beyond a simplistic community inventory in that it explores social relationships (as well as other more readily available data) in relation to the physical and economic sectors of a community. The community is viewed, in social action terms, as a social system. Sanders (1989) describes the approach as akin to "holding up a mirror before the community." In other words, local perceptions are solicited by a multidisciplinary inquiry team and cross-checked against statistical data and other available information. Finally, this information is reprocessed with the community via "town hall" type forums.

Major steps of the social reconnaissance method involve (1) assembling the study team, (2) selecting the target community/state and developing local sponsorship, (3) preparing for the field study, (4) selecting key informants, (5) lining up appointments for interviews, (6) maintaining confidentiality, (7) conducting the daily team conferences, (8) preparing notes for each interview, (9) generating a written community profile, (10) publishing and distributing the report to those who provided input, and (11) structuring a meeting for feedback with community stakeholders.

Lewin (1951) has aptly discussed the importance of conducting a force field analysis as an approach to decision making and strategic planning. Such an analysis includes pros and cons, strengths and weaknesses of a given dilemma. In the context of the social reconnaissance methodology, the perceptions held by the key informants interviewed as part of the fact-finding documentation of a community's need become dichotomous components of a force field analysis. Both potential barriers and opportunities for initiating a community-based health promotion strategy are explored in this analysis.

Catalyst for Community Change

The primary goal of the COD approach is to develop a health promotion and disease prevention model for black poor urban and rural populations. The philosophy underlying this approach is that health promotion is likely to be more successful in those populations when the community at risk identifies its own health concerns, develops its own prevention and intervention programs, and forms a decision-making board to make policy decisions and identifies resources for program implementation. This approach also develops community leadership for health promotion and advocates community health promotion. The expectation is that community organization and development for health promotion is a model that will improve the community's ability to address other important quality-of-life issues (social justice, literacy, housing, recreation, education) as well as improve the health status of its members.

Given that health behaviors are culture bound, the COD approach maintains that primary prevention efforts that address preventable disease and illness must emerge from a knowledge of and a respect for the culture of the target community. This knowledge and respect will ensure that both the community organization and development effort and any interventions that emerge are culturally sensitive and linguistically appropriate. For the poor, such an empowerment approach to health promotion is like a sleeping giant—when it rises, the historically disenfranchised will become self-reliant (Braithwaite & Lythcott, 1989).

The capacity to provide technical assistance in health promotion to the black clergy has proven to be catalytic for engaging community members in coalition activities. Community empowerment is a central theme that guides and shapes programmatic plans leading to community control over resources. This training empowers black clergy to be more effective in addressing community-based health promotion in urban and rural communities and particularly among their parishioners. The COD approach has shown positive community benefits in Georgia through linkages with the General Missionary Baptist Convention of Georgia and a small participating sample of its 861 churches. Collaboration of diverse groups to address health promotion issues is gaining momentum, but it is still a new approach. The COD approach advances the community's capacity to bring diverse groups (consumers and health and human service providers) together to share information, plan, advocate, and develop local programs for health promotion in Georgia and elsewhere in the South.

Community Organization for Empowerment

As Braithwaite and Lythcott (1989) and Braithwaite, Murphy, Lythcott, and Blumenthal (1989) note, the COD approach stresses community development and community-based health promotion intervention. Community empowerment is a central theme that guides decision making relative to all aspects of program implementation and the control of resources. The COD approach is illustrated in Exhibit 24.1. Identification of community leaders is the first step in the model. It should be noted that developing a sense of the historical evolution of the community targeted for intervention is essential. Public documents such as newspapers and organizational lists are used to identify community leaders. In addition, personal and direct contacts serve as complementary methods of identifying both formal and informal leaders. Following up on horizontal and vertical referrals (a snowball sampling approach) also helps to identify potential community members to serve on a coalition board for health promotion.

A demographic profile of the targeted neighborhood is a prerequisite to understanding the community's social niche. Further, the profile is a central factor in understanding the health needs and dynamics within the community. The demographic profile is formulated using a multiplicity of data resources. While the Census Bureau is a primary source of community data, additional sources of relevant community data include records from police departments, health departments, hospitals, local planning agencies, and social services departments. Closely related to developing the demographic profile is the identification of community resources.

The process of uncovering community resources serves to provide a more holistic understanding of the geographic area. Community resource

Exhibit 24.1. A Conceptual Model for Community Organization and Development.

- Identify community leaders
- Conduct demographic profile
- Develop community resource inventory
- Organize coalition board
- Coalition board incorporation
- Conduct community health needs assessment
- Conduct community forum
- Plan health interventions
- Provide ongoing technical assistance
- Conduct intervention evaluation

---

identification focuses on several dimensions. The first dimension is developing an inventory of the social, educational, economic, and spiritual institutions that serve as the basic infrastructure for the community. The second dimension involves locating the institutions in relation to significant community boundaries and artifacts and clarifying their relation to the target community. While legitimate and concrete resources are relatively easy to identify, less legitimate, less tangible, and less concrete resources will be virtually impossible to identify without indigenous informants. A sensitive community organizer can learn the ecology of the community by walking through the neighborhood at different hours of the day and night (both weekdays and weekends) and observing people's behavior, their gathering places, and the ebb and flow of the community. Riding through the neighborhood in a vehicle and doing a "windshield" survey can often accomplish the same objective. These strategies are instrumental components of the COD approach.

The COD approach pays meticulous attention to organizing the coalition board. While the coalition board is comprised of both health and human service providers and consumers, it is important that consumer representation not fall below 60 percent of the total coalition board member mix. Braithwaite et al. (1989, p. 59) indicate that "the rationale for initiating a consumer-dominated coalition board is based on social psychology and community organization principles. Such principles acknowledge the benefits of shared decision making, self-help, self-reliance, and reference group ownership of strategies and approaches to address one's community concerns." Braithwaite et al. (1989) further argue that it is the responsibility of the coalition board to oversee the entire process of community organization and development for health promotion. This responsibility includes conducting a community health needs assessment (a door-to-door household survey utilizing trained and paid community interviewers); convening a community forum (town hall meeting) to discuss the needs assessment data along with other data to facilitate identification of community health priorities; planning and designing the community-based health intervention; and identifying resources (including applying for funds) to support intervention projects.

Coalition board incorporation is a necessity in establishing empowerment in the community group. It is through the nonprofit incorporation status that the community group will be able to promote and pursue its own independence and continuity. With incorporation as a nonprofit organization and subsequent acquisition of Internal Revenue Service tax exempt 501(c)(3) status, the coalition is positioned to compete and qualify for grants, gifts, and other resources essential to pursuing its mission. To prepare the coalition board for such activity, comprehensive and ongoing board training in the areas identified in Exhibit 24.2 is provided.

As mentioned earlier, a community needs assessment is designed to assist the community coalition board and the community in identifying what community residents perceive as their most important health concerns. Soliciting input from residents communicates and reaffirms that they are competent in assessing issues and that their perceptions and opinions are important. This communication and reaffirmation fosters self-determination, and teaches residents that their voices can be heard by the traditional agency policy administrators and their staffs. A town hall meeting with a community forum setting allows an opportunity for the community-at-large to validate, through discussion and reaction, the findings from the community health needs assessment.

Coalition boards will typically require technical assistance in planning selected health promotion interventions. In this context an intervention is defined as a structured approach to an identified community health concern. Professional and technical assistance is provided to the coalition board in identifying and applying for various sources of funding for health intervention programs. However, it should be remembered that the coalition board members are the experts on the community and are best able to advise health professionals of necessary adaptations in health intervention models to provide maximum execution and evaluation of the intervention.

Exhibit 24.2. Coalition Board Training Areas.

- Leadership skills
- Problem solving
- Project management
- Fiscal management
- Board-staff relationships
- Conflict resolution
- Effective meeting management
- Resource development
- Resource utilization
- Selecting health interventions
- Program evaluation
- Interfacing with the media
- Networking with legislators

Public and Private Sector Initiatives in Coalition Partnerships

As mentioned earlier in this chapter, citizen participation has roots dating back to the 1960s with the Model Cities "war on poverty." Grassroots citizen involvement in decision-making boards declined during the 1970s and then was rejuvenated by selected federal agencies in the 1980s, with the Community Health Centers movement and the Area Health Education Centers program of the federal Health Resources and Services Administration. More recently, the Office of Minority Health and the Office of Substance Abuse Prevention of the Department of Health and Human Services have established major grant programs designed to fund community-based coalition partnership programs. From the private sector, the Robert Wood Johnson Foundation has initiated a multimillion dollar grant program for municipalities to combat human and community development concerns identified as "fighting back." The Kellogg Foundation has also sought to introduce the partnership concept into its grantmaking methodology and has initiated programs involving grassroots community groups with schools of medicine, public health, social work, and other health professions. These public and private initiatives reflect the belief that collaboration is essential to effective community development designed to impact the pervasive social and health disparities that separate the "haves from the have nots."

Common Pitfalls to Coalition Maintenance

Coalitions bring strange bedfellows together. Establishing coalition partnerships is a lot simpler than maintaining them. Most potential coalition members convene for different reasons. Some have hidden agendas, while others are fully committed to collaboration for achievement of a common goal. Coalitions should be aware of members who involuntarily "come to the table" (for example, because their boss sent them to the organizational meeting). While such persons may become genuinely interested in the process and goals of the coalition, they may not be fully committed, and consequently their involvement may be short-lived. A related concern involves the observation that coalition members may all have one vote but may also face political inequalities based on the influence that a particular member brings to the table. For example, the CEO of the local health department is likely to carry more weight and influence than the low-income, less articulate consumer group member. There can also be an inherent problem when a coalition is funded at the beginning of its formation. Under these circumstances, ulterior motives rooted in financial gain have a way of becoming manifest. By contrast, some coalitions have the task of growing together and seeking funding support based on participatory planning.

Factors such as distrust, impatience, and low levels of organizational maturity often serve as the nemesis of effective coalition partnerships. When several ethnic groups comprise a target community, multiculturalism is indeed a worthy goal for health education programming. Yet it can engender competition and distract from the clarity of cultural mission. It is important to define mission and purpose early in the process of organizational development. Turf problems tend to haunt interagency collaborations, especially when large bureaucratic agencies try to join forces to combat health and human service needs of local communities. Partnership efforts on a smaller scale are likely to experience similar turf protection attitudes by members not fully committed to collective planning for prevention and joint ventures for the common good. A memorandum of agreement or understanding can be a useful document for delineating the expectations and anticipated contributions of each of the coalition members. While such a document may not be legally binding, it does offer some definition to the forming of a partnership as it relates to goals, missions, purposes, and expectations.

Articles of incorporation and bylaws are instruments that commit members to a legal agreement. Such instruments take on increased importance when there is a change in an agency CEO. The concept of an agency having membership representation on a coalition board is then likely to transcend political change of the CEO or agency heads. This membership approach is particularly relevant for municipal government representation where a coalition member is subject to change as a result of a political election. For example, three months after the election in 1990, the governor of Georgia initiated a statewide freeze in spending that negatively affected an earmarked federal grant from the Office of Substance Abuse Prevention for a community empowerment project. The community-based organization was stagnated by bureaucratic red tape and consequently did not receive anticipated and committed federal funding in a timely manner due to a political shift in leadership at the highest level in state government.

Splinter grouping within a coalition is yet another divisive behavior that is common to emerging partnership coalitions intended to be broad based. Splits occur for many different reasons, but a common reason centers around historical disagreements that put members in conflict. Other common reasons why members leave coalitions include burnout, loss of interest, lack of committed time, role confusion, disagreement on issues, and divisive infighting and schisms among members. These problems can be thwarted with strong perceptive leadership from individuals who maintain credibility in multiple camps on the coalition. Sessions on conflict resolution may also circumvent schisms.

Sources of Coalition Maintenance

Some coalition partnerships have the resiliency to proceed in the face of adversity. The elements of such organizational growth are linked with evidence of strong and shared leadership where roles are clear and the power within the group is equitable and respected by its members. The presence of group-endorsed bylaws can sometimes serve as a positive instrument for defining parameters and expectations of behavior within the organization.

Given the turnover and burnout that is likely to occur, particularly among adult coalition members, young adults and teenagers are yet another source of sustaining a coalition. Involvement of teenagers and young adults as voting members of the organization serves a dual purpose. First, it is consistent with the objective of developing community-based leadership; and second, the strategy of including youth (who are the target population for many intervention programs) is a viable practice for ensuring a "youth perspective" in program planning, implementation, and evaluation. The active involvement of youth also serves as a check and balance on adults, with their adult perspective. Young adults represent the future hope for sustaining relevant health promotion initiatives through community empowerment.

Sincere participation of members in significant activities is yet another way to maintain an esprit de corps within the organization. Individuals become motivated to achieve when their efforts are appreciated and recognition is given for member contributions. Volunteerism is typically difficult to maintain in the absence of recognition and accolades for significant involvement over several years. While there is strength in diversity, cultural sensitivity is yet another important consideration, particularly when dealing with multicultural target populations and broad-based coalitions. For example, members need to be aware that in some cultures it is inappropriate to disagree publicly, while in others it is very appropriate to state disagreement and present the reasons or source of such disagreement. There also exist different cultural contexts in orientations toward time. Being on time for meetings can become a source of irritation for those who are always prompt if others are consistently late.

When coalition members can visibly see tangible and physical changes in their community, this too is a source of sustenance, since everyone enjoys being part of a positive outcome. For example, the coalition that is able to secure a major grant to develop a community cardiovascular prevention project or one that is able to have the local crack house closed and drug dealers pushed from the neighborhood is representative of a group that is likely to work cohesively. When it becomes obvious that coalition members can effect a change, create employment opportunities, and control resources for self-determination, this realization serves to sustain the momentum to coalesce for long-term community gains. In summary, the advantages of coalitions include creating greater visibility for people working together on a common goal, sharing of scarce resources for the good of the community, and strengthening referral and resource networks.

Conclusion

Organizing community-based health promotion programs in low-income areas has recently attracted the attention of both the public and private sector. This approach has been documented as one of the more progressive methods for affecting poor and medically underserved populations. It is too soon to determine its effectiveness, but feedback from residents representing several pilot communities suggests behavior changes that signal increased concern for positive life-style modifications. These changes have implications for healthier living.

The COD approach fosters community ownership of health problems and the solutions within a community. The method of involving local residents in the problem identification, problem design, and implementation builds on the community ownership concept. The COD approach emphasized within this chapter places great value on local site-specific input from grassroots, indigenous community residents on all pertinent decisions that affect the quality of life within one's community. Through communitydefined problems, community-defined solutions, and communitysanctioned and -controlled implementations of interventions, the fabric of the COD coalition movement fused by cultural sensitivity has evidenced great heuristic potential for shifting control over resources to community organizations. Participatory decision making by key community informants as a prerequisite to program planning, implementation, and evaluation can not be underestimated as a variable critical for successful health interventions. Thus creative community-driven collaborations for empowering lowincome African-American communities through coalition building and community organization remain a viable and important method of health education and health promotion (Minkler, 1990).

References

Akbar, N. (1985). *The community of self*. Tallahassee, FL: Mind Productions & Associates.

Alinsky, S. D. (1969). *Reveille for radicals*. New York: Vintage Books.

Banfield, E. C. (1961). *Political influence*. New York: Free Press.

Bennett, L., Jr. (1975). *The shaping of black America*. Chicago: Johnson.

Bernard, B. (1986). Characteristics of effective prevention programs. *Prevention Forum, 6*, 6–13.

Braithwaite, R., & Lythcott, N. (1989). Community empowerment as a strategy for health promotion for black and other minority populations. *Journal of the American Medical Association, 261*(2), 282–283.

Braithwaite, R., Murphy, F., Lythcott, N., & Blumenthal, D. (1989). Community organization and development for health promotion within an urban black community: A conceptual model. *Health Education, 20*(5), 56–60.

Centers for Disease Control. (1990, July). CDC surveillance summaries: Reports on selected racial/ethnic groups, special focus: Maternal and child health. *Morbidity and Mortality Weekly Report, 39*(3), 1–41.

Chavis, D., & Wandersman, A. (1990). Sense of community in the urban environment: A catalyst for participation and community development. *American Journal of Community Psychology, 18*(1), 55–81.

Cleage, A. B., Jr. (1989). *The black messiah*. Trenton, NJ: African World Press.

Cone, J. H. (1975). *God of the oppressed*. New York: HarperCollins.

Couto, R. A. (1990). Promoting health at the grass roots. *Health Affairs, 9*(2), 144–151.

Cruse, H. (1987). *Plural, but equal—blacks and minorities in America's plural society*. New York: Morrow.

Dewart, J. (Ed.). (1990). *The state of black America 1990*. New York: National Urban League.

Fawcett, S. B., Seekins, T., Whang, P. L., Muiu, C., & Suarez de Balcazar, Y. (1984). Creating and using social technologies for community empowerment. In J. Rappaport, C. Swift, & R. Hess (Eds.), *Studies in empowerment* (pp. 145–171). New York: Haworth Press.

Florin, P., & Wandersman, A. (1990). An introduction to citizen participation, voluntary organizations, and community organization: Insights for empowerment through research. *American Journal of Community Psychology, 18*(1), 41–54.

Freire, P. (1970). *Pedagogy of the oppressed*. New York: Seabury Press.

Freire, P. (1973). *Education for critical consciousness*. New York: Seaburg Press.

Freire, P. (1989). *Learning to question: Pedagogy of liberation*. New York: Continuum.

Garrow, D. J. (1986). *Bearing the cross: Martin Luther King, Jr., and the Southern Christian Leadership Conference*. New York: Morrow.

Georgia Council on Maternal and Infant Health. (1989). *Distribution of obstetrical care manpower report in Georgia*. (Unpublished manuscript).

Gray, S. S., Hartman, A., & Saalberg, E. L. (1985). Empowering the black family. Ann Arbor, MI: National Child Welfare Training Center.

Hale-Benson, J. (1987). *Children, their roots, cultural and learning styles*. Baltimore, MD: Johns Hopkins University Press.

Hilliard, A. G., Payton-Stewart, L., & Obedele-Williams, L. (1990). *Proceedings of the First Annual National Conference on Infusion of African and African-American Content in the School Curriculum*. Morristown, NJ: Aaron Press.

Jones, R. L. (1991). *Black psychology* (3rd ed.). Berkeley, CA: Cobb and Henry.

Katz, R. (1984). Empowerment and synergy: Expanding the community's healing resources. In J. Rappaport, C. Swift, & R. Hess (Eds.), *Studies in empowerment* (pp. 201–241). New York: Haworth Press.

Kreuter, M. W., Nelson, C. F., Stoddard, R. P., & Watkins, N. B. (1985). *Planned approach to community health*. Atlanta, GA: Centers for Disease Control.

Labonte, R. (1989). Community empowerment: The need for political analysis. *Canadian Journal of Public Health, 80*, 87–88.

LaVeist, T. A. (1992). The political empowerment and health status of African-Americans: Mapping a new territory. *American Journal of Sociology, 97*(4), 1080–1095.

Lewin, K. (1951). *Field Theory in Social Science: Selected theoretical papers*. New York: HarperCollins.

McKnight, J. (1985). Health and empowerment. *Canadian Journal of Public Health, 76,* 37–38.

Minkler, M. (1990). Improving health through community organization. In K. Glanz, F. M. Lewis, B. K. Rimer, & Associates, *Health behavior and health education: Theory, research, and practice*. San Francisco: Jossey-Bass.

National Cancer Institute, Division of Cancer Prevention and Control. (1991). *America stop smoking intervention study: The ASSIST Program*. Bethesda, MD: Author.

National Research Council. (1989). *A common destiny: Blacks and American society*. Washington, DC: National Academy Press.

Polednak, A. (1989). *Racial and ethnic differences in disease*. New York: Oxford University Press.

Rappaport, J. (1984). Studies in empowerment: Introduction to the issue. *Prevention in Human Services, 3,* 1–7.

Rawls, J. (1971). *A theory of justice*. Cambridge, MA: Harvard University Press.

Resnick, H. (1980). *Drug abuse prevention for low income communities*. Rockville, MD: National Institute on Drug Abuse.

Rotter, J. B. (1976). Some problems and misconceptions related to the construct of internal versus external control of reinforcement. *Journal of Consulting and Clinical Psychology, 43,* 56–67.

Russel-Erlich, J. L., & Rivera, F. O. (1986). Community empowerment as a non-problem. *Journal of Sociology and Social Welfare, 13,* 451–465.

Ryan, W. (1971). *Blaming the victim*. New York: Random House.

Sanders, J. (1989). Georgia reconnaissance study. *Foundation News, 30*(1), 19–24.

Short, P. F., Cornelius, L. J., & Goldstone, D. E. (1990). Health insurance of minorities in the United States. *Journal of Health Care for the Poor and Underserved, 1*(1), 9–24.

Solomon, B. B. (1976). *Black empowerment: Social work in oppressed communities*. New York: Columbia University Press.

Sommer, R. (1961). Leadership and group geography. *Sociometry, 24,* 99–110.

Swift, C. (1984). Empowerment: An antidote for folly. *Prevention in Human Service, 3,* 11–15.

Syme, S. L. (1986). Strategies for health promotion. *Preventive Medicine, 15,* 492–507.

Taylor, S. E. (1988). Internal-external control and the relationship to student verbal behavior. *Psychology: A Journal of Human Behavior, 25*(1), 37–42.

U.S. Department of Health and Human Services. (1985). *Report of the Secretary's Task Force on Black and Minority Health* (Vol. 1, Executive Summary). Washington, DC: U.S. Government Printing Office.

Wallerstein, N. (1992). Powerlessness, empowerment, and health: Implications for health promotion programs. *American Journal of Health Promotion, 6*(3), 197–205.

Wallerstein, N., & Bernstein, E. (1988). Empowerment education: Freire's ideas adapted to health education. *Health Education Quarterly, 15*(4), 379–394.

Warren, R. L. (1977). *Social change and human purpose: Toward understanding and action.* Chicago: Rand McNally.

Williams, R. (1990). Rx: Social reconnaissance. *Foundation News, 31*(4), 24–29.

25

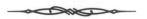

The Health
of the Black Community
in the Twenty-first Century:
A Futuristic Perspective

Stephen B. Thomas

The Bureau of the Census projects that the black population will increase from 11.7 percent of the U.S. total in 1980 to 15 percent in 2020; blacks will be nearly one of five children of school age and one of six adults of prime working age (twenty-five to fifty-four years). Rising numbers of blacks will be represented in both influential occupations and positions and among the least educated and the jobless (National Research Council, 1989). From this reference point, consider the following scenario: Over the next ten years, the black population will swell while the white baby boom generation declines. Failed by the public schools and stuck in low-paying menial jobs, black youths will become frustrated and angry. Unable to find skilled labor, industry will flee and the economy of major urban centers will crumble. By the year 2000, most blacks will live in squalid inner-city slums without local schools or hospitals and will suffer from epidemics of preventable infectious and chronic diseases. The black community will stagger in the shadow of a medical wonder world, unable to gain access to basic public health services perfected in the late twentieth century.

While this outcome is unlikely, it is not beyond the realm of possibility. In many ways the future is now for American corporations, with many of the demographic changes predicted for the work force by the turn of the century already in place. In 1987, the Hudson Institute predicted that 85 percent of all new job entrants by the year 2000 would be minorities and women. Unfortunately, most of the 645 companies surveyed in the study have yet to develop new programs to deal with the problems of recruiting, training, and managing employee diversity (Swoboda, 1990; Johnston & Packer, 1987). It is a real possibility that black youth and young adults will not benefit from the current shortage of "gold-collar" workers, people with technical skills. Young men with poor credentials, finding themselves facing low-wage job offers and high unemployment rates, frequently abandon the labor force intermittently or completely. Some choose criminal activity as an alternative to the labor market (National Research Council, 1989).

The falling employment rates among black male youth aged sixteen to nineteen and young adults aged twenty to twenty-four represent the center of our current national employment crisis. Failure of the federal government to pursue full-employment policies, the decline of older manufacturing centers, and the intense discrimination faced by young blacks represent factors over which the black community has little or no control. Society has created conditions for the production of a generation of black males who will fall through the cracks of our society. The result will be reflected in an increase in delinquent behavior, drug abuse, crime, and the failure to develop the work habits and job skills needed to succeed as adults in a technological society. These outcomes represent risk factors for the leading causes of death and illness in the black community (National Research Council, 1989).

Health Status of Black Americans

The landmark *Report of the Secretary's Task Force on Black and Minority Health* (U.S. Department of Health and Human Services, 1985) clearly demonstrated that minority groups suffer excess morbidity and mortality from preventable conditions directly related to social inequalities. The role of alcohol, tobacco, and other drug consumption must be emphasized because it contributes directly or indirectly to most of the leading causes of death in the black community.

Differences in the health status of blacks and whites have been documented in the United States as long as health data have been collected. These differences have persisted in spite of large increases in life expectancy and improvements in the health status of the general population. Manton, Patrick, & Johnson (1987) point to the following sources of these health differentials: (1) differences in life-style (for example, use of alcohol and tobacco; nutrition); (2) a lack of access to health services and a lack of health insurance; (3) poorer knowledge of health practices; (4) more hazardous occupations and environmental exposures, such as exposure of children to lead; and (5) genetic factors (for example, sickle cell trait).

Gibbs (1988) describes six social indicators used to measure the status of young black males. In each category—education, unemployment, delinquency, drug abuse, teenage parenthood, and mortality rates from homicide and suicide—the data document the serious problems many black youth in American society experience. Gibbs argues that this situation is a direct result of (1) slavery, (2) the flight of the black middle class from the inner cities, (3) discriminatory hiring practices, and (4) the conservative political climate in the United States. An inevitable consequence is excess morbidity and mortality directly related to both racial and socioeconomic inequalities.

Health status of many blacks improved as they attained middle-class status through public education and government enforcement of equal employment opportunity and entitlement laws. But our encouragement must be contained by the economic reality that since the 1970s, the economic status of blacks relative to whites has, on average, stagnated or deteriorated (National Research Council, 1989). Consequently, one can expect fewer and fewer blacks to emerge from poverty to join the middle class. The conditions of increasing economic hardships have been and will continue to be most detrimental to the fortunes of black Americans.

Lessons from History: Universal Access Is Not Enough

One must be mindful that the experience of slavery, extreme segregation, poverty, and institutional racism has shaped black history down to the present. A little more than a quarter of a century ago, 100 years after the Emancipation Proclamation of 1863, most blacks were denied the right to vote, lived in poverty, and received an inferior public school education. Historically, black Americans have been required to use the public policy process to bring about the changes necessary to win the full rights of citizenship and improve their standard of living. The best example of this process is the civil rights movement of the 1960s. Today many blacks attend universities that formerly excluded them. Blacks frequently hold professional and management positions in major corporations. Most blacks now participate in elections, and many have been elected to all but the highest political offices. It would appear that the movement of many blacks into the middle class represents victory in the struggle for full citizenship. Yet more than a century after the signing of the Emancipation Proclamation, real freedom remains elusive.

Just how true this is can best be examined from the perspective of public health. In the twenty-five-year period before 1965, persistent barriers to preventive and primary health services as well as hospital care influenced the quality of life and patterns of illness observed among blacks. Important events that led to more equal access to medical care and improved health status for blacks included (1) the Civil Rights Act of 1964; (2) Medicaid-Medicare legislation of 1965; and (3) Title VI of the Civil Rights Act, which prohibited racial discrimination in any institution receiving federal funds, thus giving hospitals a powerful incentive to alter their practices (National Research Council, 1989). In spite of increased access to personal health care services, black Americans continue to have disproportionately large numbers of premature and excess deaths, compared to the white majority.

The landmark *Black Report* in Great Britain demonstrated that after decades of universal access to health services, health inequalities not only persist but are increasing (McBeath, 1991). In response to this evidence, William McBeath (1991), executive director of the American Public Health Association, emphasized the importance of access to medical care, and a better standard of living—assuring nutritious foods, basic education, safe water, decent housing, secure employment, and adequate income. It has been demonstrated that these are the prerequisites of a healthy life-style. In the absence of these prerequisites, the health status of black Americans will continue to be cause for righteous indignation well into the twenty-first century.

Where Do We Go from Here?

From the mountain of social and economic inequality, black Americans must carve out a foundation on which to securely stand and demand the promise of public health. The history of the federal government's role in health is characterized by an unfocused approach with little continuity. The harsh reality is that it is generally impossible to find any form of health policy that is not a threat to some participant in the health arena. As Evans (1982, p. 329) notes, "It would be naive in the extreme to assume that all participants are wholly, or even primarily, committed to a struggle against disease and death." Brown (1978, 1979) argues that inoculations were highly cost effective, that health education was a necessity, and that the mass media could be used to reinforce individual cost-benefit efforts in health promotion. Yet, "each of these [is] opposed to our present system of health care cost reimbursement" (1978, p. 2). According to Neubauer and Pratt (1981), to acknowledge the political nature of health is to recognize the political forces for whom illness is economically beneficial. Subsequently, this economic incentive will be reflected in public policy "either as active opposition to specific legislation or to programs at the formulation or implementation stage, or as the ability to fix the boundaries of the political agenda" (p. 225). The authors further state that in this society, the most important aspects of the "health problem" are fundamentally political (as opposed to "economic" or "social" or "scientific"). To accept this is to acknowledge that some organized interests are dependent on illness as a direct or indirect outcome of what they do. It is little wonder that no consistent program of prevention can be launched in this country. It is within this context that personal behavior change efforts without an equal or greater emphasis on policy change are tantamount to blaming the victim (Brown, 1978, 1979; Evans, 1982).

Excess deaths attributed to alcohol, tobacco, and drug abuse are directly tied to federal policy decisions. Tobacco and alcohol are legal drugs heavily promoted to black Americans. There is clear evidence that alcohol and tobacco companies have targeted blacks as a major market to direct sophisticated advertisements and community support campaigns to. The pages of respected black publications from *Ebony Magazine* to the official publication of the National Association for the Advancement of Colored People (NAACP) are littered with alcohol and tobacco advertisements. Additionally, during a convention of black newspaper publishers in 1987, Henry Brown, vice president of Anheuser Busch, said that "corporations placing beverage and tobacco advertising in black-owned media should not be criticized for supporting the community when many major advertisers give nothing back to blacks" ("Making History," 1987, p. 3A). Few if any black health professional organizations have demonstrated clear opposition to black media's promotion of alcohol and tobacco products. The federal government's response has been slow and has been complicated by irrational regulatory policy. An example of irrational federal policy is the fact that the Department of Agriculture delivers price supports to tobacco producers at the same time that the Department of Health and Human Services is mounting a campaign against cigarette smoking (Thomas, 1990; Thomas, Duncan, & Gold, 1987).

In 1990, Dr. Louis Sullivan, Secretary of Health and Human Services, presented to the nation *Healthy People 2000: National Health Promotion and Disease Prevention Objectives* (U.S. Department of Health and Human Services, 1990). Healthy People 2000 is a comprehensive strategic plan designed to focus our national health resources on prevention in its broadest sense. This shift away from medical technology is driven by economic forces that demonstrate that our nation can no longer afford not to invest in prevention. Consider the following:

- Smoking, the single most preventable cause of death and illness in the United States, costs our health care system more than $65 billion annually.
- AIDS is an almost entirely preventable disease. The annual cost of treating all diagnosed AIDS patients, about $4.3 billion in 1990, could climb as high as $13 billion by 1992.
- The yearly cost of treating alcohol and drug abuse is at least $16 billion. The total economic impact of alcohol and drug abuse, including not only treatment but premature death, accidents, crime, and lost productivity, is more than $110 billion annually.

Healthy People 2000 acknowledges that medical care alone will not eliminate the devastating impact of chronic disease, the high rate of infant mortality, the burden of homicide and violence, or any of the other health problems that have a disproportionate impact on the black community. It is a major initiative that provides a foundation for a rational health policy. It begins with three broad national health goals for the decade: increase the span of healthy life for Americans, reduce health disparities among Americans, and achieve access to preventive services for all Americans.

These are worthy goals that, if achieved, will improve the health status of all black Americans. Unfortunately, enthusiasm for Healthy People 2000 is diminished because it includes no specific proposals on how to achieve its laudable goals. It does not call for a national health program with universal medical insurance coverage and comprehensive benefits. It may be described as a massive jigsaw puzzle to be assembled at the community level, with only limited support from the federal government.

The entire policy is based on the assumption that we as individuals can control our health destinies in significant ways. It is true that risk factors such as smoking, alcohol consumption, and lack of exercise are under our control.

Yet health policy that expects an individual to overcome the political forces that support alcohol and tobacco production—as well as the forces of corporate advertising designed to promote tobacco and alcohol consumption—is unrealistic. Health policy that expects an individual to overcome economic barriers to gain access to medical care is unreasonable. To expect individual black Americans to overcome the multiple factors that contribute to their persistent health disadvantage is to ensure that a large segment of the black community will not get to the promised land of Healthy People 2000.

One must be mindful that the ethnicity of an individual is not an independent risk factor. In other words, blacks do not have higher morbidity and mortality rates compared to whites because they are black. The relationship between poor health and socioeconomic status has been well documented. People with the least education, people who live in the least desirable neighborhoods, and people who work at the least prestigious jobs are all more likely to die earlier than people on the other end of these scales. This is why disease prevention policies that assign primary responsibility to individual men and women are unjust (Tesh, 1988).

Our country must create a health care system that meets the needs of poorly served, underserved, and never-served segments of society. Blacks are overrepresented among these population segments. They are no less worthy than anyone else of being treated with human dignity and receiving the health care that should be a full right of citizenship. The World Health Organization (1981a, 1981b) resolved that by the year 2000, all citizens of the world should attain a level of health that will permit them to lead a socially and economically productive life. Public policy designed to meet this goal must ensure that essential health services be made accessible to everyone; be delivered in ways acceptable to individuals, families, and communities; require full participation of individuals receiving services; and be provided at a cost the community can afford (World Health Organization, 1981a).

According to WHO, essential health services should include but not be limited to the following (1981a):

1. Basic environmental sanitation
2. Adequate supply of safe water
3. Promotion of proper nutrition
4. Control of local endemic disease (for example, lead poisoning, drug addiction, violence)
5. Health education
6. Family planning services
7. Maternal and child care
8. Immunization against major diseases
9. Treatment for common diseases and injuries

From this perspective, improving the health status of blacks must go beyond personal health service delivery and address the biological, environmental, and life-style determinants of health. Public health professionals must be free from the constraints imposed by the traditional public health model of host and agent in a single-cause, single-effect relationship. They must operate from a comprehensive concept of health that recognizes the multiple causes and multiple effects of risk factors associated with the leading causes of excess death in the black community (that is, poverty, smoking, infant mortality).

A Framework for Social Action

The health field concept, used by Lalonde (1974) to formulate strategies for improving the health of Canadians, could well serve as a platform for the development of effective health promotion and disease prevention programs in the black community. According to Terris (1984), the first official statement of policy that acknowledged the start of a new era in public health was the Lalonde Report. This new era was described as the second epidemiologic revolution, which like the first epidemiologic revolution, was geared toward conquering infectious diseases.

The essence of the Lalonde Report is the health field concept, according to which the determinants of health can be broken up into four broad domains: (1) human biology, (2) environment, (3) life-style, and (4) system of health care organization (see Figure 25.1). These four domains were identified through an examination of the causes and underlying factors of sickness and death in Canada. Briefly stated, the human biology domain encompasses the health outcomes directly derived from human biology (for example, genetics, growth, aging). This domain is characterized by limited corrective intervention by the individual or community. The environment domain includes all the factors related to health that are external to the human body (such as safe food and water, effective sanitation, noise pollution, safe social environment). This domain is characterized by limited individual control and relatively greater community control over corrective intervention. The life-style domain deals with individual decisions that have an impact on health (for example, seat belt use, substance abuse, stress management, physical fitness). This domain is characterized by a maximum of individual corrective intervention and limited community control. The system–of–health care–organization domain includes public and private institutions devoted to delivery of health services (for instance, medical care, dental care, nursing homes, pharmacy services, mental health services). This domain has received the most attention and money, on the assumption that these services will bring about major improvements in the health status of the American population. It is characterized by minimum potential for individual intervention and maximum potential for corrective sociopolitical intervention.

Each domain of the health field concept can be further refined as

Figure 25.1. Domains of the Health Field Concept.

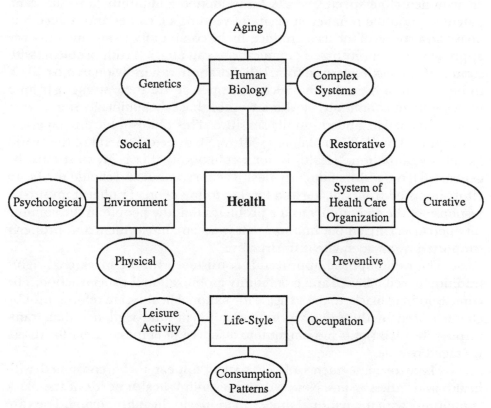

Source: Dever, 1976, p. 55. Reprinted by permission of Kluwer Academic Publishers.

follows: (1) environment includes social, psychological, and physical components; (2) life-style includes consumption patterns, leisure activity, and occupation; (3) human biology includes complex internal systems, maturation and aging, and genetic inheritance components; and (4) system of health care organization includes restorative, curative, and preventive components (Dever, 1991).

The health field concept can be used by human service organizations, in a process of risk factor analysis, to identify health promotion and disease prevention priorities in their community. The individuals in the community can participate in the determination of which risk factors are associated with selected domains of the health field concept. For example, smoking behavior is a function of life-style consumption patterns where the individual has maximum potential for corrective intervention. One solution would be for the health care delivery system to provide smoking cessation programs for individuals seeking services. This approach relies on individual choice and access to affordable, convenient service.

Smoking behavior is also a function of the availability of tobacco products in the physical and social environment. One solution from this environmental perspective would be to mount community advocacy campaigns to limit the number of cigarette vending machines and reduce billboard advertising of tobacco products in the community. Using this advocacy approach, community-based organizations can attack health problems with strategies and tactics derived from collaboration with individuals most likely to benefit from the solution. Such strategies derive their strength from a philosophy of community health advocacy that is scientifically sound, ethnically acceptable, and culturally sensitive. This philosophical perspective was captured by Halfdan Mahler (1981, p. 8), director-general of the World Health Organization: "Health is not a commodity that is given. It must be generated from within. Similarly, health action cannot and should not be an effort imposed from outside and foreign to the people; rather it must be a response of the community to the problems that the people in the community perceive, carried out in a way that is acceptable to them and properly supported by an adequate infrastructure."

The philosophical approach is consistent with the black civil rights tradition of self-reliance and community mobilization for social action. The contribution of blacks to the struggle for national health care reform must be characterized by the same vision, commitment, and vigilance that transformed the civil rights movement into a source of empowerment for disadvantaged people.

Mainstream segments of our society appear to be consumed with health and fitness issues. Now is the time to link health needs of the black community with the national preoccupation with healthful living. The case must be made that regardless of race or social class, we have a common destiny. Staying healthy must be a national priority so that we can work to make a living as well as make life worth living. There is increasing evidence that wide public support is mounting to address many of the major health problems facing blacks. Jacob (1987) reported on a national poll the Gallup Organization conducted for the Joint Center for Political Studies; the poll found surprising agreement between blacks and whites on the major problems confronting the nation. Although white Americans continued to believe that civil rights was not a major problem, respondents of both races identified unemployment, drug abuse, and the high cost of living as the three most important issues; both ranked crime, health care, and the quality of public education among the top ten. This provides evidence for the possibility of increased interracial cooperation on issues that disproportionately affect the health status of the community. From this common destiny, a vision of health for all black Americans could begin with a shared pledge on the part of society to:

- Forge a future—with all being born healthy to parents who want them and who have the time, the means, and the skills needed to bring them up and care for them properly

- Forge a future—with all being educated in societies that endorse the basic values of healthy living and encourage individual choice and allow it to be exercised
- Forge a future—with all being assured the basic requirements for health and being protected effectively against disease and accidents
- Forge a future—with all living in a stimulating environment of social interaction, free from the fear of war, with full opportunities for play and satisfying economic and social roles
- Forge a future—with all growing old in a society that supports the maintenance of their capacities for a secure, purposeful retirement, offers care when care is needed, and finally allows them to die with dignity (World Health Organization, 1981b; McBeath, 1991).

Conclusion

The health status of the black community is tied to the role black Americans play in the nation today and the role they will play in the future. The evidence clearly points to the central importance of jobs for men and women at pay levels that permit families to live above the poverty line. Today, the great majority of black Americans contribute to the political, economic, and social health of the nation. However, the increasing high school dropout rates, the growing thousands of young black men who have not participated in the labor market (many are in prison or dead), and the increasing teen pregnancy rate contribute to negative consequences that can nullify the civil rights gains of the past thirty years. Blacks will not be able to attribute such degradation to overt racism alone. They will instead be faced with the reality that through benign neglect, an entire generation of blacks were unable to walk through the open doors of opportunity because they were ill-prepared to function in a technological society.

The battleground for freedom must be shifted from the arena of constitutional justice to the arena of public health justice. The promise of public health for the future of black Americans must be directed toward societal goals that maximize human potential and minimize risk factors inhibiting that potential. The mission of public health is to create conditions that foster good health; the substance of public health should involve organized community efforts aimed at the prevention of disease and promotion of health (Shannon, 1990; Institute of Medicine, 1988). From this perspective, community activism, community development, and social action become legitimate tools needed to attack such complex health issues as infant mortality, violence, drug abuse, and AIDS. As the American public becomes increasingly aware of the black community's health predicament, there will be opportunity and danger. The opportunity is to deal comprehensively rather than haphazardly with the problem as a whole—to see it as a social catastrophe brought on by years of economic deprivation and to meet it as other disasters are met, with adequate resources. The danger is that health problems will be attributed to some innate weakness of black people and used to justify further neglect and to rationalize continued deprivation.

Once black Americans shift the focus of their struggle for freedom from the arena of constitutional justice to the arena of public health justice, the 1970s image of a black family unable to purchase a home in the white section of town because of the color of their skin is replaced by the 1990s image of a black family unable to secure primary health care because they have no insurance. The 1950s image of a black man unable to gain lodging because of his race is replaced by the 1990s image of a black male selling crack because he cannot read well enough to secure meaningful employment. In the 1960s, the mass media brought pictures into every American household depicting freedom marchers being attacked by vicious police dogs. The moral conscience of our nation was stimulated and helped to create the interracial coalitions responsible for passage of the 1964 Civil Rights Act. Pictures of crack babies hanging onto life by a thin thread have the power to stimulate our moral conscience and prepare a foundation for the interracial coalitions needed to achieve the promise of health for all by the year 2000. It is from the standpoint of this conception of public health as social justice that the black community can once again serve as the best measure of our nation's true greatness.

References

Brown, J. (1978). *The politics of health care.* Cambridge, MA: Ballinger.

Brown, R. (1979). *The Rockefeller medicine men: Medicine and capitalism in America.* Berkeley: University of California Press.

Dever, A. (1976). Epidemiological model of health policy analysis. *Social Indicators Research, 2,* 55.

Dever, A. (1991). *Community health analysis: Global awareness at the local level* (2nd ed.). Germantown, MD: Aspen Systems.

Evans, R. (1982). Retrospective on the "New Perspective." *Journal of Health Politics, Policy, and Law, 7*(2), 325–344.

Gibbs, J. T. (Ed.). (1988). *Young, black, and male in America: An endangered species.* Dover, MA: Auburn House.

Institute of Medicine. (1988). *The future of public health.* Washington, DC: National Academy Press.

Jacob, J. (1987). Black America 1986: An overview. In J. D. Williams (Ed.), *The state of black America* (pp. 7–14). New York: National Urban League.

Johnston, W., & Packer, A. (1987). *Workforce 2000: Work and workers of the 21st century.* Indianapolis, IN: Hudson Institute.

Lalonde, M. (1974). *A new perspective on the health of Canadians.* Ottawa: Canadian Department of Health and Welfare.

McBeath, W. (1991). A public health vision. *American Journal of Public Health, 81*(12), 1560–1565.

Mahler, H. (1981). The meaning of health for all by the year 2000. *World Health Forum, 2*(1), 5–22.

Making history: Woman elected president of the National Newspaper Publisher's Association (1987, June). *Columbus Call and Post*, p. 3A.

Manton, K., Patrick, C., & Johnson, K. (1987). Health differentials between blacks and whites: Recent trends in mortality and morbidity. *Milbank Quarterly, 65* (Suppl. 1), 129–199.

National Research Council. (1989). *A common destiny: Blacks and American society*. Washington, DC: National Academy of Sciences.

Neubauer, D., & Pratt, R. (1981). The second public health revolution. *Journal of Health Politics, Policy, and Law, 6*(2), 205–228.

Shannon, I. (1990). Public health's promise for the future: 1989 presidential address. *American Journal of Public Health, 80*(8) 909–912.

Swoboda, F. (1990, July 20). The future has arrived, survey finds: Growing numbers of minority workers, other predictions in place now. *Washington Post*, pp. F1, F4.

Terris, M. (1984) Newer perspectives on the health of Canadians: Beyond the Lalonde report. *Journal of Health Policy, 5*(3), 327–337.

Tesh, S. (1988). *Hidden arguments: Political ideology and disease prevention policy*. New Brunswick, NJ: Rutgers University Press.

Thomas, S. (1990). Community health advocacy for racial and ethnic and minority populations in the United States: Issues and challenges for health education. *Health Education Quarterly, 17*(1), 15–19.

Thomas, S., Duncan, D., & Gold, R. (1987). Roll call voting behavior of the U.S. Senate on selected health legislation 1973–1982: Implications for health education. *American Journal of Health Promotion, 2*(2), 22–36.

U.S. Department of Health and Human Services. (1979). *Healthy people: Surgeon General's Report on Health Promotion and Disease Prevention* (PAS Publication No. 79-55071A). Washington, DC: U.S. Government Printing Office.

U.S. Department of Health and Human Services. (1985). *Report of the Secretary's Task Force on Black and Minority Health* (Vol. 1, Executive Summary). Washington, DC: U.S. Government Printing Office.

U.S. Department of Health and Human Services. (1990). *Healthy people 2000: National health promotion and disease prevention objectives*. Washington, DC: U.S. Government Printing Office.

World Health Organization. (1981a). *Global strategy for health for all by the year 2000*. Geneva: Author.

World Health Organization. (1981b). *Targets for health for all by 2000*. Geneva: Author.

AFTERWORD

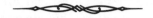

This book is perhaps the best attempt to date to comprehensively describe the health status of African Americans or blacks in America. The writers who appear in these pages are on the front line of the struggle to improve the health of African Americans, and they are intimately involved with the specific issues about which they write.

By almost any measure, the health status of African Americans is a cause for grave concern. While there has been slow, continuing progress, especially since the mid 1960s and the advent of Medicaid and Medicare, two grim facts mar that progress. First, the gap in health status between African Americans and the majority population is wide and it is not closing. Second, new and exacerbating challenges to the health of all Americans in the 1980s (for example, AIDS and violence) had a disproportionate impact on African Americans, so that for the first time in this century, their life expectancy experienced years of decline.

The writers gathered here have illustrated, with a clarity previously unequaled, the complexity of African-American health status and issues in the black community. Whether the health problems of African Americans are viewed from the perspective of etiology, presentation/expression, access to care, response to care, or natural history, they are complex and require a broad-based, comprehensive approach. The need for multidisciplinary strategies to define and maintain or restore the health of African Americans is a theme dramatically restated throughout this volume.

As long as our highly sophisticated health care system in America encourages narrow training and education of health professionals and discourages the team approach to public health, health care, and research, it cannot and will not adequately address the health needs of African Americans. Similarly, the dominant role of poverty in the health status of African Americans condemns medical services to failure unless they are accompanied by comprehensive social services. Nor will health services that are driven by one's ability to pay — out of pocket, by insurance or governmental

programs that cover less than half of those in poverty, and at that inadequately—be accessible or responsive to the needs of African Americans.

In the debate over health care reform, these authors take the position
that, despite its sophistication, the system of health care in America is failing
all of its people. However, it is failing African Americans miserably. The lack
of emphasis on comprehensiveness, the lack of incentives for preventive
intervention, the barriers to access, and the underrepresentation of African
Americans and other minorities in the health professions all combine to
create what the American Medical Association recently referred to as a
"racist" health care system—a system that disproportionately fails African
Americans and other minorities.

So where do we go from here? The contributors to this book have not
only described and analyzed the health status of African Americans, but they
have made valuable recommendations for improvement. We must find a way
to implement these recommendations as we continue to search for strategies.
Four recurring themes of the book stand out:

1.   In order to enhance the health of African Americans, we must work to
     improve socioeconomic status. Retired medical educator Dr. Alfred
     Haynes, former dean and president of Charles R. Drew Post-Graduate
     Medical School, reminds us about the accuracy of the adage "Poverty
     kills." This theme is acknowledged in many of the chapters.
2.   The knowledge, attitudes, and behavior of African Americans must be
     targeted and enhanced in order to close the health gap as we know it.
     There is still a difference between reality and vision. While reality defines
     our situation, it is vision that drives and guides us to realize our best
     futures. The Meharry "I Have a Future" program for African-American
     teenagers from housing projects (chosen by President Bush as the 404th
     Point of Light) attacks teenage pregnancy, violence, drug abuse, and
     early school dropout by improving the attitudes of young people toward
     the future.
3.   We as a nation must give proper emphasis and support to those things
     that we know work in improving the health status of African Americans
     and others. These include Headstart programs, the Women, Infants, and
     Children (WIC) program, and prenatal care and immunizations, to
     name a few. The continued underfunding of these programs while
     billions of dollars are spent on high technology of questionable value is
     one of America's greatest health care dilemmas today.
4.   The verbal commitment that we as a nation have made to health care as a
     right must now be matched by health care reform that, at a minimum,
     assures universal access to care, removing all financial and adminis-
     trative barriers. If access to quality basic health care for all must come at
     the expense of elective, "high-tech" care for a few, so be it. It is time to bite
     the bullet.

Finally, I am convinced that the health of African Americans will be enhanced when larger numbers of African Americans are participants in the health care system as providers. A study by S. N. Keith, R. M. Bell, A. G. Swanson, and A. P. Williams, reported in the *New England Journal of Medicine* in 1985, showed that minority physicians are more likely than their non-minority counterparts to serve in underserved communities, to serve the poor, and to serve other minorities. Furthermore, the education and training of more African-American youth for health science careers will, in and of itself, be therapeutic for those young people and for their families and communities.

But one might ask, "Whose responsibility is it to improve the health status of African Americans?" I am reminded of the story (author unknown) involving four young people named Everybody, Somebody, Anybody, and Nobody. There was an important job to be done and Everybody knew that Somebody would do it and Anybody could do it, but Nobody did it. Somebody got angry because he knew it was Everybody's job. Everybody knew that Anybody could do it, but Nobody realized that Everybody would not do it. So, in the end, Everybody blamed Somebody when Nobody did what Anybody could have done.

We can all improve the health of African Americans, and we must all join in to do this important job.

August 1992

David Satcher
President, Meharry Medical College
Nashville, Tennessee

NAME INDEX

A

Adams, J. M., 91
Aday, L. A., 160
Adebimpe, V. R., 231
Adragna, N., 95
Aiken, L. H., 112
Airhihenbuwa, C. O., 268, 269, 270, 272, 277
Ajzen, I., 273
Akbar, N., 25, 139, 174, 269, 271, 323
Alan Guttmacher Institute, 42, 215, 303
Albright, N., 47
Albright, T., 47
Alcohol, Drug Abuse, and Mental Health Administration, 132
Aldous, J., 270
Alexander, K. L., 241
Alinsky, S. D., 323
Allen, W., 271
Allen, W. R., 4
Allison, A. C., 194
Altman, E., 151
American Association of Retired Persons, 222, 223
American College of Preventive Medicine, 250
American Psychiatric Association, 21
Anderson, N. B., 95
Anderson, R. M., 129
Anderson, W. F., 228
Aneshensel, C. S., 149
Annest, J. L., 179, 180
Antonovsky, A., 13, 149
Antunes, G., 25
Apostolides, A. Y., 96
Apostte, R. A., 241
Aranda, J., 99

Armor, D. J., 241
Arnold, M. S., 129
Aronoff, R., 282, 283, 291
Artz, L., 263
Asante, M. K., 244, 270, 271
Association of American Medical Colleges, 282, 283, 285
Awad, G. A., 28

B

Bachrach, L. L., 148
Bakalar, J., 82, 83, 84
Bakeman, R., 57
Baker, F. M., 23, 28, 231
Baker, S. P., 133
Baldwin, J. A., 270
Ball, R. M., 318
Baltrop, D., 184
Banfield, E. C., 323
Banks, A., 195
Baquet, C. R., 106, 108, 111, 112, 113
Barancik, J. I., 132
Barker, J. C., 232
Barrett, S. A., 22, 24, 28
Barrios, N., 195
Bassuk, E. L., 148, 150
Bastien, J. W. , 262
Beaglehole, R., 98
Beauregard, K., 16
Becker, M. H., 100, 160, 247
Beet, E. A., 194
Beevers, D. G., 93
Bell, C. C., 6, 22, 23, 77
Bell, P., 80
Bell, P. B., 65, 66, 74
Bell, R. M., 283
Bell, Y. R., 270

Bellinger, D., 187
Benjamin, L., 24
Bennett, L., Jr., 241, 324
Bennett, M.B.H., 152
Berenson, G. S., 91, 94, 95
Berk, M. L., 242
Berman, S. H., 248
Berman-Rossi, T., 150
Bernard, B., 324
Bernstein, E., 323
Bernstein, J., 13, 232
Besdine, R. W., 228
Beverly, C., 81, 86
Billick, I. H., 179
Billingsley, A., 152, 214
Birch, H. C., 212
Black, E., 151
Bland, I., 22, 23
Blaustein, M. P., 95
Blendon, R. J., 112
Blum, R. W., 307, 308
Blumenthal, D., 130, 328, 329, 330
Bone, L. R., 263
Boone, M. S., 175
Boston Commission on Safe Public
     Schools, 133
Bowlby, J., 156
Boyd, J. H., 232
Boyer, R., 148
Boyle, E., Jr., 93
Braithwaite, R., 129, 176, 270, 322, 323,
     325, 328, 329
Brass, W., 228
Brenner, M. H., 232
Breton, M., 150
Brisbane, F., 86
Brooks-Gunn, J., 207
Bross, D., 170
Brown, B. S., 26
Brown, C., 138, 139
Brown, D. R., 21, 30
Brown, G. W., 150
Brown, J., 341
Brown, R., 341
Brunswick, A. F., 30
Buerki, R. C., 263
Buescher, P. A., 171, 172
Bullard, R. D., 5
Bureau of Alcohol, Tobacco and Fire-
     arms, 134
Burke, J. D., 232
Burnham, L., 218
Burnham, V. R., 257
Burton, B., 262
Burton, L. M., 210, 211
Bush, T., 59
Butler, F. R., 225

Butler, P. A., 16
Butler, R. N., 227

C

Cafferats, G. L., 268
Canessa, M., 95
Cannon, M. S., 24
Caprio, R. J., 184
Cardwell, J., 111
Carey, R. M., 290
Carter, A., 133
Carter, J. H., 23, 26
Carter, A., 70, 71
Cartoof, V. G., 307
Carty, L. A., 21, 22, 24, 231
Cates, W., 302, 303
Centers for Disease Control, 6, 67, 43, 55,
     56, 58, 123, 124, 125, 126, 127, 132,
     174, 179, 315
Centerwall, B., 133
Chamberland, M., 59
Chao, L. M., 262
Charney, E., 180, 184
Chavis, D., 322
Chavkin, W., 150
Chen, Y., 224
Child, R. C., 259, 263
Children's Defense Fund, 170, 307, 317
Chisholm, J. J., 179
Christensen, P. B., 262
Clausen, J. A., 27
Clayton, L. A., 106, 111
Cleage, A. B., Jr., 323
Cleary, P. D., 22, 27
Cockerham, W. C., 25
Cohen, M. B., 150
Cole, L. C., 178
Collier, W., 111
Colombo, T. J., 257
Comer, J. P., 22, 213
Commission on Minority Participation in
     Education and American Life, 242
Committee on an Aging Society, 223
Community Services of New York, 316
Cone, J. H., 323
Conn, R. H., 262
Consensus Conference, 202
Cooke, C. J., 257, 262, 263
Coombes, J., 319, 320
Cooper, R., 223, 227
Copeland, E., 36
Copeland, E. J., 28
Corder, L., 225
Corey, C. R., 112
Cornelius, L. J., 326
Cornu, G., 195
Cottingham, C., 213

Cowan, M., 195
Crayton, B., 70
Crockett, M. S., 150
Cromwell, J., 230
Cronin, C., 40
Cruse, H., 324
Cubbeddu, L. X., 99
Cullen, J., 113
Cuoto, R. A., 324
Current, A. A., 179
Curriden, M., 41

D

Dailey, T., 317
Dalhaus, A. A., 259
Dash, L., 39, 41
Davidow, B., 179
Davidson, M., 226
Davies, N. E., 317
Davis, J. M., 184, 185
Davis, K., 225, 230, 231, 242
Dawson, D., 273
Deeds, S. A., 273
Delano, B. G., 262
Dennis, R. E., 140
Derryberry, M., 249
Desmond, S. M., 273
Deutschle, K. W., 258, 259
Dever, A. L., 344
Dewart, J., 323
Diabetes Surveillance Report, 123
Dietz, P. E., 133
Dittes, N., 303
Dobson, A., 225
Dohrenwend, B. P., 25, 149
Dohrenwend, B. S., 25, 149
Donovan, P., 303
Du Bois, W.E.B., 243, 250, 301
Duncan, D., 342
Dunham, H. W., 25
Dunn, F. G., 99

E

Eaton, W. W., 21
Ecland, B. K., 241
Edelman, M. R., 268
Edwards, B. K., 108, 109
Egbert, L. D., 231, 242
Egbuono, L., 242
Eisman, S., 307
Ellerbrock, T., 59
Ellis, K., 68
Emerson, M. R., 309
Eng, Y., 179
Entwisle, G., 96
Erfurt, J. C., 96

Erikson, E., 139
Evans, J., 66, 80
Evans, R., 341
Evans, W. J., 269
EVAXX, Inc., 111
"Experts Find," 283
Eyre, H. J., 109–110

F

Family Health International, 310
Farber, M., 200
Farfel, M., 180
Farhquhar, J., 137
Faris, R.E.L., 25
Farley, R., 4
Fassel, D., 83
Fawcett, S. B., 324
Fay, R., 10
Felder, L. H., 317
Fielding, J. E., 98
Filardo, T., 148
Fischer, P., 232
Fischhoff, J., 199
Fishbein, M., 273
Fishma, L. E., 269
Flaherty, J., 151
Flamembaum, W., 99
Florin, P., 322
Floyd, R. L., 172
Fodor, J. T., 249
Forrest, J. D., 301, 302, 303, 305, 306, 307
Foster, T. A., 91, 94, 95
Fox, E. L., 256, 259, 262
Fox, E. R., 148
Freeborn, D. K., 257
Freeman, H. E., 112
Freeman, H. P., 233
Freire, P., 129, 322, 323
Freis, E. D., 98, 99
Frerichs, R. R., 91, 94, 95
Frey, W. H., 9
Frisch, R., 47
Fuglesang, A., 273
Funnell, M. M., 129
Furstenberg, F. F., 207, 208, 209, 210

G

Gagnon, A. J., 262
Gaitz, C. M., 25
Gallagher, J., 41
Gallegos, K. V., 65, 73
Galloway, J. R., 259, 262
Gambert, S. R., 228
Gamshadzahi, A., 111
Garrow, D. J., 323
Gary, L. E., 20, 24, 30

Gaston, M. H., 195, 201
Gavin, J. R., III, 126–127
Gaviria, M., 151
Geiss, L. S., 126
Gelles, R., 37, 40
Georgia Council on Maternal and Infant Health, 326
Georgia Department of Human Resources, 44
Gerstein, D., 75
Gewirtz, M., 179
Gibbs, J. T., 339
Gibbs, T., 108
Giblin, P. T., 263
Gibson, R. C., 223, 232, 233
Gigandet, J., 231
Gilliam, A., 148, 150, 151, 152, 155
Gillum, B. S., 96
Gillum, R. F., 91, 93, 96
Glanz, K., 268
Glasgow, D. G., 208
Glock, C. Y., 241
Goddard, L. L., 65, 76
Gold, R. B., 16, 302, 305, 342
Goldenberg, R. L., 167
Goldstone, D. E., 326
Gong, Y. L., 262
Gordon, C., 25
Gosset, V. R., 68, 70
Gourdine, R. M., 208, 211, 212, 214
Grant, L. D., 179, 184, 185
Gray, B. A. 29
Gray, S. S., 321
Green, A., 98
Green, L. W., 247, 268, 273, 277
Greenwald, P., 108, 113
Griffith, E.E.H., 6
Griffiths, W., 277
Grim, C. E., 93
Grimes, D., 303
Grinspoon, L., 82, 83, 84
Gross, T. P., 151
Grosser, C. F., 260, 263
Guardado, S., 305
Guigli, P. E., 150
Gunby, P., 273
Gunnoe, C., 180
Gunter, E. P., 172
Gussow, D. D., 212
Gutman, H., 208
Guttentag, M., 8

H

Hale, C. B., 13
Hale-Benson, J., 323
Halfner, D. P., 248
Hall, E. T., 270

Hallinan, C., 273
Hames, C. G., 96
Hamlyn, J. M., 95
Hammack, F. M., 210
Hanft, R. S., 269
Hankey, B. F., 108, 109
Harburg, E., 96
Hargreaves, M., 111
Harlin, V., 133
Harper, M. S., 226
Harrington, M., 256
Harris, E., 231
Harris, T., 150
Hartman, A., 321
Hartman, R., 40
Harwood, J., 75
Hauenstein, L. S., 96
Hauser, P. M., 223
Hausman, A. J., 135, 141
Haywood, J. L., 229
Hebel, J. R., 96
Heller, B. R., 263
Helms, J. E., 270
Henderson, W. G., 98
Henshaw, S. K., 302, 303
Herrick, J. B., 192, 194
Hersey, J. C., 273
Heyden, S., 96
Hill, R. B., 152, 214, 241
Hilliard, A. G., 29, 323
Hirsch, M. B., 309
Hobgood, J., 259, 263
Hochbaum, G. M., 160
Hodgson v. Minnesota, 304, 308
Hoff, W., 259, 262
Hollander, R., 151
Hollifield, J. W., 99
Holmes, T. H., 149, 150–151
Holt, B., 250
Horibe, H., 91
Horm, J. W., 108
Houston, E., 22, 23
Howard, C., 27
Howell, E. L., 225
Hsu, L., 95
Humbert, J., 195
Hyer, K., 227
Hypertension Detection and Follow-up Program Cooperative Research Group, 90, 92, 99

I

Institution of Medicine, 3, 10, 12, 171, 347
Israel, B. A., 149, 151
Itano, H. A., 194
Iverson, D. C., 273

J

Jackson, A. M., 269, 270
Jackson, D., 180
Jackson, J., 229
Jackson, J. J., 28
Jackson, J. S., 31, 223, 232, 242
Jackson, R., 57, 98
Jacob, J. E., 268, 344
James, S. A., 94, 229
Jaynes, G. D., 4, 170
Jessor, R., 139
Jessor, S. L., 139
John E. Fogarty International Center, 247, 250
Johnson, C. J., 133
Johnson, D. W., 208
Johnson, L., 74
Johnson, V. E., 72, 74
Johnston, W., 338
Joint Center for Policy Studies, 133
Joint National Committee, 98, 99
Jolly, P. W., 262
Jones, A. C., 269
Jones, B., 22, 23
Jones, B. E., 29
Jones, D. J., 20
Jones, E., 207
Jones, E. E., 24
Jones, R. L., 250, 323
Jordan, R., 178
Joselow, M. M., 184
Joseph, J., 247
Joyce, T. J., 307
Juane, J., 195

K

Kapantais, G., 6, 15
Karlqvist, S., 262
Kasarda, J. D., 9
Katz, R., 130, 325
Kaufman-Kurzrock, R. D., 273
Kaul, B., 179
Kegeles, S. S., 248
Keil, J. E., 93
Keith, S. N., 283
Kelso, R. R., 259, 262
Kendrick, J. S., 172
Kenney, A. M., 16
Kent, J., 259, 260, 262, 263
Kerner Report Updated, The, 79, 80
Kesie, B., 262
Kessel, S. S., 170
Kessler, B., 180
Kessler, R., 151
Kessler, R. C., 26
Kilcrease, D. T., 262

Kindler, A. R., 28
King, L., 82
King, L. M., 271, 273, 275, 276
King, M. L., Jr., 301
Kinney, T., 200
Kirkpatrick, D., 195
Kirschenbaum, S., 258
Kitagawa, E. M., 223
Klein, L., 167
Kleiner, R., 270
Kleinman, J. C., 170
Klerman, L. V., 307
Knight, J. W., 148
Knittel, R. E., 259, 263
Knutson, A. L., 277
Kolder, V., 41
Konotey-Ahulu, F.I.D., 192
Koop, C. E., 134
Korchin, S. J., 24
Kosby, M., 200
Kozol, J., 159
Kraegel, J. M., 231
Kramer, B. M., 26
Krejci, J. W., 231
Kreuter, M. W., 247, 268, 273, 326
Krischer, J. P., 170
Kristal, A., 150
Kumanyika, S., 273
Kumar, A., 262

L

L., 75
Labonte, R., 324
Ladner, J. A., 152, 208, 209, 210, 211, 212, 213, 214, 217, 218, 219
Lalonde, M., 344
Lam, J., 148
Lane, R. E., 181
Lang, N. M., 231
Langer, T. S., 147
Lansdown, R., 180
Larson, L. C., 171
Last, J. M., 4
Lauriat, A. L., 148
LaVeist, T. A., 322
Lawson, I. R., 228
Lawson, W. B., 231
Lazarus, R. S., 158
Leffall, L. D., 4
Lenihan, A. J., 171
Leonard, P., 269
Lerner, N., 195
Leventhal, H., 248
Levine, D. M., 257
Leviton, A., 180, 181
Levt, D. R., 269
Levy, F., 241

Lewin, K., 327
Lewis, F. M., 268
Lilley, J. L., 95
Lin-Fu, J. S., 180
Linn, M. W., 149
Linn, S., 181
Lloyd, J., 111
Lloyd, S. M., 282
Locke, B. Z., 24
Long, E. C., 262
Louis Harris & Associates, 302
Lovell, A. M., 150
Lumb, J., 57
Lyles, M. R., 23, 26
Lynch, K. B., 282, 292, 294, 295
Lynch, R. B., 295
Lythcott, N., 129, 176, 270, 322, 323, 325, 328, 329, 330

M

McAdoo, H. P., 152, 208, 214, 218
McBeath, W., 340, 347
McCord, C., 233
McCormick, M. C., 167, 170
McCray, E., 57
McFadden, G. M., 258
McGee, G., 74
McKnight, J., 325
MacMahon, S. W., 98
Mahaffey, K. R., 180
Mahler, H., 344
"Making History," 341
Manderscheid, R. W., 22, 24, 27, 28
Manton, K. G., 232
Margulis, H. L., 184
Markowitz, D., 195
Marks, J. S., 242
Marsa, L., 215
Marshall, O. M., 79, 86
Martin, E., 212, 218
Martin, J., 212, 218
Mashalaba, N. N., 262
Maslow, A. H., 158
Massey, M., 110
Materson, B., 98, 99
Mathur, Y. C., 262
Matney, W. C., 208
Matomora, M. K., 263
Maurer, K., 91
Mayberry, C., 70
Media General/Associated Press, 302
Mejia, A., 263
Mentzer, W., 195
Meyer, P., 93
Meyer v. Nebraska, 304
Meyers, A., 257, 262, 263
Michael, S. T., 147

Mielke, H., 180
Milazzo-Sayre, L. J., 27
Milburn, N., 148
Miller, R. L., 282
Miller, S. M., 230
Miller, W., 223
Minkler, M., 330
Missouri Department of Health, 307
Mitchell, J., 56
Mitchell, J. B., 230
Mitchell, T., 151
Mitlar, I. B., 180
Mitteness, L. S., 232
Mocan, N. H., 307
Mondanaro, J., 150
Monheit, A., 16
Monson, R., 111
Moodie, A. S., 259, 262
Moore, B. J., 262
Moore, F. I., 263
"More Blacks," 292
Morgan, S. P., 208
Morrell, V., 317
Morris, D. W., 262
Morton, R. D., 212, 213, 214
Mosher, W., 302
Moynihan, D. P., 208, 214
Muhlenkamp, A. F., 149
Mullan, F., 257
Mullen, P. D., 273
Mullen, P. P., 172
Muller, C., 269
Mullooly, J. P., 257
Murphy, F., 129, 328, 329, 330
Murphy, R. S., 180
Myers, H. F., 30, 229, 271, 273, 275, 276
Myers, L. W., 28

N

Nakano, K., 111
National Association for Perinatal Addiction Research and Education, 173
National Association for the Advancement of Colored People (NAACP), 302
National Black Women's Health Project, 48–49
National Cancer Institute, 48, 108, 117, 326
National Center for Health Statistics, 14, 27, 29, 35, 41, 98, 111, 112, 123, 141, 179, 185, 273, 302
National Commission to Prevent Infant Mortality, 170, 171, 173
National Family Planning and Reproductive Health Association et al. v. Sullivan, 306
National Institute on Drug Abuse, 66, 67, 75

National Institutes of Health, 124, 127
National Research Council, 6, 59, 241, 321, 338, 339, 340
National Urban League, 79
National Vital Statistics System and National Health Interview Survey, 226
Needleman, H. L., 179, 180, 181, 182
Neel, J. V., 194
Neighbors, H. W., 27, 242
Nelson, C. F., 326
Nelson, M. D., 171
Neubauer, D., 341
New Jersey School Board, 217
New York v. Sullivan, 305
Nickens, H. W., 4, 282
Nishiura, E. N., 197, 204
Nobles, W. W., 26, 65, 76, 86, 270
Noren, J. J., 4
Norton, D. G., 214
Norton, R. N., 98

O

Obedele-Williams, L., 323
Oberlander, L. B., 259
O'Conner, D. J., 95
O'Connor, E., 319, 320
Office for Substance Abuse Prevention, 80, 81
Office of Environmental Affairs, 181, 187
Office of National Drug Control Policy, 67, 68, 69
Office of Policy and Planning, 207
Office of Substance Abuse Prevention, 71
O'Hare, W. P., 8, 224
Ohio v. Akron Center for Reproductive Health, 304
Okie, S., 224
Olmeda, E. L., 27, 28
Olsen, L. K., 269
Orient, J. M., 262
Otten, M. W., Jr., 242
Ouellet, R. P., 96
Overby, L., 151
Oxtoby, M., 59

P

Packer, A., 338
Packman, S., 195
Paltiel, F. L., 147
Parsons, M., 41
Parham, T. A., 270
Parker, S., 270
Parks, A. G., 232
Parron, D. L., 27, 28
Partridge, K. B., 273
Passel, J., 10

Pathy, M. S., 227
Pauling, L., 194
Payton-Stewart, L., 323
Pearce, D., 152
Pechacek, T. F., 109–110
Pederson, A. M., 28
Pennsylvania Department of health, 172
Petersdorf, R. G., 282, 283
Piazza, T., 241
Pineiro, O., 270
Planned Parenthood Federation of America, 305, 308
Planned Parenthood Federation of America v. Agency for International Development, 309
Planned Parenthood Federation of America v. Bowen, 305
Planned Parenthood Federation of America v. United States Department of Health and Human Services, 306
Pless, I. B., 184
Pliner, A. J., 307
Polednak, A., 321, 324
Population Crisis Committee, 310
Population Reference Bureau, U.S. Department of Labor, 13
Poussaint, A. F., 20, 21, 23, 36
Powell-Griner, E., 6, 15
Pratt, R., 341
President's Commission on Mental Health, 22, 24, 28
Price, J. H., 273
Price, R., 151
Primm, B., 86
Prineas, R. J., 91
Proctor, E., 269
Prothrow-Stith, D., 133, 135, 141
Public Health Service, 121, 125, 130

R

Rabin, P. V., 232
Rabinowitz, M. B., 179, 181
Rabins, P. V., 231
Rahe, R. H., 149, 150–151
Randall-David, E., 130
Rappaport, J., 321
Rawls, J., 323
Raymond, C., 281
Ready, T., 282
Reda, D., 98
Reed, W., 187
Regier, D. A., 232
Reis, P., 36
Report of the National Advisory Commission on Civil Disorders, 187
Resnick, H., 324
Resnick, M. D., 307
Rhode Island Department of Health, 249

Rice, M., 242
Richardson, T. M., 76
Ries, L.A.G., 108, 109
Riessman, C. K., 231
Rimer, B. K., 268
Rimm, E. B., 98
Ringen, K., 112
Rist, M. C., 216
Rivera, F. O., 322
Robbins, B. M., 231
Robbins, P. R., 248
Roberts, J., 91, 180
Robinson, B., 231
Robinson, J. G., 10, 106, 111
Robles, E. F., 195
Roca, R. P., 231
Rochat, R W., 302, 303
Roe v. Wade, 304
Rogers, G., 259, 262
Rontz, M. J., 231
Ropers, R. H., 148
Rosen, A., 269
Rosenberg, M. L., 27, 151
Rosenfield, S., 231
Rosenstein, M. J., 27
Rosenstock, I. M., 160, 248, 273
Rosenthal, E., 21, 22, 24, 231
Roth, L., 148
Rothenberg, R., 60
Rothman, I. L., 231, 242
Rotter, J. B., 323
Rounds, K. A., 149, 151
Rowe, J. W., 223, 226, 227, 228
Rowley, P. T., 195
Royal Commission on Environmental Pollution, 181
Rubin, G., 262
Rubin, L. 148
Ruiz, D. S., 23
Russel-Erlich, J. L., 322
Russell, L., 318
Russell, R. D., 248
Russo, R. M., 257
Rust v. Sullivan, 305
Ryan, W., 322, 232

S

Saalberg, E. L., 321
St. Pierre, R. W., 269
Salber, E. J., 262, 263
Saldo, B. J., 232
Sanders, J., 326, 327
Saunders, E., 90, 91, 100
Sayles, J. A., 149
Sayre, J. W., 184
Schatzkin, A., 223
Schiff, I., 47

Schoen, C., 225
Schoenbaum, S., 181
Schoenborn, C. A., 170, 172
Scott, B., 69, 70
Scott, J., 25
Scott, M., 148, 151
Scragg, R., 98
Seabron, C., 150
Secord, P. F., 8
Secretary of Health and Human Services, 78
Seligman, M., 151
Selik, R., 60
Selye, H., 158
Shaef, A. W., 83
Shannon, I., 347
Shapiro, S., 170, 232
Shier, D. R., 179
Shindell, S., 4
Shook, D. C., 262
Shopland, D. R., 109–110
Short, P. F., 16, 326
Shouse, T. W., 212, 213
Siegel, J., 226
Siegel, J. E., 317
Simpson, C., 282, 283, 291
Simpson, N., 112
Singer, S. J., 194
Singh, B., 99
Singh, S., 16, 301, 302, 305, 306
Sliepcevich, E. M., 249
Smith, C. H., 259, 260, 262, 263
Smith, D., 273
Smith, E. J., 28
Smith, M. A., 179, 184, 185
Smith, S. H., 26
Sobell, M. B., 65
Society for Women's Health Research, 46
Solomon, B. B., 321
Solomon, H. S., 95
Somervell, P. D., 25
Sommer, R., 324
Sonnenschein, M. A., 24
Sors, A. J., 179
Sparer, G., 112
Spivak, H., 135, 141
Spurlock, J., 26
Stalgaitis, S., 263
Stamfer, M. J., 98
Starfield, B. H., 170, 242
Stark, T., 307
Steinhauer, M., 223
Steinmetz, S., 37, 40
Stepto, R. G., 212
Sterling, M., 259
Stewart, B., 231
Stewart, J. B., 271
Stewart, J. C., 263

Stoddard, R. P., 326
Stokes, J., 4
Stone, R. A., 95
Storer, D. J., 231
Straws, M., 37, 40
Stringham, P., 137
Sudman, J. R., 316
Suelyle, M., 241
Sullivan, L. W., 226, 267
Sullivan, J. F., 217
Sussman, L., 21
Svigir, M., 258
Swanson, A. G., 283
Swift, C., 322
Swoboda, F., 338
Syme, S. L., 323
Szasz, T. S., 23

T

Taking Our Bodies Back, 47
Talbott, G. D., 65, 73, 82
Tallon, J. R., 317
Taylor, S. E., 30
Terris, M., 344
Tesh, S., 343
Teutsch, S. M., 242
Thomas, C. S., 22
Thomas, G. E., 241
Thomas, J., 197
Thomas, S., 342
Thomas, S. B., 148
Thorpe, K. E., 317
Tietze, C., 302
Tlasek, M. E., 231
Torrens, P. R., 16
Torres, A., 303, 307
Troup, J., 151
Trussel, J., 42
Trussell, J. T., 303
Turner, K. S., 282
Tyroler, H. A., 94, 96

U

Ulbrich, P. M., 26
Urbanowicz, M. A., 180
U.S. Bureau of the Census, 7, 8, 9, 10, 24, 307
U.S. Congressional Budget Office, 224
U.S. Department of Health and Human Services, 4, 6, 14, 15, 39, 46, 106, 110, 111, 114, 153, 165, 166, 226, 241, 243, 244, 249, 267, 281, 284, 290, 305, 321, 339, 342

V

Varju, L., 263
Vermylen, C., 195
Veterans Administration Cooperative Study Group on Antihypertensive Agents, 90
Viau, A., 262
Voors, A. W., 9, 94, 95
Vostal, J., 184

W

Wagenknecht, L., 110
Wagner, M., 41
Wallerstein, N., 323
Wallsich, L. S., 303
Wandersman, A., 248, 322
Wang, M. Q., 269
Wara, W., 195
Warheit, G. J., 26
Warren, R. C., 242
Warren, R. L., 323
Warren, S. E., 95
Watkins, N. B., 326
Watson, D. W., 65
Webber, L. S., 91, 94, 95
Weber-Burdin, E., 148
Webster v. Reproductive Health Services, 304
Weissman, M., 133
Weitzman, M., 137
Wells, I. C., 194
West, M., 93
Wetterhall, S. F., 126
Whitely, P., 57
Whitfield, C. L., 75
Whitten, C. F., 197, 199, 204
Wilcox, B. L., 149
Wilenksky, G. R., 242
Wilkinson, D., 256
Will, J. C., 126
Willet, W. C., 98
Williams, A. P., 283
Williams, B. A., 76
Williams, D. H., 30
Williams, J.R.M., 4
Williams, L. S., 150
Williams, R., 326
Williams, R. L., 26
Williams, R. M., 170
Williams, S. J., 16
Williamson, D. F., 242
Willie, C. V., 26
Wilson, J. F., 273
Wilson, L. A., 228
Wilson, W. J., 42
Wolfgang, M. E., 132, 140
Womble, M., 86

Women's Health Care Forum, 38
Wood, S. J., 232
Woode, M. K., 282, 292, 294, 295
Woodlander, S., 241
Woods, K. L., 93
Woolhandler, S., 227
World Health Organization Regional Office for Europe, 40
World Health Organization, 174, 226, 310, 343, 347
Worth, D., 44
Wortman, C., 151
Wright, J. D., 148
Wyshak, G., 47

Y

Yankauer, A., 13
Yates, S., 307
Young, M.A.C., 247
Yule, W., 180

Z

Zabin, L., 309
Zahniser, C., 172
Zambrana, R. E., 153
Ziegler, J. E., 249
Zimmerman, R. J., 26
Zoller, G., 133

SUBJECT INDEX

A

Abortion: and adolescent pregnancy, 306–309; as "genocide," 311; and government funding, 303; legislation, 302–303, 307–309; and sickle cell disease, 197–199; and Supreme Court rulings, 304–305. *See also* Contraception; Family planning; Reproductive freedom

Access to care. *See* Health care access

Access to Care Model, 160

Acquired immune deficiency syndrome (AIDS): and adolescent pregnancy, 215; and AIDS-related complex, 55; black-to-white ratio of, 56–59; and epidemic of fear, 61; and excess mortality, 15; and Haitian immigrants, 56; and Hispanics, 58; and HIV, 55–56; and homosexuality, 43–44, 60–62; and infant mortality, 172; and IV drug use, 59–60, 67; and mortality, 43; public health programs for, 61; and sociology, 60–61; symptomology/origins of, 55; and women, 44. *See also* Human immunodeficiency virus (HIV); Sexually transmitted disease (STD)

Addiction, 64, 83. *See also* Alcoholism; Chemical dependency; Drug abuse

Adolescent pregnancy: and abortion, 306–309; and AIDS, 215; causes of, 42, 209–210; and drug abuse, 68, 215–216; and education, 210; medical consequences of, 212; and poverty, 206; programs/policies for, 216–218; psycho-socio-medical problems of, 212–215; race effect of, 42, 208; rates of, 207; and sexual revolution, 208;

social consequences of, 208–212; and socioeconomic status, 209–210. *See also* Adolescents

Adolescents: developmental tasks of, 138; drug abuse of, 66; high-risk, 140; narcissism in, 139; normal behavior in, 138; and peer pressure, 139; and racism, 139; violence prevention for, 135–137. *See also* Adolescent pregnancy

African Americans: age composition of, 7; and AIDS, 56–59; and alcoholism, 79–81; birth/fertility rates of, 11–12; culture of, 269–271; demographic processes of, 10–16; education level of, 242; experience in U.S., 241–244; families, 211–212, 218; gender composition of, 7–8; health care access, 340–341; health disparities in, 4, 244–246; health status of, 242–243, 268–269, 339–340; homeless, 10; household composition of, 8; income level of, 242; mortality of, 4, 6, 12–16, 243–244; population increase of, 338; and poverty, 8–9, 112–113, 121; and public health programs, 61–62; sociodemographic characteristics of, 7–10; socioeconomic status of, 8–9; state/regional distributions of, 9–10; and unemployment, 339. *See also* Race effect

Aid to Families with Dependent Children (AFDC), 16, 148

AIDS-related complex (ARC), 55. *See also* Acquired immune deficiency syndrome (AIDS)

Alcoholics Anonymous, 74, 75, 84, 85–86

Alcoholism: and African Americans, 79–81; defined, 83–84; etiology of, 82–83; health/social dangers of, 79; and homelessness, 148; and infant mortality, 172–173; and men, 79; prevention approaches to, 68–69; problem description, 81–82; and self-help groups, 74–75; and social development, 87–88; and social policy issues, 88; treatment of, 83–87; and women, 28, 38. *See also* Chemical dependency; Cirrhosis; Drug abuse; Substance abuse intervention; Substance abuse prevention; Substance abuse treatment

American Cancer Society, 47, 115

American College of Obstetrics and Gynecology, 198

American Diabetes Association, 125

American Medical Association, 64

American Public Health Association, 269

Association of American Medical Colleges, 283

Association of Black Psychologists, 198

B

Blacks. *See* African Americans

Boston Childhood Lead Poisoning Prevention Program, 188

Boston Commission for Safe Schools, 134

C

Cancer: alcohol-related, 46–47, 79; and attitude, 111–112; and biological factors, 112; black-to-white ratio of, 106, 108–109; breast, 47–48, 108; cervical, 47, 108–109, 113; and clinical trials, 117; contributing factors to, 109–111; data collection on, 106–108; and diet, 111; education and services for, 118; and the elderly, 227; and environmental agents, 111; incidence rates of, 108–109; and intervention networks, 115–116; and knowledge, 111; lung, 48, 108–109, 113; and medical resources, 112; and mortality, 106–109; national intervention plans for, 113–114; national outreach efforts for, 114–118; and population-based studies, 116; and poverty, 112–113, 224; research on, 117; and research training, 117–118; and smoking, 109–110; and socioeconomic factors, 112–113; survival rates of, 109

Cancer Information Service, 118

Cancer Prevention and Clinical Research in the Underserved Populations initiative, 117

Cancer Prevention Awareness Program, 118

Cardiovascular disease: black-to-white ratio of, 90–91; and diabetes, 126; and the elderly, 227–228; and mortality, 90; and women, 46, 90. *See also* Hypertension

Centers for Disease Control (CDC), 55, 56, 61, 67, 124, 125, 179, 326

Chemical dependency: and addiction, 64, 83; and culture, 65–66; as disease, 64–65; extent/effects of, 66–68; and interventions, 72–74; prevention of, 68–72; psychological aspects, 65; treatment of, 74–75. *See also* Drug abuse; Substance abuse intervention; Substance abuse prevention; Substance abuse treatment

Children: and environmental circumstances, 216; and health insurance, 316–317; homeless women with (study), 153–155; and lead poisoning, 180; and sickle cell anemia, 200–202. *See also* Infant mortality

Cirrhosis: mortality rates of, 79. *See also* Alcoholism

Coalition building: and coalition maintenance, 331–333; community, 325–327; and empowerment, 323–327; and health promotion, 325–327; and public/private sector, 331

Community: change in, 327–328; and citizen participation, 323; and empowerment, 321–325; and health promotion, 324–325; organization and development (COD), 321, 326–331, 334

Community-based programs: and Centers for Disease Control, 61; for diabetes, 130–131; for drug abuse, 38, 70; for hypertension, 101, 257, 260–261; and Native Americans, 258–259; for preschool preventive care, 257; results of, 261–262; for spousal abuse, 37; for tuberculosis, 258. *See also* Community health workers; Public health programs

Community Clinical Oncology Programs, 117

Community health workers: defined, 255–256; and health education/promotion, 262–263; roles/services of, 256–259; training of, 259–260. *See also* Community-based programs

Consumer Products Safety Commission, 180

Contraception: and far right, 305–306; legislation regarding, 302–303. *See also* Abortion; Family planning; Reproductive freedom

Cork Institute on Alcohol and Other Substance Abuse, Morehouse School of Medicine, 86

D

D.C. Cancer Control Consortium, 115
D.C. Commission on Public Health, 115
D.C./NCI Cancer Initiative, 115
Depression: and elderly, 231; and women, 149, 150-151
Diabetes: and amputation, 126; black-to-white ratio of, 123-124; and cardiovascular disease, 125; and cerebrovascular disease, 125; and community-based programs, 129-130; complications of, 122, 124-126; defined, 121-123; and diet, 122; education about, 125; and the elderly, 227, 228; genetic component in, 122-123, 125; and insulin-dependence, 122-123; and kidney disease, 125-126; maturity-onset, of youth, 122-123; and men, 122, 124; and mortality, 124; national conferences on, 124-125; and pregnancy, 123; prevention of, 128-129; research directions in, 126-129; and vision disorders/blindness, 126; and women, 45-46, 122-123, 124
Diagnostic and Statistical Manual of Mental Disorders (DSM-III), 21, 231, 232
Disease prevention. *See* Health education; Health promotion
Division of Diabetes Translation, 124
Drug abuse: adolescent, 66; and AIDS, 59-60; and community-based programs, 38; and homelessness, 148; and infant mortality, 173; self-help groups for, 74-75; and teenage pregnancy, 68, 215-216; and women, 38. *See also* Alcoholism; Chemical dependence; Substance abuse intervention; Substance abuse prevention; Substance abuse treatment
Drug Abuse Warning Network, 67

E

Education: and adolescent pregnancy, 210; and diabetes, 126; and empowerment, 323; medical, 283-293. *See also* Health education
Elderly: assessment of, 231-232; black-to-white ratio of, 222, 226; health care access/utilization of, 228-229; health care policy recommendations for, 229; and health insurance, 225; health issues of, 226-228; income of, 225; life-expectancy of, 225-226; male, 29; mental health of, 231-232; and mortality, 14; and poverty, 224-225; quality of life of, 223; resources of, 233-234; rural, 232; statistics regarding, 222-223; and unemployment, 225, 232-233
Elisa HIV test, 55-56
Empowerment: and coalition building, 323-324, 325-327; community, 321-325, 328-331; definitions, 324-325; and education, 323; and health, 325-327; and powerlessness, 322; and women, 151-152, 301
Environmental Protection Agency, 188-189
Epidemiologic Catchment Area (ECA), 25
Exercise/fitness, 45, 346

F

Families: African American, 211-212, 218; in cultural context, 213; life-styles of, 210-212, 214; and stress, 214
Family planning: international, 309-310; and Title X of Public Health Service Act, 305-306. *See also* Abortion; Contraception; Reproductive freedom
First National Conference on Black Women's Health Issues, 35, 36

G

Gender: demographics of, 7-8; and mental health, 26-29. *See also* Men; Women
Government programs. *See* Community-based programs; Public health programs

H

Health: of African Americans, 242-243, 268-269, 339-340; black/white disparity in, 4; and culture, 130-131; defined, 4; determinants, 344; models, 272-273; and socioeconomic factors, 147; vision, 346-347. *See also* Mental health; Reproductive health
Health and Nutrition Examination Survey (1972-74), 91
Health Belief Model, 160
Health care: access to, 316-317; and creaming, 230; and homeless women, 153, 154; long-term, 229-230; national, 318, 319; policies/practices, 230; and targeting, 230
Health care access: for African Americans, 340-341; barrier to, 326; for the elderly, 228-229; in Great Britain, 340;

and health insurance, 316–317; for the homeless, 153; for the mentally ill, 21–24; and racism, 269

Health care interventions: cultural basis, 269–271; PEN-3 model, 271–277. *See also* Health education; Health promotion; Substance abuse intervention

Health care policy: and access to care, 316–317; and adolescent pregnancy, 216–218; and alcoholism, 88; and the elderly, 229; and essential health services, 343; and Medicaid, 317; politics of, 341; principles of, 318–319; reform proposals for, 317–318; and smoking, 136, 345–346; in social action framework, 344–347; and violence, 134–135. *See also* Public health programs

Health care professionals: education of, 283–293; and race effect, 269, 281–284

Health Careers Opportunity Program, 283

Health education: and cancer, 118; and community health workers, 262–263; definitions, 247; and fear arousal approach, 248; and influencing behavior, 247–248; and learning theory, 249; principles of, 250–252; program development, 249; program evaluation, 249–250; and sickle cell disease, 196–198; targets of, 267; and threat avoidance approach, 248–249. *See also* Health care interventions; Health promotion

Health insurance: and access to care, 316–317; and children, 316–317; and the elderly, 225; and financial barriers, 326; and unemployment, 16. *See also* Medicaid; Medicare; Supplementary Security Income (SSI)

Health promotion: and coalition building, 325–327; and community, 324–325; and health field concept, 344–345; national objectives of, 342; PEN-3 model for, 271–277. *See also* Health care policy; Health education

Health Promotion Resource Center, Morehouse School of Medicine, 326

Health workers. *See* Community health workers

Healthy People 2000, 114, 167, 342, 343

Heart disease. *See* Cardiovascular disease

Homeless women: and depression, 151, 154–155; and health care system, 153, 154; incidence of, 148; and interventions, 150; research directions, 159–160; S-5 intervention model, 155–159; and self-esteem/self-efficacy, 156; and self-health action, 158; and stress, 152,

156–157; and support networks, 152–153, 156; Washington, D.C. (study), 153–155

Homelessness: and alcoholism/drug abuse, 148; incidence of, 148; and interventions, 150; and mental health, 21; and poverty, 148; and race effect, 10; research on, 148; and self-esteem, 151–152; and stress, 149

Homicide, and men, 132. *See also* Violence

Howard University Cancer Center, 115

Hudson Institute, 338

Human immunodeficiency virus (HIV): and AIDS, 55–56; antibody tests, 55–56. *See also* Acquired immune deficiency syndrome (AIDS)

Hypertension: and alcohol abuse, 98; community-based treatment centers for, 101; and compliance, 100–101; control of, 96–97; demographics of, 90–91; and diet, 98; drug therapy for, 99–100; and environmental theory, 96; epidemiology of, 91–93; genetic factor in, 93–94; hormonal/physiological factors in, 94–96; and smoking, 98; treatment of, 97–100. *See also* Cardiovascular disease

I

Indigenous community health workers. *See* Community health workers

Infant mortality: and AIDS, 44; black-to-white ratio of, 165–170; causes of, 167–170; demographics of, 166–167; and drug abuse, 173; and fetal alcohol syndrome, 172–173; and lead poisoning, 184–185; and low birthweight, 167–170; and maternal health, 41–42; and maternal nutrition, 171–172; and maternal prenatal care, 39–42, 170–171, 175–176; and maternal risk factors, 171–175; and maternal smoking, 172; national reports on, 171; risk factors in, 11–12; and sexually transmitted disease, 173–175; as social problem, 41; statistics on, 13, 165

Institute for the Advanced Study of Black Family Life and Culture, 86

Institute of Medicine, 171

Institute on Black Chemical Abuse, 86

J

Johns Hopkins University East Baltimore hypertension project, 260–261

K

Kaiser Family Foundation, 326

L

Lead poisoning: airborne, 183–184; asymptomatic, 181–183; black-to-white ratio of, 180; and Boston prevention program, 188–189; as child health problem, 181–183; and children, 180, 182; detection/management of, 179; effects/symptoms of, 181, 184–185; and infant development/mortality, 184–185; and IQ, 184; paint-based, 183; prevention of, 179, 185–186; silent, 182; soil-/dust-based, 184; sources of, 179–180, 183–184
Links, Inc., 115

M

Malnutrition, 44–45. *See also* Nutrition
Maryland Hypertension Program, 96
Medicaid, 16, 225, 229–231, 317. *See also* Health insurance
Medical schools: minority programs in, 283–284; minority representation in, 282–283; University of Virginia minority program, 284–292
Medicare, 17, 225. *See also* Health insurance
Men: and alcohol-related illness, 79; and diabetes, 123; elderly, 29; and health, 339; and homicide, 132; and homosexuality, 43–44, 60–62; and hypertension, 97; and incarceration, 43–44; and mental health, 28–29; mortality rates of, 12–13, 15–16; and support networks, 29; and violence, 133
Mental health: and alien culture diagnosis, 24–25; in cultural context, 22; defined, 20; and the elderly, 231–232; and gender, 26–29; and labeling, 22–23; and racism, 24–25; research in, 30–31; and social support networks, 149–150; and socioeconomic status, 25–26; trends in, 20–21; utilization/treatment of, 21–24
Mortality: African American, 4, 6, 12–16, 243–244; AIDS-related, 43; of cancer, 106–109; of diabetes, 125; of the elderly, 14, 222–223; and excess deaths, 14–16, 243–244, 341; of heart disease, 90; and life expectancy, 13; and poverty, 223. *See also* Infant mortality

N

Narcotics Anonymous, 74
Nation of Islam, 70, 84
National Advisory Council on Civil Disorders, 187
National Association for Sickle Cell Disease, Inc., 196, 198, 202–203
National Association for the Advancement of Colored People (NAACP), 86
National Association of Black Social Workers, 198
National Association of Children of Alcoholics–Adult Children of Alcoholics, 86
National Black Alcoholism Council, 86
National Black Leadership Initiative on Cancer, 114
National Black Women's Health Project (NBWHP), 49
National Cancer Act (1971), 107
National Cancer Advisory Board, 114
National Cancer Control Research Network, 115
National Cancer Institute, 107, 114, 116, 117, 118
National Center for Health Statistics, 36, 43, 47, 107, 124, 244
National Commission to Prevent Infant Mortality, 171
National Diabetes Advisory Board, 124
National Diabetes Data Group, 124
National Drug and Alcoholism Treatment Survey (1987), 67
National Health and Nutrition Examination Survey (NHANES), 35
National Health Interview Survey, 107
National Household Survey on Drug Abuse (1988), 66
National Institute of Diabetes and Digestive and Kidney Disease, 125
National Institutes of Health, 194, 196, 201, 202, 203–204, 284
National Medical Association, 115, 198
New World Community of Islam in the West, 70
Northeastern Ohio Trauma Study, 133
Nutrition: and cancer, 111; and cardiovascular disease, 95, 98; and diabetes, 123; and malnutrition/undernutrition, 44–45; maternal, and infant mortality, 171–172

O

Oakland Parents in Action program, 70–71
Office of Minority Health, 45, 115, 125

P

PEN-3 health education model: advantages of, 277; application of, 275–277; cultural basis for, 269–271; description, 271–275; and other health models, 272–273

Physician Data Query system, 118

Planned Approach to Community Health (PATCH) program, 326

Poverty: and adolescent pregnancy, 206; and African Americans, 8–9, 121; and cancer, 112–113, 224; and education, 210; and the elderly, 224–225; and homelessness, 148; and mortality, 223

Pregnancy. *See* Adolescent pregnancy; Reproductive health

Prenatal care. *See* Women: prenatal care

Primary Prevention of Cancer in Black Populations, 116

Prisons: and AIDS, 43–44; population increase in, 134

Public health programs: and adolescent pregnancy, 216–218; and African Americans, 61–62; for AIDS, 61; for cancer, 113–118; for diabetes, 130–131; for sickle cell anemia, 196; and smoking, 135; and violence, 134–135. *See also* Community-based programs

Public Health Service, 115

R

Race effect: and adolescent pregnancy, 42, 208; and AIDS, 56–59; and birth/fertility rates, 11; and cancer, 108–109; and cardiovascular disease, 90–93; and diabetes, 124–125; and elderly health care, 230–231; and health care professionals, 269, 281–284; and homeless women, 147–148; and homelessness, 10; and infant mortality, 166–170; and lead poisoning, 180, 186–187; and mental health, 20–24; and mortality rates, 12–16; and sickle cell anemia, 193–194; and socioeconomic status, 8–9, 21; and violence/homicide, 134. *See also* African Americans

Racism: and chemical dependence, 65–66, 79–80; and health care delivery system, 269; and lead poisoning, 187; and mental health, 21, 24–25; and stress, 24–25; and violence, 139–140; and women, 36

Reproductive freedom: defending, 310–311; and empowerment/autonomy, 301–302; health impact of, 302–303; legislation regarding, 302–303; threats to, 302, 303–306. *See also* Abortion; Contraception; Family planning

Reproductive health: and cancer, 47–48; cultural issues of, 39; and diabetes, 45–46; and infant mortality, 13, 39–42; and prenatal care, 39–40; and sexually transmitted disease, 42–43; and teenage pregnancy, 42; U.S. vs. European policy on, 41; and women's concerns, 38–39

School Based Youth Services Program (New Jersey), 217

Science Enrichment Program, 118

Second National Health and Nutrition Examination Survey, 179

Secretary's Task Force on Black and Minority Health, 6, 14, 46, 121, 166, 243, 244

Self-help groups. *See* Support networks: self-help groups

Sexism, 36

Sexually transmitted disease (STD): and education, 42–43; and HIV infection, 59; and infant mortality, 173–175. *See also* Acquired immune deficiency syndrome (AIDS)

Sickle cell anemia: drug therapy for, 194–195; etiology of, 192–193; gene therapy for, 195–196; genetic basis for, 193; genetic counseling on, 196–198; government role in, 204; health care response to, 201; health/mental health consequences of, 199; and national/community organizations, 196; newborn screening for, 201–203; and prenatal diagnosis/abortion, 197–199; and quality of life, 200, 204; and race effect, 193–194; research on, 194–196, 203–204; and service needs, 199–201; and sickle cell trait, 193, 194, 196–198; transplant therapy for, 195; treatment of, 194–196, 200, 203–204; and unemployment, 200; and West Africans, 194

Smoking: and cancer, 109–110; and hypertension, 98; an infant mortality, 172; intervention networks, 116; public health strategies for, 135, 345–346

Socioeconomic status: and adolescent pregnancy, 209–210; and cancer, 112–113; and health, 269; and health care, 229–230; and mental health, 25–26; and race effect, 8; and social class, 8; and women's health issues, 147

Spousal abuse: community-based treatment centers, 37; and women, 36–37. *See also* Violence

Stress: and coping behavior, 149; family,

214; and homelessness, 149; and racism, 24–25; and sickle cell anemia, 199; and women, 27–28, 35

Stroke, 90, 126. *See also* Cardiovascular disease

Substance abuse intervention: defined, 72; failure of, 73–74; principles of, 72–73; and treatment, 72

Substance abuse prevention: for alcohol abuse, 68–69; and community-based programs, 70; confrontational approach to, 69; and elementary school programs, 70–71; goals of, 68; planning guide for, 71; research on, 68–69; and social skills/self-esteem, 70

Substance abuse treatment: and behavior therapy, 84; and chemical dependency, 74–75; and cognitive behavior therapy, 84; and detoxification, 74–75, 84–85; and drugs, 85; and group therapy, 85–87; research in, 86; and self-help groups, 74–75; social development approach to, 87–88; and twelve-step programs, 75, 85–87

Supplementary Security Income (SSI), 225. *See also* Health insurance

Support networks: and cultural patterns, 152; and elderly men, 29; and self-help groups, 74–75; and substance abuse prevention, 74–75, 85–87

Surveillance, Epidemiology, and End Results Program, 107

T

Teen Outreach (Missouri), 217

Teenage pregnancy. *See* Adolescent pregnancy

Title X, Public Health Service Act, 305–306

U

Unemployment: and African Americans, 339; and the elderly, 225, 232–233; and health insurance, 16; and sickle cell anemia, 200; social costs of, 232–233

United Way, 196

University of Oklahoma Health Sciences Center, 127

University of Virginia School of Medicine Medical Academic Advancement Program: community support for, 295; consortium, 293–294; and continuing education, 294–295; funding of, 292–

293, 294; I, 285–288; II, 288–292; student tracking system, 295

Urban League, 86

U.S. Bureau of Labor Statistics, 281

U.S. Bureau of the Census, 9, 121, 224, 338

U.S. Department of Health and Human Services, 68, 79, 106, 114, 121, 125, 166, 342

V

Violence: adolescent, 135–141; family/friend, 133–134; "get tough" approach to, 134; glamorous view of, 135; and health care role, 140–142; incidence of, 132–133; and labeling, 140–141; prevention of, 134–138; and public health strategies, 134–135; and victims, 140–141; and women, 37–38. *See also* Homicide; Spousal abuse

Violence Prevention Curriculum for Adolescents, 135–136

Violence Prevention Project, Boston Department of Health and Hospitals, 135, 137

W

Washington, D.C., homeless women with children (study), 153–160

Western Blot test, 56

Women: and abuse, 36–37; and AIDS, 44, 59–60; and alcoholism, 28, 38, 47; and cancer, 47–48; and depression, 149, 150–151; and diabetes, 45–46; and drug abuse, 38; and empowerment, 151–152, 301; and exercise, 45; and family planning, 174; and fertility/birth rates, 11–12; and heart disease/hypertension, 46; and malnutrition, 44–45; and mental health, 27–28; mortality rates of, 12–13, 16; and prenatal care, 39–42, 170–171, 175–176; and racism/sexism, 36; and reproductive health issues, 38–39; and self-help groups, 49; and socialization, 213; and stress, 27–28, 35, 149. *See also* Gender; Homeless women; Reproductuve freedom; Reproductive health

World Health Organization Advisory Group, 226, 346

Y

Year 2000 Objectives for the Nation, 118, 127–128